GERONTOLOGY
for the Health Care Professional

GERONTOLOGY
for the Health Care Professional

WALTER C. CHOP, MS, RRT
CHAIRMAN
Department of Health Services
Southern Maine Technical College
South Portland, Maine

REGULA H. ROBNETT, MEd, MS, OTR/L, BCN
ASSISTANT PROFESSOR
Department of Occupational Therapy
University of New England
Biddeford, Maine

 F. A. DAVIS COMPANY • Philadelphia

F. A. Davis Company
1915 Arch Street
Philadelphia, PA 19103

Printed in the United States of America

Last digit indicates print number: 10 9 8 7 6 5 4 3 2 1

Publisher: Jean François Vilain
Senior Editor: Lynn Borders Caldwell
Developmental Editor: Christa Fratantoro
Production Editor: Stephen D. Johnson
Cover Designer: Louis J. Forgione
Cover Concept: Regula H. Robnett

As new scientific information becomes available through basic and clinical research, recommended treatments and drug therapies undergo changes. The authors and publisher have done everything possible to make this book accurate, up to date, and in accord with accepted standards at the time of publication. The authors, editors, and publisher are not responsible for errors or omissions or for consequences from application of the book, and make no warranty, expressed or implied, in regard to the contents of the book. Any practice described in this book should be applied by the reader in accordance with professional standards of care used in regard to the unique circumstances that may apply in each situation. The reader is advised to check product information (package inserts) for changes and new information regarding dose and contraindications before administering any drug. Caution is especially urged when using new or infrequently ordered drugs.

Library of Congress Cataloging in Publication Data

Gerontology for the health care professional / [edited by] Walter C. Chop, Regula H. Robnett.
    p.   cm.
  Includes bibliographical references and index.
  ISBN 0–8036–0398–3
  1. Aged—Health and hygiene. 2. Gerontology. 3. Geriatrics. 4. Aging. I. Chop, Walter C. II. Robnett, Regula H.
  [DNLM: 1. Geriatrics. 2. Aged. 3. Aging—physiology. WT 100 G3753 1999]
  RA564.8.G466 1999
  618.97—dc21
  DNLM/DLC
  for Library of Congress   99-10900
                                                                 CIP

Dedication

*To my wife, Gail, and children
Jenny, Chris, and Alex for their
love and patience. Also to my
father, Walter, and the memory
of my mother, Olga.*

Walter C. Chop

*To my wonderful family, Steve,
Dylan, Rhiannon and Grosi
(Marta H. Gibbs), for their
love and support.*

Regula H. Robnett

PREFACE

The elderly have always made up the majority of patients/clients cared for by health care professionals. Their conditions are some of the most challenging to treat in that they often have multisystem involvement. Yet, many health care providers have had little or no training in the physical and psychosocial factors that relate to this unique segment of the population.

Gerontology is the study of aging in all its aspects: biological, psychological, and social. Geriatrics, the study of diseases of the elderly, is included under this umbrella. The recently released Pew Health Professions Commission Report, *Healthy America: Practitioners for 2005,* recommends improved educational preparation for all allied health professionals who will be working with older patients. With the current "graying of America" and 80 million baby boomers (those born between 1946 and 1965) heading into their 40s and 50s, few will not be working with elderly patients/clients soon. Practically the only exceptions are the medical fields of pediatrics and obstetrics.

An American Society of Allied Health Professions (ASAHP) task force report on gerontology recommended more interdisciplinary education and collaboration among health care providers. The Pew Commission's Report also contains specific education suggestions. This text, unlike many others, reflects these recommendations. We have solicited chapter authors and contributors from a wide range of health professions, making the text generic in nature.

We present an introductory approach to the aspects of aging and an overview of pertinent issues involved in caring for the elderly patient/client. Our intent is to make the text short and concise yet complete and thorough in its coverage of the chapter topics. Some chapters, by the nature of the subject matter (e.g., Chapter 3, Physiology and Pathology of Aging), present more in-depth coverage of material. Other chapters, such as Chapter 2, Social Aspects of Aging, tend to address many issues only briefly because of the preponderance of material and anecdotal examples under each subheading.

Throughout the book we have attempted to make the information as student friendly as possible. Chapter authors write with the presumption that they are addressing individuals with little or no background in gerontology. We did, however, presume that the student had a basic prerequisite knowledge of anatomy and physiology, psychology, and perhaps some background in nutrition and pharmacology. Pedagogical features such as behavioral objectives, key terms, review questions, and learning activities were added to facilitate learning and enhance comprehension.

We hope that these features will prove helpful and that the reader will find this information useful.

Walter C. Chop, MS, RRT
Regula H. Robnett, MS, OTR/L

ACKNOWLEDGMENTS

So many individuals contribute to the successful completion of a textbook. We would like to thank those who have helped us in our endeavors with compiling, writing, and reviewing *Gerontology for the Health Care Professional.*

We would first like to thank our talented contributors who made it possible for us to truly produce a textbook representative of all allied health professionals.

Our heartfelt thanks also go to the following people:

- Those who let us reprint their photographs: JoAnn Pagano, Im Sik Im, Paul Kim, Darby Northway, Jim Harrison, Gary Bonnacorso, Mary Harper, Elderhostel, and the Sun City Poms.
- Those who permitted us to photograph them: Connie Pettit, Marge Bennett, Elsie Wood, Brockie Sweetland, and Alexander Chalmers.
- Those who allowed us to use their work: Nicholas Allen, David Ames (*Age and Aging*), Ann Wasson (*Aging Arkansas*), and Allyn and Bacon.
- Coastal Manor, Schoellkopf Health Center, and Black Bear Medical for allowing us to use their facilities for photographs.
- Our colleagues at work for their support including Dennis Leaver and Susan Nestor of Southern Maine Technical College and Janice Beal, Barbara Schwarzlander, Judy Kimball, Glen Ellen Roth, and Debbie Dewitt of the University of New England.
- Paul Kleyman, Editor, *Aging Today,* for helping us to make connections with some very important people.
- The F. A. Davis Company, especially Lynn Borders Caldwell, Marianne Fithian, and Christa Fratantoro, for believing in our product, prodding us along the way (as needed), and guiding us every step of the way.
- And finally, thank you to all of our reviewers for their constructive comments, with special thanks to our chapter reviewers Oliver J. Drumheller, EdD, RRT, Bonnie Deister, MA, MS, BSN, RN, CMA-C, Marilyn L. Blaisdell, MA, OTR/L, and Melinda D. Sissel, COTA/L.

If we inadvertently left anyone out, please forgive us.

Walter and Regi

ix

CONTRIBUTORS

SUSAN CLAYBROOK, MEd, RRT
Speech Language Pathologist
Belgrade, Maine

LIZ DELANO, MS, EMT-P
Educational Coordinator
Southern Maine Emergency Medical Services
South Portland, Maine

SALLY DOE, MS, RTR
Program Director, Radiography
Southern Maine Technical College
South Portland, Maine

PAUL D. EWALD, PhD
Associate to the Chancellor
Antioch University
Yellow Springs, Ohio

BETSY GRAY, MSW, CCSW
Clinical Assistant Professor
School of Social Work
University of New England
Biddeford, Maine

JOYCE L. MacKINNON, EdD, PT
Associate Dean for Academic Affairs
School of Allied Health Sciences
Indiana University/Purdue
  University at Indianapolis
Indianapolis, Indiana

NANCY MacRAE, MS, OTR/L, FAOTA
Associate Professor
Department of Occupational Therapy
University of New England
Biddeford, Maine

THOMAS D. NOLIN, Rph, MS
Doctoral Student
University of Pittsburgh
School of Pharmacy
Pittsburgh, Pennsylvania

NANCY RICHESON, CAS, MA, CTRS
Graduate Lecturer
University of Nebraska
Omaha, Nebraska

DAVID A. SANDMIRE, MD
Assistant Professor
Department of Life Sciences
University of New England
Biddeford, Maine

EDWARD F. SAXBY, JR., JD
Elder Law Attorney
Toole and Saxby, P.A.
Portland, Maine

NANCY SMITH, MSN
Chair, Department of Nursing
Southern Maine Technical College
South Portland, Maine

LOUISE D. WHITNEY, MS, RD
Nutrition Matters
Lansing, Michigan

REVIEWERS

REBECCA R. BAHNKE, OTR/L
Program Director
Occupational Therapy Assistant Program
Parkland College
Champaign, Illinois

J. NILE BARNES, BS, NREMT-P
Assistant Professor
EMS Technology
Austin Community College
Austin, Texas

MARILYN L. BLAISDELL, MA, OTR/L
Assistant Professor
Occupational Therapy Assistant Program
Becker College
Worcester, Massachusetts

MELANIE A. CIESIELSKI, RRT
Educator
Respiratory Care Program
Forsyth Technical Community College
Winston-Salem, North Carolina

BONNIE DEISTER, MA, MS, BSN, RN, CMA-C
Chairperson and Assistant Professor
Medical Assisting and Paramedic Departments
Broome Community College
Binghamton, New York

MARTHA DeSILVA, MEd, RRT
Program Director of Respiratory Care
Massasoit Community College
Brockton, Massachusetts

TERRY DeVITO, RN, MEd, EMT-P, CEN
Assistant Professor and Coordinator
Paramedic Program
Capital Community College
Hartford, Connecticut

OLIVER J. DRUMHELLER, EdD, RRT
Senior Medical Educational Specialist
Respironics
Pittsburgh, Pennslyvania

BRUCE FEISTNER, MSS, RRCP
Program Director/Associate Professor
Respiratory Care Program
Dakota State University-Science Center
Madison, South Dakota

MICHAEL FUGATE, MEd, RT(R)
Lead Didactic Faculty
Radiography Program
Santa Fe Community College
Gainesville, Florida

WILLIAM GALVIN, MSESd, RRT, CPFT
Assistant Professor
School of Allied Health
Program Director
Respiratory Care Program
Teaching and Administration Faculty
TIPS Program
Gwynedd-Mercy College
Gwynedd Valley, Pennsylvania

LIANE HEWITT, MPH, OTR
Chair, Occupational Therapy Department
Program Director and Assistant Professor
Occupational Therapy Assistant Program
Loma Linda University
Loma Linda, California

MARTY HITCHCOCK, CMA, AAS
Program Director
Medical Assisting Program
Gwinnett Technical Institute
Lawrenceville, Georgia

DEBRA LIERL, MEd, RRT
Program Chair of Respiratory Care
Coordinator EMT Program
Cincinnati State Technical and Community College
Cincinnati, Ohio

HOLLY LOOKABAUGH-DEUR, PT, GCS, MHS
Clinical Specialist in Geratric Physical Therapy
CEO, Generation Rehab
Muskegon, Michigan

CAROL A. MARITZ, MS, PT
Program Director and Assistant Professor
Physical Therapist Assistant Program
MCP/Hahnemann University
Philadelphia, Pennsylvania

SANDRA D. OSTRESH, MEd, RT(R)
Program Director and Professor of Radiologic Technology
Quinsigamond Community College
Worcester, Massachusetts

BARBARA ROM, MS, OTR/L
Program Coordinator
Occupational Therapy Program
Green River Community College
Auburn, Washington

MELINDA D. SISSEL, COTA/L
Instructor
Department of Occupational Therapy
Shawnee State University
Portsmouth, Ohio

CONTENTS

7

8

9

10

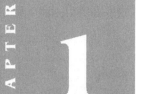

I refuse to take seriously society's idea
that at the arbitrary age of 65 I am
suddenly a lamp going out.
Roger S. Mills
(quoting an elder in History of
Elder Hostel, 1993)

Demographic Trends of an Aging Society

Walter C. Chop

CHAPTER OUTLINE

America, An Aging Society
Global Aging
Gender and Age
Race and Aging
Geographic Distribution:
   Where U.S. Elderly Live

Marital Status
Economic Status
Health Care
Long-term Care
Summary

 BEHAVIORAL OBJECTIVES

Upon completion of this chapter, the reader will be able to:

1. Describe why the "graying of America" is occurring.
2. Identify the fastest growing segment of the population.
3. Discuss life expectancy in terms of gender.
4. Contrast aging by races in the United States.

5. Identify the states where the largest number of individuals older than 65 live.
6. Discuss the elderly in context of their lifestyles (married or living alone).
7. Contrast the economic status of those older than 65 in terms of race and marital status.
8. List disease conditions the elderly are most likely to experience.
9. Discuss health care expenditures for those older than 65 and the demand placed on the health care system by them.
10. Describe pertinent issues involving the long-term care of the elderly.

KEY TERMS

Age cohort	Medicare
Baby boom generation	Old-old
Demographics of aging	Social Security
Elderly, elders	Third agers
Long-term care	Young-old
Medicaid	

🔲 AMERICA, AN AGING SOCIETY

The graying of America began accelerating as the first of the **baby boom generation** (those Americans born between 1946 and 1964) turned 50 years of age in 1996. From that time on, one American will turn 50 years of age every 7 seconds for the next 18 years. This will have dramatic consequences for all aspects of our society, especially our health care system.

In 1900 only 4 percent, or 1 in 25 Americans, were older than 65 years of age. The population of those older than 65 numbered 3.1 million in 1900. As of 1994, this same age cohort numbered 33.2 million, representing 12.7 percent of the total population. To put this in perspective, the population of those older than 65 has increased by more than 2 million people (7% of the population) since 1990, while the younger than 65 age group increased by only 4 percent (Fig. 1–1).

Growth of the older than 65 cohort will continue to increase as baby boomers begin turning 65 in 2010. This will cause yet another rise in the elderly segment of the population.

Projections for the year 2030 estimate that 22 percent or 70.2 million, Americans will be older than the age of 65. To get a true feel for the demography of changing America, note the baby boom bulge on the population chart in Figure 1–2. One can easily envision the top-heavy appearance of this same chart 25 years from today.

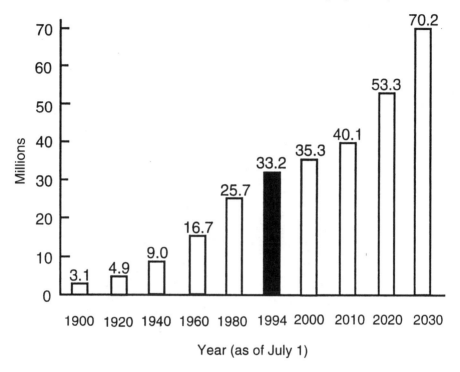

Note: Increments in years on horizontal scale are uneven.

FIG. 1–1. Number of persons in millions 65+: 1900 to 2030. (Reprinted from 65+ in the United States. U.S. Department of Commerce, Economics and Statistics Administration, Bureau of the Census, Washington, DC, 1996.)

An even more dramatic aging trend exists among those older than 85 years of age, often referred to as the old-old. This age cohort is expected to triple in size between 1986 and 2030 and be nearly seven times larger in 2050 than in 1980.[1] The number of those elderly exceeding 100 years of age is also dramatically increasing. It is expected that the numbers in this age group will reach 100,000 by the year 2000.

Looking beyond the **demographics of aging,** let us now consider what the term old age implies to us. "Old age" is a difficult and complex concept to grasp, as our idea of aging is constantly changing. What we thought of as old in the 19th century is considered middle age now. Policy makers have used the age of 65 as a marker in establishing policies affecting the elderly. Some biologists, however, tell us that a person's biological age is more im-

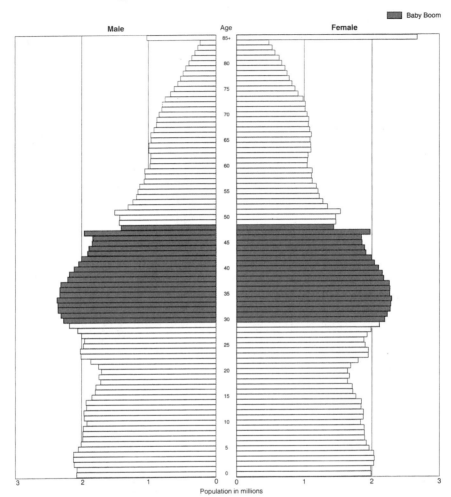

FIG. 1–2. Population by age and sex: July 1, 1994. (From the U.S. Bureau of the Census.)

portant than the person's chronological age when determining an individual's health status.[2] Bernice Neugarten was the first to coin the term **young-old**, which denotes relatively healthy, and financially independent, elders of any age, although usually those between 55 and 74 years of age.[3] The so-called **old-old** usually refers to those older than age 75 whose activities are often limited by functional disabilities. The French have a similar method of categorizing the elderly. They use the terms **third-agers**, or *elder*, when referring to those persons 65 to 85 years of age. Their "old-old" refer only to those individuals older than age 85.

   Whatever classification of aging one chooses to use is a matter of preference as long as one realizes the limitations and variations implied by the term
old age. The salient point to note is that there is a great amount of variability
among "old agers." While many individuals moving into the "third age" and
beyond are of sound mind and body as well as financially secure, others in
this same age cohort are experiencing functional declines as well as health
care or financial needs.

▨ GLOBAL AGING

As of 1990, 28 countries had more than 2 million persons older than 65, and
12 additional countries had more than 5 million. China had the largest number of individuals older than 65, with 63.4 million elders. The United States
had the world's second largest population of those older than 65, with 31.6
million (1990). The entire elder population of the world will increase dramatically between 1995 and 2030. The **elderly** population in Canada and
Japan will double over this time, while in the United States it will increase
by 90 percent.[4]

▨ GENDER AND AGE

Today in the United States, and throughout most countries in the world,
women can expect to live, on average, 7 years longer than men. As of 1990,
life expectancy was 79.3 years for women and 72.6 years for men. Life expectancy projections for 2020 are 81.8 for women and 74.9 for men.[4] This
gender difference in life expectancy persists throughout the aging process.[1]
In fact, among those 85 to 89 years old, there are only 43.7 men for every
100 women (Fig. 1–3).[5] This greater longevity in women is due to the fact
that heart attacks, cancer, and stroke—the major killer diseases—are, or have
been, more common in men. Other factors influencing female longevity may
have to do with women's greater sensitivity to changes in their body condition, which make them more likely to seek out earlier medical intervention.
Women may also handle stress better and have better social support systems
than their male counterparts.

▨ RACE AND AGING

The aging baby boomer generation will contain a far greater racial and ethnic mix than any generation that preceded it. This is due to both increasing
immigration from nonwhite countries and a lower fertility rate among the
white population.[5] The U.S. Census Bureau predicts that nonwhite populations will account for approximately half (47.3%) of the U.S. population by
2050.[5]

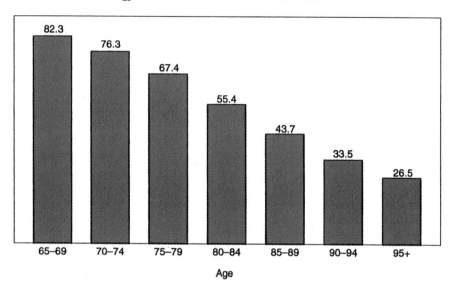

FIG. 1–3. Number of men per 100 women by age: 1994. (From U.S. Bureau of the Census. Data consistent with U.S. Population Estimates by Age, Sex, Race, and Hispanic Origin: 1990 to 1993, Population Paper Listing-8 [PPL-8], 1994.)

Life expectancy for nonwhite Americans is less than it is for whites. African-American men and women currently live on average 6 and 5 years less, respectively, than their white counterparts. However, if a black person of either sex lives to age 65, their life expectancy is much closer to whites than it was at birth.[1] Other ethnic minorities in the United States, including Mexican-Americans and Native Americans, have life expectancies lower than African-Americans.[4] Even with their relatively low percentages, minority persons older than age 65 are growing in numbers at a faster rate than their white counterparts. It is projected that minority populations will represent 25 percent of all the elderly people by 2030, up from 14 percent in 1990[6] (Fig. 1–4). Examining this further, we see individuals older than 65 in specific ethnic groups increasing between 1990 and 2030 by the following percentages: Caucasians, 93 percent; Hispanics, 555 percent; African-Americans, 160 percent; Native Americans, 231 percent; and Asians and Pacific Islanders, 693 percent.[5] It should be noted that Native Americans have the shortest life expectancy of any minority group (45–50 years of age) and also have the lowest standard of living.[7]

As noted previously, besides an overall increase in the number of older Americans, there will also be a more heterogeneous mix of ethnic and cultural backgrounds. This will require health care providers to become more culturally sensitive, acquiring new skills to better recognize and respect cul-

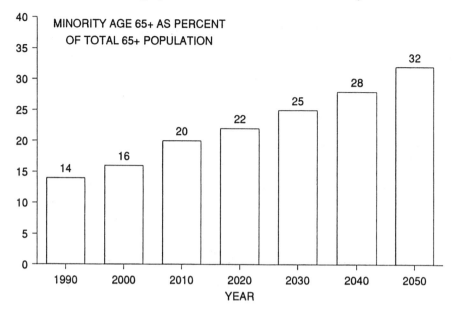

FIG. 1–4. Growth of the minority elderly population: 1990 to 2050. (Figures computed by Donald G. Fowles, U.S. Administration on Aging, from data in U.S. Bureau of the Census, Projections of the Hispanic Population: 1983–2050, by Gregory Spencer. Current Population Reports Series P-25 No. 995 [November 1986], and in U.S. Bureau of the Census, Projections of the Population of the United States by Age, Sex, and Race: 1988 to 2080, by Gregory Spencer. Current Population Reports Series P-25, No. 1018 [January 1989].)

tural differences. Health care professionals will also need to understand the diseases, disorders, and concerns more common not only to a specific age group but to particular ethnic groups as well (Table 1–1).

In some elderly minorities, social factors may play a role in reinforcing negative health patterns and behavior. These factors can account for the short life spans of certain minorities, as in the case of African-Americans. Yet this same minority can expect to outlive their white counterparts if they live to age 80. At this point a racial mortality crossover phenomenon occurs in which life expectancy for blacks exceeds that of whites.

🔲 GEOGRAPHIC DISTRIBUTION: WHERE U.S. ELDERLY LIVE

As of 1994 approximately half (52%) of the U.S. elderly population lived in nine states: California, New York, Florida, Pennsylvania, Texas, Illinois, Ohio, Michigan, and New Jersey. California had more than 3 million Amer-

TABLE 1–1. *Top Ten Chronic Conditions for People Older Than 65, By Age and Race: 1989 (number per 1,000 people)*

Condition	65+	Age 45–64	65–74	75+	White	Race (65+) Black	Black as % of white
Arthritis	483.0	253.8	437.3	554.5	483.2	522.6	108
Hypertension	380.6	229.1	383.8	375.6	367.4	517.7	141
Hearing impairment	286.5	127.7	239.4	360.3	297.4	174.5	59
Heart disease	278.9	118.9	231.6	353.0	286.5	220.5	77
Cataracts	156.8	16.1	107.4	234.3	160.7	139.8	87
Deformity or orthopedic impairment	155.2	155.5	141.4	177.0	156.2	150.8	97
Chronic sinusitis	153.4	173.5	151.8	155.8	157.1	125.2	80
Diabetes	88.2	58.2	89.7	85.7	80.2	165.9	207
Visual impairment	81.9	45.1	69.3	101.7	81.1	77.0	95
Varicose veins	78.1	57.8	72.6	86.6	80.3	64.0	80

Source: National Center for Health Statistics: Current Estimates from the National Health Interview Survey, 1989. Vital Health Stat 10, No. 176, October, 1990.

icans older than 65, with Florida and New York containing more than 2 million each and the remaining six states all having more than 1 million.[8]

Florida in 1994 registered 18.4 percent of its population as older than the age of 65. On a percentage basis, other states with large elderly populations include Rhode Island (15.6%), Iowa and West Virginia (15.4%), Arkansas (14.8%), North Dakota and South Dakota (14.7% each), Connecticut (14.1%), and Massachusetts, Missouri, and Nebraska (14.1% each) (Fig. 1–5).

States experiencing a dramatic increase in their older than 65 populations between 1990 and 1994 include Nevada (30%), Alaska (27%), Arizona and Hawaii (15% each), Utah (13%), and New Mexico, Wyoming, and Colorado (12% each) (Fig. 1–6). This trend seems to indicate, for the most part, a continued movement toward warmer states, with the exception of Alaska and the Rocky Mountain states of Utah, Wyoming, and Colorado. It also points out the apparent appeal of living in less densely populated states, some of which also have lower costs of living. Older individuals moving to these states are generally affluent and well-educated and often have existing ties to these new areas such as family, friends, or previously purchased retirement property. Many are also seeking escape from metropolitan life to the relative safety and comfort of rural or small town USA.

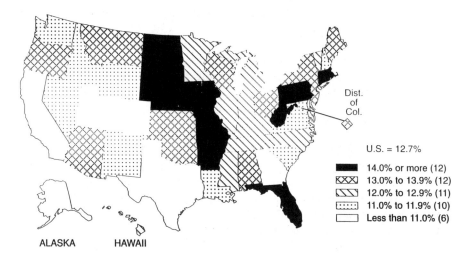

FIG. 1–5. Persons 65+ as percentage of total population: 1994. (Reprinted from 65+ in the United States. U.S. Department of Commerce, Economics and Statistics Administration, Bureau of the Census, Washington, DC, 1996.)

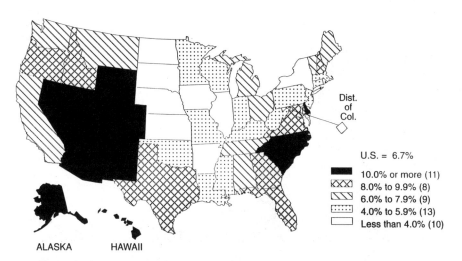

FIG. 1–6. Percentage increase in population 65+: 1990 to 1994. (Reprinted from 65+ in the United States. U.S. Department of Commerce, Economics and Statistics Administration, Bureau of the Census, Washington, DC, 1996.)

In general, older Americans have a tendency to change residences less frequently than their younger counterparts. The result of this has led to an increased "graying" of certain communities. A number of counties have elderly populations exceeding 20 percent of the whole population. Many of these counties are located in the predominantly agricultural nation's heartland, where older persons have stayed on while the youth have moved on.

▨ MARITAL STATUS

In 1994, 77 percent of elderly men were married, compared with only 43 percent of women (Fig. 1–7). What accounts for this, in large part, is the fact that women outlive men, thus increasing the ratio of widows to widowers. There were five times as many widows (8.5 million) as widowers (1.7 million) in 1994. Half of all women older than 65 years of age are widows. Although divorce in the older population has remained relatively low (6% in 1994), it is expected that this will increase dramatically with the aging of the baby boom generation.[1] Divorce rates are somewhat higher in the older African-American population, occurring 18 percent in men and 9 percent in women.

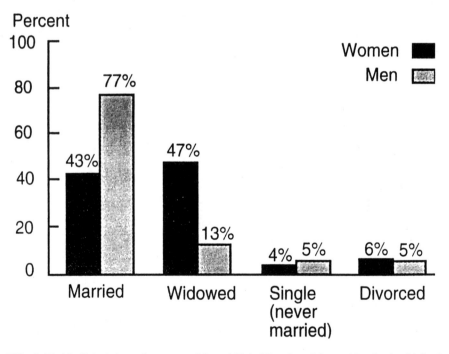

FIG. 1–7. Marital status of persons 65+: 1994. (Reprinted from 65+ in the United States. U.S. Department of Commerce, Economics and Statistics Administration, Bureau of the Census, Washington, DC, 1996.) An additional 3% of men and 2% of women, or 708,000 older persons lived with nonrelatives.

⊠ ECONOMIC STATUS

The economic status of elderly Americans is more varied than in any other age group. Looking solely at income, persons 65 and older, on average, receive less than those younger than 65. In 1989 the median income of families headed by persons older than 65 was $22,806, compared with the median income of $36,058 in families whose head was age 25 to 64 (Fig. 1–8). Even more significant is the median income of elderly people living alone versus those ages 25 to 64 living alone: $9422 and $20,277 respectively. These figures may be somewhat misleading, however, as the elderly have greater tax advantage, often have their home mortgage paid off, and are covered by Medicare insurance.[9]

Sources of income for those 65 and older in 1992 were as follows: **Social Security** (40%), asset income (21%), public and private pensions (19%), earnings (17%), and all other sources (3%).[9]

As of 1994, poverty levels for the elderly were about the same as it was for those age 18 to 64—11.7 percent and 11.9 percent, respectively. In terms of race, poverty figures for those older than 65 show 10 percent of whites at the poverty level, compared with 27 percent of African-Americans and 23 percent of Hispanics. Older women had approximately twice the poverty rate of

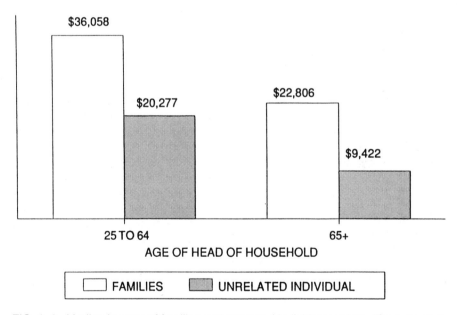

FIG. 1–8. Median income of families and unrelated individuals: 1989. (From the U.S. Bureau of the Census. Unpublished data from the March 1990 Current Population Survey.)

older men (15% to 7%). Since 62 percent of those older than 85 years of age are women, many of whom are widows, their economic hardships are likely to intensify. Single elders were more likely to be poor (23%) than older persons living in families (6%). More than half of older African-American women who lived alone in 1994 fell below the poverty level.[8]

🔲 HEALTH CARE

In a 1993 assessment of general health, 72 percent of those persons 65 and older claimed their health was good to excellent. This compares with individuals younger than 65, 92 percent of whom considered their health to be good to excellent.[8] There was no significant degree of difference between the genders. However, only 56 percent of elderly African-Americans rated their health as good to excellent.

The majority of elderly persons have at least one chronic condition. In 1993, the following conditions (per 100 elders) were present: arthritis (49), hypertension (35), heart disease and hearing impairments (31 each), orthopedic impairments (18), cataracts and sinusitis (15 each), and diabetes, tinnitus, and visual impairments (10 each).[8] Heart disease, cancer, and stroke account for 7 of every 10 deaths among those older than 65. Alzheimer's disease, confirmed on autopsy, is the leading cause of cognitive impairment in the elderly.

Those 65 and older visit a physician, on average, eight times per year as compared with three visits per year in the younger than 65 cohort. Activity of elderly persons is limited or restricted on an average of 34 days per year as a result of illness or injury, as reported in 1993. They are also hospitalized three times as often and stay approximately 50 percent longer than those younger than 65. The elderly, although constituting only 12.7 percent of the U.S. population, accounted for more than one third of all hospital stays and nearly half the days of care in hospitals in 1993.[8] Health care expenditures are also unbalanced. Most health care dollars are spent toward the end of the one's life. In 1987, health care for elders accounted for 36 percent of the total personal health care dollars spent. These health care expenditures totaled $162 billion, averaging $5560 per older individual, which was approximately four times the health care costs for persons younger than 65.[8] In 1987, two thirds (63%) of health care expenditures for the elderly came from federally funded programs. They include **Medicare** ($72 billion), **Medicaid** ($20 billion), and other programs ($10 billion). Persons younger than 65 drew only 26 percent from these government-sponsored programs.[8]

It has been estimated that by the year 2025, nearly two thirds of the U.S. health care budget will be devoted to services for the elderly.[10] This will place incredible demands on the health care system and its professionals. The question remains as to whether we will be ready to handle this staggering demand for health care services, to say nothing of affording the astronomical costs!

LONG-TERM CARE

As of 1988, approximately 6.9 million persons older than the age of 65 required long-term care. It is estimated that by the year 2000 this number will increase to 9 million, and by 2040, owing to the aging baby boom generation, it is projected that 18 million individuals older than 65 will need long-term care.[1] Since 1966, when Medicare and Medicaid were introduced, the percentage of elderly requiring nursing home care has doubled from 2.5 to 5 percent.

In the population of those older than 85, one in four need to be placed in nursing homes. As this represents the fastest-growing segment of the population, the demand for nursing home beds will increase dramatically. Right now the number of nursing home beds is increasing by only half the rate at which this **age cohort** is increasing. Projections indicate that the number of nursing home residents will likely increase from 1.5 million in 1990 to 2.1 million in 2005 and 2.6 million by 2020.[1]

Elders who find themselves in **long-term care** facilities will, on average, use their life savings within 1 year. At that point they become eligible for Medicaid. Considering the sharp increase in need, the question that begs asking is, where will the funds come from to continue support of this program? This presents another problem for our ever-aging society, especially considering the ongoing debates to cut health care benefits such as Medicare.

As a result of the trend to get patients out of the hospital and back home as soon as possible, home health care has seen a dramatic increase. Expenditures for home health services were $7.9 million dollars in 1990. This is expected to increase to $19.8 billion by the year 2020.[1] The advantage of home care is that it allows one to remain in the community, which can be more beneficial than living in a long-term care facility from both a personal as well as financial perspective. A policy change that will affect delivery of both long-term and home care is the prospective payment system (PPS). This will require health care providers to become more productive and efficient in delivery of elder services in alternative settings.

SUMMARY

The demographics clearly indicate that the United States, as a nation, is growing older. On January 1, 1996, one American began turning 50 years of age every 7 seconds. This aging baby boom generation will effect massive societal changes. These changes will occur in terms of gender, race, geography, marital status, economics, and health care. The number of women will surpass those of men, with African-Americans, Hispanics, Native Americans, Asians, and Pacific Islanders aging by a greater percentage than whites. Some states will have close to an equal number of individuals younger and older than age 65. Social Security and other government entitlement programs are likely to be stretched to the breaking point, if they have not already broken. The health care system, perhaps most of all, will experience demands never previously encountered.

Health care professionals will be at the forefront of this aging tidal wave as it washes over, and through, our health care systems. Although hospital admissions and length of stays are on the decline as of 1996, this may not be the case in 2010 to 2030 as baby boomers descend upon health care institutions. Even without dramatic increases in hospital admissions, long-term care and home care are expected to experience a dramatic rise in patient volume. It is not unrealistic to expect that two out of three health care professionals will be working in either long-term care or home care in the future. The majority of the patients in these settings will be elderly. Therefore, it would benefit health care professionals to have an understanding of trends and projections as they relate to the "graying of America."

REVIEW QUESTIONS

1. As of January 1, 1996, one American will turn 50 every _____ for the next 18 years.
   A. 7 minutes
   B. 7 seconds
   C. Hour
   D. None of the above

2. The fastest growing segment of the population consists of individuals:
   A. 1–18 years of age
   B. 24–40 years of age
   C. 30–50 years of age
   D. 50–65 years of age
   E. Older than 85 years of age

3. The young-old, according to Bernice Neugarten, refers to those:
   A. 45–55 years of age
   B. 55–74 years of age
   C. 65–75 years of age
   D. 60–80 years of age

4. Women can expect to live, on average, _____ years longer than men.
   A. 2
   B. 5
   C. 7
   D. 10

5. Which ethnic group of those older than 65 is expected to increase at the most rapid rate between 1990 and 2030?

   A. African-Americans
   B. Native Americans
   C. Whites
   D. Hispanics
   E. Southeast Asians

6. As of 1994, the state that had the largest percentage of its population older than 65 was:

   A. Rhode Island
   B. California
   C. North Dakota
   D. Florida
   E. None of the above

7. In 1994 widows exceeded widowers by:

   A. 50%
   B. 100%
   C. 200%
   D. 500%

8. Poverty levels for the elderly in relation to those 18–64 are:

   A. Equal
   B. Greater by 50%
   C. Lesser by 25%
   D. Lesser by 50%

9. Elders account for what percentage of total personal health care expenditures?

   A. 10%
   B. 27%
   C. 36%
   D. 50%

10. When an elderly person in a long-term care facility expends their life savings, which of the following plans provides for their continued care?

    A. Medicaid
    B. Medicare
    C. Social Security
    D. All of the above

LEARNING ACTIVITIES

1. List what you believe will be some trends set by the baby boomer generation as it ages.

2. Design an elder community in a United States location. What factors would you consider in the design? Where would you place this community?

3. Which health care services and/or products are likely to be required by an aging population?

4. What will be possible roles and responsibilities of future health care professionals in long-term care facilities and home care?

5. Visualize yourself and your friends as older than 65 years of age. Where will you be living? What will you be doing? What will be your hobbies/roles? What will society be like?

🔲 REFERENCES

1. U.S. Senate Special Committee on Aging, American Association of Retired Persons, Federal Council on the Aging, and U.S. Administration on Aging: Aging America, Trends and Projections, 1991 ed. U.S. Department of Health and Human Services, Washington, DC, 1991.

2. Hayflick, KI: How and Why We Age. Ballantine Books, New York, 1994.

3. Neugarten, B: The rise of the young-old. In Gross, R, et al (eds): The New Old: Struggling for a Decent Aging. Doubleday Anchor, Garden City, NY, 1978, p 47.

4. Oriol, W: The demographics of an aging revolution. In Preparing for an Aging Society: Changes and Challenges. National Council on the Aging, Washington, DC, 1992.

5. Hollman, FW: U.S. Population Estimates, by Age, Sex, Race and Hispanic Origin: 1989. (Current Population Reports Series, p-25, no. 1057). U.S. Bureau of the Census, Washington, DC, March, 1990.

6. Spencer, G: Projections of the Population of the United States, by Age, Sex, and Race: 1988 to 2080. (Current Population Reports Series, p-25, no. 1018). U.S. Bureau of the Census, Washington, DC, January, 1989.

7. Aiken, LR: Aging, An Introduction to Gerontology. Sage, Thousand Oaks, CA, 1995.

8. American Association of Retired Persons: A Profile of Older Americans: 1995 AARP, Administration on Aging, U.S. Dept. of Health and Human Services, 1995.

9. Grad, S: Income of the Population 55 or Older, 1994. Social Security Administration Office of Research and Statistics, Washington, DC, January, 1996.

10. Chop, W: Resources for an aging population. RT: The Journal for Respiratory Care Practitioners 8(1):25, December/January, 1995.

In old age, wandering on a trail
of beauty, lively may I walk.
It is finished in beauty.
Navajo Nightway Chant

Social Aspects of Aging

Walter C. Chop

 BEHAVIORAL OBJECTIVES

Upon completion of this chapter, the reader will be able to:

1. Discuss trends in ethnic aging.
2. Define ageism, and state examples of myths that promote it.

3. Discuss the media's portrayal of the elderly.
4. Describe political involvement of the elderly, including their organizations and activities.
5. Describe retirement as well as various attitudes and feelings of individuals toward it.
6. Discuss some of the diverse lifestyles of the elderly.
7. Describe the "late life" crisis experienced by many elderly couples.
8. Contrast types of relationships between aging parent and adult child.
9. Describe sibling relationships in later life.
10. Discuss the importance of friendships to an aged individual.
11. Identify the five major categories of grandparents according to Neugarten and Weinstein.
12. State the major sources of income for persons older than 65.
13. Describe the role of good nutrition in maintaining a number of body functions and slowing the decline of aging.
14. Discuss the importance of fitness and exercise to the aging body.
15. Identify reasons why health promotion and disease prevention programs are so beneficial to aging individuals.
16. Describe issues related to health care financing as they affect the elderly.

KEY TERMS

Ageism	Medicaid
American Association of Retired Persons (AARP)	Medicare
	Mediterranean diet
Baby boom generation	Myths of aging
Ethnic aging	National Council of Senior Citizens
Grandparenting	Retirement
Gray Panthers	Senior Volunteer Corps
Health promotion/disease prevention	Social Security
	Structural lag
Late life crisis	Third age

ETHNIC AGING

Culturally, aging, as well as treatment of the elderly, is often determined by the value systems of an **ethnic** group. This also may determine the way the older person views the process of aging as well as the manner in which he or she adapts to growing older.[1] Some ethnic groups view the elder as an authority figure who resides in a position of power within the family and community. Other ethnic groups take an almost opposite view and see the elder in terms of added responsibility, if not burden, to family and society.

African-American elderly, as the largest ethnic minority in the United States, have lagged behind whites in terms of social and economic status. Many elderly African-Americans must continue working because of lower Social Security benefits.[2] On a more positive note, African-Americans, in general, have extensive kin networks and also tend to have better coping skills than their white counterparts.[2] Black elders often provide help to young family members and neighbors. Community institutions, such as the church, are very important sources of physical and emotional support.

Aged Hispanics in the United States make up the second largest ethnic minority and the fastest growing ethnic group. According to 1990 U.S. Census projections, Hispanics will outnumber African-Americans by the year 2030.[7] Mexican-Americans, who make up 60 percent of the Hispanic population, generally have close relationships and more contact with their children and thus greater family solidarity than their white counterparts.[1] Like African-Americans, Hispanic elderly tend to be socioeconomically less well off than older whites and most other ethnic elders. Hispanic elderly also have a greater propensity toward developing diabetes as well as for contracting an infectious disease.[1]

Native American elderly fall into the lowest socioeconomic category. The following social and economic indicators clearly illustrate this:

- 57 percent have incomes barely covering expenses
- 28 percent are partially to totally blind
- 64 percent have less than an eighth grade education
- 56 percent live in housing that is more than 30 years old and often substandard[1]

In 1982 the Indian Aging Network was established to help address some of these problems. This organization also reinforces the concept that the knowledge and wisdom of the elders is needed in order to preserve Native American culture and history.[1]

Asian-American older persons make up a small but rapidly growing fraction of the elderly population in the country. As a group they tend to be somewhat better off, by most social indicators, than other elderly minority groups. Family life and a respect for the knowledge and wisdom of the elder are central to Asian culture.[2] This has, however, decreased somewhat with modernization and integration into American society.

Japanese-American elderly are the most well off of Asian elders economically, socially, and in terms of life expectancy. They also have the highest educational expectations for their children.

As with other Asian-American groups, Chinese elders also strive to maintain and strengthen their cultural heritage. Family life is central to their existence. Many Chinese elders live with their children, because less than half are covered by Social Security, never having had paid employment in this country.[1]

More recent immigrant arrivals include Vietnamese and other Southeast Asians. Their numbers are, in fact, growing faster than any other Asian group. Approximately 75% of Vietnamese elderly live with their extended families. Many have never worked in this country, and, as is the case with many Chinese elders, therefore are not entitled to Social Security benefits.

🔳 AGEISM

In addition to racism and sexism, we must now add **ageism** to our list of "ism's." This term was coined by Dr. Robert Butler in 1969 in an article entitled "Ageism: Another Form of Bigotry."[3] Butler defined ageism as a systematic stereotyping of, and discrimination against, people who are old. The relationship of old age with ageism is similar to that of skin color with racism and gender with sexism. Dr. Butler states that ageism perpetuates the notion of a gender gap. In doing so it reflects a revulsion and distaste on the part of the young and middle-aged for growing old, disease, disability, uselessness, and death.[3] Ageism also categorizes older persons as senile, rigid in thought and manner, as well as old-fashioned in morality and skills. It perpetuates the attitude of the younger generation seeing older people as different from themselves. Thus, they subtly may cease to identify elderly individuals as human beings.

Since Dr. Butler first wrote about ageism, there has been some gradual improvement in attitudes toward the elderly. This has, in part, been fostered by greater public education, increased media attention, and the appearance of more positive role models, especially in the recent movies "Fried Green Tomatoes" and "Driving Miss Daisy." This, however, has done little to reverse the deeper undercurrents that run below the surface of ageism. Cited here are just some examples of myths that promote the continuation of ageism:

- The majority of old people (older than 65) are senile (have defective memory or are disoriented or demented) (see Chapter 4).
- The majority of old people have no interest in, nor capacity for, sexual relations (see Chapter 7).
- The majority of old people feel miserable most of the time.
- The majority of old people are unable to adapt to change.
- It is difficult for the average old person to learn something new.
- In general, old people tend to be pretty much alike.[4]

Another **myth of aging** conjures an image of the elderly entering into a kind of "Fantasy Land" where every experience is "rosy" and "carefree." Then there is the overly sympathetic image of the "poor old dear" who can do little to care for himself or herself. Negative connotations are also implied when one refers to an unfamiliar elderly person as "honey," "dear," or by his or her first name without asking his or her preference. This "infantilizing" the elderly increases dependency rather than fostering independence. Although this is more subtle, it is another form of ageism and should be avoided.

Research has shown that health care professionals are significantly more negative in their attitudes toward older patients than toward young ones.[5] This suggests that stereotyping of elderly patients by health care professionals may serve as a justification for not attending to their needs. Health providers may also have this attitude because the older patient reminds them of their own mortality and eventual demise.[5]

Many negative terms have been used to describe the elderly. These include "geezer," "old hag," "fogey," "old duffer," "dirty old man," "fossil," "old goat," "battle ax," "out to pasture," and "over the hill" to name a few. Other negative images center on the elderly as "greedy geezers" who have more than their "fair share of advantages and tend to siphon off public money that should be going to poor children.[6] This attitude is reflected in the cover of the rock group Megadeath's CD entitled "Youthanasia," where one sees an old woman ("hag") hanging the young out to dry on a clothesline.

Much has been written regarding attitudes toward older workers. They are thought to be ridged, inflexible, and incapable of learning new skills. It should, therefore, come as no surprise that the most common type of economic discrimination against the elderly is employment or working discrimination.[4] This discrimination may prevent an older person from being hired. Work discrimination against elders is obvious when older workers are asked to take early retirement, even seduced into it by a tempting retirement package, the so-called golden parachute. Until 1967 retirement was compulsory for workers who reached 65 years of age, regardless of their health or ability. Here again we see another myth of aging that implies there is a general loss of ability that begins occurring around age 65 or earlier. However, in healthy adults there exists no sudden or general loss of ability at age 65 or any other age.[4] Any losses that may occur generally do so gradually over a number of years. Even some disorders considered inevitable as we age (such as visual and hearing disturbances) may be reversible or amenable to treatment.

It is interesting to note the findings of a survey that shows that 80 percent of adults believe that most employers discriminate against older workers, and 61 percent of employers agreed that they do this.[7] This discrimination ignores several advantages to having older workers as employees, such as lower rate of absenteeism, less turnover, lower accident rate, less alcoholism and drug addiction, and more job satisfaction and company loyalty.[4]

THE MEDIA'S ATTITUDE TOWARD THE ELDERLY

The media play a major role in perpetuating age stereotyping. Generally they portray the elderly as "more comical, stubborn, eccentric and foolish than other characters."[5] They are also depicted as "narrow-minded, in poor health, foundering financially, sexually dissatisfied and unable to make decisions."[5] Although we do see older individuals on entertainment and other special programming, it is unusual to see a realistic portrayal of an older person on television. This treatment by the media appears inconsistent when considering that older adults watch television more than any other age group (averaging more than 40 hours a week).

Commercials tend to portray elderly at their worst—when they have some kind of physical ailment. We see older actors in commercials for laxatives, skin moisturizers, gas elimination medications, analgesics, and hair coloring products, just to name a few. This would not be as detrimental to the image of the older adult if we also saw the elderly in other types of commercials advertising general use products. If all goes well, this will change as advertisers begin to realize that a steady increase in those older than 65 will continue for the foreseeable future. They may also realize that many of these elders have dollars to spend.

POLITICAL INVOLVEMENT

One third of those who vote in both local and national elections are older than 55, with the average age of the American voter being 47.[5] This will increase with the aging of the **baby boom generation.** In fact, when "Boomers" advance into their fifties and sixties, they will set the political agenda and dominate election outcomes.[8] The elderly generally wield more clout at nominating conventions as a result of their increased degree of involvement. Elders tend to be involved in politics more out of a sense of fulfillment than a means to a concrete end. They generally enjoy political participation but are often disillusioned regarding the potential outcome.

There exists a misconception that the elderly tend to vote more conservatively. This is false. Elderly people generally vote along lines almost identical to the voting pattern of the rest of the population.[8] They even comprise the same proportion of party organizations as the general population.

The **American Association of Retired Persons (AARP)** boasts having 35 million members, plus more than 1000 employees in its Washington, DC, headquarters and 10 regional centers.[9] If the AARP were an independent nation in numbers, it would be the 30th largest nation in the world (with only slightly fewer people than Argentina).[8] The major mission of the AARP is to disseminate information and support research on aging. They do not sponsor political action committees (PACs). They do, however, provide their members with information on legislation that may affect them, such as health care information, proposed changes to Social Security, or pending legislative action. The AARP strongly encourages social reform. Their 1992 vision statement was titled "Toward a Just and Caring Society."

A more "militant," but much smaller, organization of elderly persons is the **Gray Panthers.** It has approximately 75,000 members with chapters in 30 states.[9] The Gray Panthers was founded by Maggie Kuhn, who along with six other women designed its organizational structure. The catalyst for these women coming together was their forced retirement at 65 years of age. The first issue taken on by the fledgling organization, however, was not age discrimination, but rather opposition to the war in Vietnam. The Gray Panthers did not want to be perceived as an organization that was only dedicated to fighting ageism. Philosophically the Panthers believe that "gray power" should be on the cutting edge of social change by working with other organizations and "establishing intergenerational bonds necessary for real social change—the continuity of life."[9] The Gray Panthers continue to work for affordable and adequate housing for all, the elimination of homelessness, and the promotion of innovative work concepts that include flexible work/retirement schedules (job sharing, flex time, shorter work week) for all.[9]

In the 1970s the Gray Panthers mobilized people to expose and document nursing home abuse in their own communities. Around the same time, they were also instrumental in the enactment of the Age Discrimination Employment Act, which raised mandatory retirement age from 65 to 70. In 1990, they fought to add the intergenerational amendment to the Older American Act, which decries discrimination of any age group.[9]

Another politically active elder organization is the **National Council of Senior Citizens,** which primarily focuses on political and legislative issues. The organization maintains a Congressional voting record that scores legislators as to how they vote on issues. This record is mailed to half a million persons annually.

Overall, the political power of the elderly is unrivaled by any other group. "What the gray lobby wants, it usually gets."[8] Some examples of this political success are listed here:

> 1965—Medicare and Medicaid enacted
> 1967—Age discrimination in employment made illegal
> 1972—Social Security indexed to inflation
> 1978—The age of mandatory retirement for most workers pushed back to 70
> 1986—Mandatory retirement, at any age, eliminated for almost all workers.[8]

Caution to those politicians voting against legislation "friendly" to the elderly. The elderly are, and will continue to be, a strong force with which to reckon.

RETIREMENT

Before the industrial revolution, **retirement** as a phase of life did not exist. Individuals worked until they either became disabled or too infirm to do otherwise. They generally died shortly afterward. If they did survive to a "ripe old age," they were usually supported by family or by some charitable organization such as the local church. It was only in 1889 that Chancellor Bismarck of Germany established retirement for individuals reaching age 65. He chose the age of 65 as the beginning of retirement by adding 20 years to the then normal life expectancy of 45 years.[10] Other European countries soon followed with similar retirement systems. In 1935 the United States was the first country to establish a nationalized pension system for those older than 65.[10] Although life expectancy has increased dramatically since the turn of the century, 65 has remained the average retirement age in most Western countries. Individuals who retired in 1900 spent only 3 percent of their lives in retirement. This accounted for only a few years of their total life. Today the average retiree spends 25 to 30 percent, or 20 to 35 years, in retirement. This accounts for more additional years of life than were ever available in all human history.

Perhaps by eliminating the term *retirement* and replacing it with a more positive or proactive term, some of the social stigma attached to retirement, such as loss of status and function, diminished contact with others, and a decrease in income, can be reversed. One such term suggested by G. P. Mulley, is **Third Age.**[11] The first age is childhood and preparation for work; the second is employment and family raising; this is followed by the third age; and the fourth and final stage is dependence.[11] Although a somewhat more positive term than retirement, third age still seems to "pigeonhole" an individual into a preassigned age bracket.

Matilda and John Riley, pioneers in the field of social gerontology, call for a structural revolution in our attitudes toward working and retirement (Fig. 2–1). They believe that we should have a non-age-differentiating society where there are no established ages for school, work, or retirement. This mirrors their conviction that the dynamism of aging has been outrunning the dynamism of structural change.[12] They refer to this problem as a **"structural lag"** in which an imbalance exists between the number of individuals age 65 and older and the availability of productive and fulfilling role opportunities for them in order to recognize and develop these capacities.[12] What they envision is an age-integrated society in which individuals of all ages can enter and leave educational systems, work roles, and leisure endeavors throughout the life span (Fig. 2–2). A study from Great Britain and the United States found that more than 80 percent of individuals in their sixties were fully mobile, mentally alert, and in overall good health, thus still fully able to work.[11]

With the retirement years making up a larger portion of one's life, a number of issues need to be addressed. What will persons do with all their newfound leisure time? Will some individuals look at it as a period of regression or boredom, or perhaps just a period for "killing time"? Others may even ex-

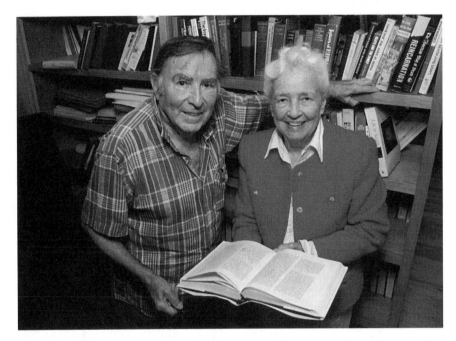

FIG. 2–1. Matilda and John Riley, pioneers in the field of social gerontology. (Courtesy of Gary Bonaccorso, The Times Record, Brunswick, Maine)

perience a sort of anxiety-neurosis. In his book *Learn to Grow Old,* Tournier states that "we have been trained for work and not for leisure."[13] The philosopher Montaigne put this another way: "Work first, play later."

Tournier stresses the need to prepare for retirement when we are still in middle age. This can be accomplished in part by developing hobbies or spare-time occupations. However, Tournier adds that even hobbies that have given us a few hours pleasure after work may not be enough to sustain us when, after retirement, it is the only thing left to fill our lives.[13] It seems clear that in addition to hobbies or interests we need to formulate a new mindset when approaching retirement. In *Growing Old Disgracefully: New Ideas for Getting the Most Out of Life,* the authors state that it is necessary to "clear out old messages."[14] This, they say is first done by exorcising your demons and discarding old patterns that get in your way. They also state that it is important to have role models—individuals who have reached old age maintaining a positive attitude.[14]

A 1991 survey on productive aging conducted by Harris and associates arrived at the following conclusions:

1. Individuals must prepare for longer and more productive lives. Forty percent of older respondents expressed interest in furthering their education

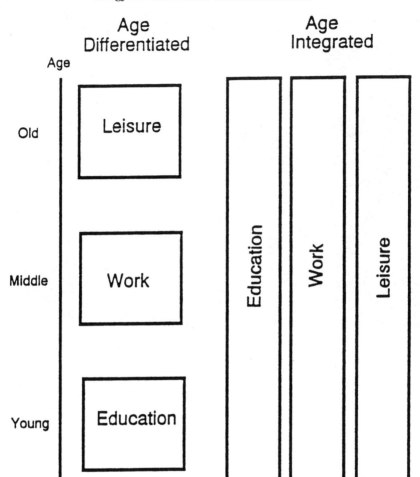

FIG. 2–2. Ideal types of social structures. (Adapted from Riley, M, and Riley, J: Age integration and the lives of older people. Gerontologist 34:111, 1994, with permission.)

or training. An even higher percentage wanted more education or training if this was provided "on the job."

2. Employers need to encourage older workers to participate in life-long learning and training. This can be accomplished more readily by the creation of flexible workplaces and work hours.

3. Educational institutions must become more aware of the needs of older learners. Elders are encouraged to see the relevance of educational endeavors. Self-paced instruction and physical environment are important considerations in elderly education.[15]

One researcher described retirement in terms of the following three phases: disenchantment phase, reorientation phase, and termination phase.[16] It should be noted that one does not necessarily progress through all three phases. The disenchantment phase, in which one realizes that retirement is not what was expected, is followed by the reorientation phase, which involves acceptance and adjustment to the retirement role. Finally, sometimes the termination phase occurs, in which depression, illness, and/or disability convert one's role or status into that of care receiver or patient.[16]

The dream of a carefree retirement can be deceptive. Numerous studies, especially in men, have found that depression, illness, and death increase fairly dramatically within 3 to 5 years after retirement. This may come as no surprise, because work satisfaction is the best predictor of longevity. Many of us define ourselves by the work we perform, for example, "I am a teacher" or "salesperson" or "computer technician." We sometimes find it difficult to look at ourselves without thinking in terms of our career titles. Our very identity is often linked to our professional life, without which many of us would perceive a loss of purpose and/or prestige.

Men who continue to have high career goals suffer most from anxiety and other detrimental symptoms after retirement. Traditionally this loss of identity following retirement has been experienced by men more often than women. This is in part due to the fact that all the earlier studies looked at the effect of retirement exclusively on men. Women were studied only as to the effect that their husband's retirement had on them. A few studies report that women who retire experience a greater loss of self, and accompanying depression, than men. These were, for the most part, women who put all their energies in job or career in place of marriage or children. In general, most women did not experience this post-career anxiety/depression syndrome.

White men tend to cope less well with retirement. Those between the ages of 70 and 74 commit suicide at a three times higher rate than nonwhites and a five times higher rate than women of the same age.[16] Although persons older than 65 make up only 11.5 percent of the population, they account for 25 percent of all suicides. Again, this occurs much more frequently among men than women, with an approximate 10:1 ratio among those 65 and older.[16]

Retirement can also be viewed in a more positive light. For example, Robert Allison, former CEO of Doe-Anderson of Louisville, Kentucky, states "My 3 years of retirement have been the best years of my life. Not once has the thought ever crossed my mind that I'd like to be back running the agency."[17] When asked by his friends what he would find to do each day, Allison decided to come up with some suggestions for a happy retirement. They are summarized as follows:

- Be married to someone you have fun being with.
- It is better if you both are in good health.

- Have enough resources so as not to drastically reduce your lifestyle.
- Don't overcommit yourself.
- Don't anticipate being called by your former employer for counsel and advice.
- Recognize and accept that your situation has changed and perhaps so will some of your friends.
- Cut the cord with your former employer.
- Be personally and publicly supportive of your former employer or place of employment.
- Don't wait for others to make things happen, initiate your own actions.
- Do something to pump up your adrenalin once in a while.[17]

LIFESTYLES OF THE ELDERLY

The elderly, like any group of individuals, are incredibly diverse. Ken Dychtwald, president of Age Wave Inc., states that "No age group is more varied in personal background, physical abilities, personal styles, social needs, or financial capabilities than today's older population. While some older people are dreadfully sick and waiting for death, some are fit and training for marathons. Some wait in breadlines for a warm meal. Others have condos in Vail and yachts in Tahiti."[8] Dychtwald suggests that this diversity should be acknowledged in social policy as well as governmentally sponsored programs.

The question that should be asked is: What is deemed meaningful to the elderly individual? For some elders this entails spending time with grandchildren. Others such as the mall walkers, senior center card players, and "get together for lunch bunch" find meaning in personal interactions with their friends. Some prefer to continue working, like John and Matilda Riley, mentioned earlier. Matilda, age 82, is a senior social scientist at the National Institute on Aging; John, age 85, is a consultant and researcher.[18] Others would rather spend their time on the golf course or on a boat.

Some elders are determined to challenge themselves in pursuit of some activity that few, regardless of age, would choose to follow. Mary Harper, a 79-year-old great-grandmother, is one person who rose to such a challenge (Fig. 2–3). In 1994, she became the oldest person to sail across the Atlantic single-handedly. Although she broke a rib in severe weather, she later said "the whole trip was worth it just to see the waves." In answer to why she did it alone, she explained that "it was something she wanted to do. . . . but didn't want to be responsible for a crew."[19] Another elder who has refused to settle down to "quiet old age" is Corena Leslie, who sky-dived 3 days before her 90th birthday.[20]

Other elders, such as Jacob Landers, launch themselves into second ca-

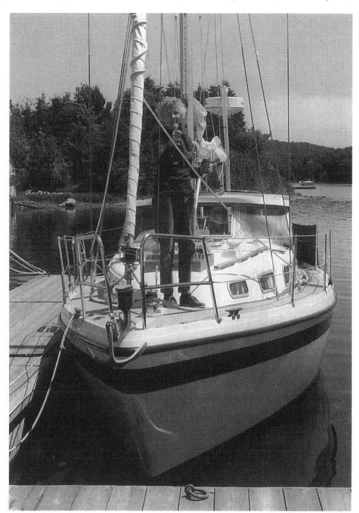

FIG. 2–3. Mary Harper, the oldest person to sail across the Atlantic Ocean single-handedly. (Courtesy of Mary Harper.)

reers. Landers entered law school at 67 without ever having previous thoughts of becoming a lawyer. He had already completed several careers, including that of a teacher, administrator, and consultant. Each time he retired from one he found himself getting restless and decided to begin a new career. On one particular Thanksgiving, while talking with his daughter who was a law student at that time, he said he wished he could also go to law school. His daughter said, "Why don't you?" That was all it took to launch him into yet one more career. When their conversation was finished, he told her he would apply to law school the following Monday. Today Landers is a staff attorney at the Brookdale Center on Aging at Hunter College in New York City. Most of his work involves lobbying for the elderly on cases that involve retirement guidelines, **Social Security,** and **Medicare.**[8] These may seem to be unusual cases, but all over the country on a regular basis we hear of "ordinary" people doing extraordinary things during their so-called old age.

Large numbers of the elderly devote many hours to volunteering. According to Tom Endres, acting director of National Senior Volunteer Corps, "Older Americans are a reservoir of talent, experience and energy." Communities are eagerly tapping into this source of person power to help combat a number of societal ills. The **Senior Volunteer Corps** is actually an umbrella organization that encompasses three programs: Retired Senior Volunteer Program (RSVP), Foster Grandparents, and Senior Companions.[21]

Many elders believe what Margaret Ratz has stated: "If you have mental stimulation, you have life."[9] Ms. Ratz is a member of the Plymouth Harbor Retirement Community of Sarasota, Florida, where longevity among its residents is greater than the national average. This unique community encourages individuals to get involved in a myriad of activities, which include electing representatives from each apartment cluster to serve on the board of residents that governs Plymouth Harbor. Residents also pool their resources in supplying volunteer lecturers on just about every topic imaginable. People at Plymouth Harbor appear more involved, interested, and perhaps "more alive" than the stereotypical portrayal of retirees.[9] One is reminded of the movie "Cocoon," in which elders in a retirement community come in contact with large egg-shaped pods from outer space and are instantly rejuvenated in their interests and pursuits. As Ralph Waldo Emerson states in his poem "Immortality" (1885): "It is not length of life but depth of life."

FAMILY AND SOCIAL ROLES

THE AGING COUPLE

Relationships that last into old age have usually experienced and, if all went well, overcome many crises. A **late life crisis** is also to be expected. For some couples this is just another of life's transitions that they have shared together. Others, however, find it to be a time of deep soul searching, wondering what the future of the relationship will be like. This is especially true if the crisis occurs in the decades of the fifties and sixties, when it usually coincides with the empty nest syndrome and/or retirement.[22]

If a couple successfully weathers this late life crisis, their feelings for each other can actually become enriched and strengthened. However, a problem can occur when the partners experience their late life crises at different times. This can occur not only for couples whose age differences are fairly significant but also for couples who are the same chronological age but on different personal time tables.

There are those couples who are not destined to grow older together. Maybe they have stayed together for the sake of the children, or perhaps they became absorbed in work or other activities so they would not have to deal with their underlying relationship issues. There are also couples who are closely connected but not emotionally in touch. They may even be genuinely fond of each other but view their relationship as more a business partnership than marriage.[22] A "marriage of convenience" is similar to this, in which each partner does "his or her own thing." Sometimes one or both partners in this type of relationship engages in an extramarital affair, which can often bring about the final unraveling of the marriage.[22]

Although some relationships worsen or dissolve with age, others actually get better and experience a sort of renewal or rebirth. Late life can be the most satisfying years of a marriage for the couple who even through difficult times, and certainly through great mutual frankness, have come to accept each other for who he or she is.[13]

AGING PARENT AND ADULT CHILD

Relationships between aging parents and adult children tend to be as varied as spousal relationships. Generally there exists a fair degree of involvement between the generations. Older parents very often provide help and support both emotionally and financially, when possible. Ideally this should be done "without strings attached." Unfortunately, in some instances, strained relations can develop between parent and child. Verbal finger pointing—unfair fighting with "you never" or "you always" statements—can upset relations, as can favoritism toward certain siblings. Sometimes parental disapproval of lifestyle or friends can bring about disharmony. Disappointment coupled with shame may cause one to "keep up appearances" and place the son's or daughter's feelings second.[22] If affection and communication remain open between parent and adult child, parental and adult child psychological well-being is enhanced.[23]

Aging baby boomers may find they have less time to spend with their children as demands of aging parents occupy more of their time.[8] Increasing numbers of adult children will become caregivers to their aging parents. In fact, approximately 80 percent of the elderly will receive care from their families at some point in their lives.[8] It is estimated that the average American woman can expect to spend more time caring for an aging parent than she did caring for her children.[8] As these boomers become a "sandwich generation," their frustration often mounts, sometimes leading to elder neglect and even abuse.

SIBLINGS

Approximately 80 percent of older persons have living brothers and/or sisters.[24] As we age, sibling relationships become more important.[22] More effort may be made to visit siblings, even if this requires traveling greater distances, in old age than in middle age. Sibling relationships are especially important in the lives of older persons who never married.[24]

Sibling rivalries, however, can and often do persist into old age. In some cases they may lie dormant and resurface in later life.[22] An aging, sick parent can sometimes intensify unpleasantness between older siblings as previous rivalries resurface. Many sibling relationships are also shattered by the contesting of a parent's will.

FRIENDS

Friendships from early life often continue into old age, in part, as a result of individuals who have "shared history." Deep, personal bonds with friends often mean more to elders than casual family ties or involvement with social groups.[9] Research over the past two decades has concluded that friends are more important to the psychological well-being of the elderly than family members.[23] The relationship between friendship and psychological well-being is not clear, but there does appear to be a connection. Elders feel loss when separated from old friends and often seek out new friends.[23] Friends often provide elders with support in time of need or crisis. Assisting in emergencies and providing needed transportation, care during illness, and comfort during bereavement are examples of such support.[23]

Older women generally have more friends than older men. They also place more value on the friendships and talk about them more, while men tend to be more passive about their friendships.[24] It should come as no surprise that employed women, and those who are socially active, tend to have more friends than those who neither work nor are socially involved.[23]

Friendships tend to be retained into later life if they begin in middle life. This seems to increase with one's socioeconomic status.[24] Older persons are generally selective of their friends, tending toward establishing friendships with those of the same gender, similar social and economic status, and from the same town or community.[24] Elders engage in the role of being a friend indefinitely; often longer than the role of spouse, worker, or organization member. Although the number of friends generally decreases with age, some elderly actually report an increase in their number of friends. Most elders experience a feeling of loss with the death of a friend, but learn to accept it as an inevitable part of growing old. However, almost all elderly believe that replacing lost friends is very difficult.[24]

GRANDPARENTING

Of the 72 million individuals in the United States in 1996 older than 45, nearly 50 million were grandparents.[8] It is estimated that there will be 98 million grandparents by 2002.[25] Approximately 18 million, or half, of the individuals older than 65 are great-grandparents.[8] Families now, and into the next millennium, may include grandparents, great-grandparents, and even some great-great-grandparents.

More than 25 years ago Bernice Neugarten and Karol Weinstein described five major types of grandparents:

- Distance figures
- Fun-seekers
- Surrogate parents
- Formal
- Reservoirs of family wisdom

These **grandparenting roles** certainly are not "carved in granite." As generational relationships change, so too do these roles often change. One of a grandparent's most important roles is that of caregiver. This consists of everything from babysitting and parenting to providing financial support for college tuition or a deposit on a house. If grandparents are better off financially than their children, they generally become supportive financially. They may provide money for a much-needed vacation or new car. It is estimated that grandparent spending accounts for 25 percent of dollars spent on toys in the United States.

Besides providing financial support, grandparents sometimes step in to take care of grandchildren when parents are physically or sexually abusive or if parents become addicted to drugs or are otherwise no longer able to parent. Grandparents can also act as mediators when conflicts arise between parents and children. When parents divorce, grandparents can offer support, comfort, consolation, and sometimes financial assistance to their grandchildren. Divorce, however, can also force grandparents out of their grandchild's life. Many grandparents fight back for visiting rights via organizations such as the Foundation for Grandparenting and Grandparents-Children Rights, Inc.

Arthur Kornhaber, M.D.,[25] author of *Contemporary Grandparenting* and *Grandparent Power,* created the Foundation for Grandparenting to nurture and lobby for intergenerational relationships. This foundation even offers a summer camp and conference center for grandparents and grandchildren in Roquette, New York. Kornhaber's studies have shown that children raised by grandparents tend to be more "well rounded". They also have a greater respect for the past. They are more likely to speak more than one language, perform better in school, and have a good sense of family and family values.

Closeness with grandchildren is often related to how as parents, they, and their children felt about each other and interacted while their own children were growing up.[22] Bonds between generations may become stronger when parents see their own parents in the role of grandparent, spending time with their children. Sometimes grandparents or adult children choose to maintain a distance, not only geographically, but also physically. They may have other priorities such as work or leisure. But more often grandparents welcome interactions with grandchildren as a chance to relive their early years, without the stresses and responsibilities experienced with their own children the first time around. A new grandchild can be like a blood transfusion, which may reawaken for the older couple the early days of their own marriage and early parenting.[22]

There even exist Adopt a Grandparent/Grandchild programs. One such program was created at the University of Pittsburgh.[8] These programs can be excellent for kids without grandparents or elders without grandchildren. Others become "foster grandparents" through youth centers or other community organizations. Whatever the case may be, grandparenting remains one of the most rewarding and fulfilling experiences of later life.

🔲 FINANCIAL STATUS OF THE ELDERLY

The importance of financial security in "old age" cannot be overemphasized. Most elderly men and women have worked a good portion of their lives to establish a pension or so-called nest egg from which to draw during their later years. It should therefore come as no surprise that elders signal a rallying cry every time mention is made of reducing Social Security or Medicare benefits. "Saving for a rainy day" was an adage that many lived by, especially those who lived through the Great Depression. This interferes sometimes with the willingness to spend money on luxuries for themselves or even on what others may deem necessary for their well-being (e.g., home safety adaptations, assistive technology, and the like).

The median income for persons older than 65 in 1994 was $15,250 for men and $8950 for women. Household median income for families headed by persons older than 65 was $26,512 in 1994 (Fig. 2–4). Nonfamily (persons living alone or with nonrelatives) elder households had a median income of $11,504.[26] African-Americans and Hispanics reported lower median incomes in all the aforementioned categories. Elderly median net worth (assets minus liabilities) was $86,300 in 1994. This was well above the national average of $37,600 for all age groups.[26]

The major source of income in 1994 for individuals older than 65 was **Social Security.** Although it is listed under retirement benefits, it is certainly the outstanding figure in this category.[26] Next highest source of income was earnings, at 18 percent, followed closely by asset income at 17.6 percent.[26] Private pensions, or annuities, and government employee pensions accounted for 9.7 percent and 8.4 percent, respectively, with all other means accounting for 4.2 percent (railroad, 0.6%; public assistance, 0.9%, and other, 2.7%).

Although more elderly have achieved financial security than ever before, there still exist 3.7 million individuals older than 65 living at the poverty level.[26] This accounts for 11.7 percent of persons older than 65 (about the same

Family households with head 65 +

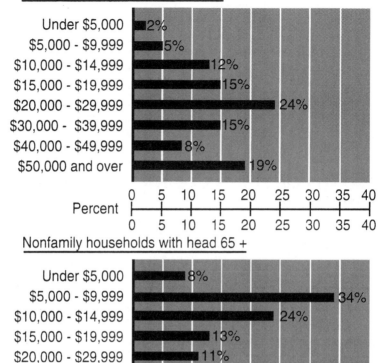

$26,512 median for 11.2 million family households 65 +

$11,504 median for 10.1 million nonfamily households 65 +

FIG. 2–4. Percentage distribution by income: 1994. (Reprinted from 65 + in the United States. U.S. Department of Commerce, Economics and Statistics Administration, Bureau of the Census, Washington, DC, 1996.)

as the rate for persons 18 to 64, which is 11.9%).[26] It has been shown that once older persons exhaust their resources, they are unlikely to generate the income necessary to improve their economic status or to leave assistance programs.[27] Individuals older than 65 also have more difficulty reentering the job market than their younger cohorts. Besides diminished employment opportunities, they are also least likely to benefit from inheritance. Many are often left to fend for themselves, living off their meager pension or Social Security benefits, which are barely adjusted for inflation. In addition to having lower incomes, the elderly spend a much larger portion of their total expenditures on health care and housing than their younger low-income counterparts.

Elderly black and Hispanic women, especially if they are unmarried, have an even more difficult time financially than their white counterparts. Approximately 54 percent of older black women living alone were living at the poverty level in 1994.[26] This should come as no surprise, because many held low-skill, low-wage jobs as a result of inadequate education as well as discrimination in the labor market.[28] It needs to be kept in mind that Social Security benefits, meager as they may be, will continue to be an important source of income for black and Hispanic women.

HEALTH PERSPECTIVE OF THE ELDERLY: AN OVERVIEW

This section on health perspective of the elderly contains an overview of topics that are covered in greater depth elsewhere in this text. As a result of improvements in health care, better diet, and more emphasis on exercise, Americans are entering the "sunset" years healthier than ever before. Aging needs to be differentiated from disease. Studies by the National Institute on Aging point out that many of the health problems of old age are not due to aging but rather to improper care of and use of one's body over the years. If one's body has been subjected to overeating, toxins (such as cigarette smoke or alcohol), lack of adequate exercise, and poor nutrition, it should come as no surprise that in old age one will have more medical problems.

NUTRITION

This is a brief overview of nutrition in the elderly; it is covered in greater depth in Chapter 5.

Although we purport to be a nation of plenty, 25 percent of persons older than 65 suffer from some form of malnutrition.[29] Poverty, although the major cause of malnutrition, is far from the only factor. It is estimated that 40 percent of all nursing home patients and 50 percent of all hospital patients are malnourished.[29] This, in large measure, is due to the fact that few doctors are trained to recognize malnutrition in the elderly. Some of the reasons for elderly malnutrition, besides poverty, include depression, lack of mobility in getting to the grocery store, unbalanced diet, problems with chewing or swallowing, chronic illness, and certain medications that suppress appetite.[29] Also, lack of physical ability and energy to cook and feed themselves compounds their problems.

It appears that poor nutrition may play a role in the progressive decline of several body functions with aging. Associated with aging is progressive decline in energy, lean body mass, and protein intake. Many elderly consume less than the recommended dietary allowances (RDA) for calcium, iron, zinc, copper, thiamin, riboflavin, folate, and vitamins B_{12}, B_6, and D.[30] Research clearly points out the need for alteration of RDA in many elderly individuals and that RDA intake of vitamins based on age alone may be misleading.[31]

It also appears that a number of age-related changes such as loss of bone density, atherosclerotic lesions, opacification of eye lens, a blunted immune system, and certain carcinomas can be slowed by nutritional interventions or hastened by improper nutrition.[31] Besides promoting an increase in healthy aging with improved quality of life, a delay in the onset of diseases could save billions in health care dollars.

Much has been written regarding the benefits of the so-called **Mediterranean Diet.** This diet is rich in carbohydrates, fiber, and monounsaturated fat, which translates into a diet consisting of olive oil, whole-grain breads, soups, beans, vegetables, and fruits. Wine, usually red, is also consumed in moderation at mealtimes. Several studies have shown lower rates of heart disease in persons following this diet.[32] It was also concluded that it is never too late to start eating a healthy diet. In fact, other studies support the fact that diets consisting of fruits, vegetables, and olive oil contribute to longevity, even among those individuals who have already reached age 75.[32]

FITNESS AND EXERCISE

The old adage of "use it or lose it" is very applicable when it comes to making a case for exercise in the older person. A number of studies have shown that exercise that increases aerobic capacity increases the number of synapses between brain neurons, thus increasing mental speed.[33] One study also found that physically fit elderly produced more alpha waves, a pattern associated with calmness even under pressure, and displayed sharper peaks and valleys in their waves, which signifies the ability to block out distractions.[33]

The ideal exercise program for individuals older than 60 should emphasize exercises that increase strength, flexibility, and endurance.[34] It should be initiated only after consultation with a medical specialist. Low-impact activities such as walking, swimming, or bike riding are ideally suited for most elderly. Exercise should be preceded by stretching and should be increased in gradual increments. An exercise "prescription" from a physician is a good way to begin, especially for those who have been away from exercise for any length of time. Ideally, in order to achieve an aerobic workout, activity should be fairly brisk. Again, an elderly person needs to be reminded not to exceed his or her ability level. Many hospitals, colleges, and community organizations now have exercise programs especially tailored to the elderly individual.

HEALTH PROMOTION AND DISEASE PREVENTION

In 1990 a document entitled *Healthy People 2000* was released by the U.S. Public Health Service. The intent of this report was to reduce preventable death and disability for Americans by the year 2000. Healthy People 2000 focused on three major goals:

1. To increase the span of healthy life
2. To reduce health disparities
3. To achieve access to preventive services[35]

The report emphasized the need for vitality and independence with aging. It should be noted that Healthy People 2000 is health-oriented, not disease-oriented, and takes into account socioeconomic, lifestyle, and other nonmedical related influences that can affect one's health.

The common complaints associated with aging include joint stiffness, weight gain, fatigue, loss of bone mass, and loneliness. These can all be slowed, prevented, or eliminated by **health promotion disease prevention** activities.[34] Activities should focus on exercise, stress management, nutrition, and substance abuse control. Educational sessions first need to be conducted before initiating any of the aforementioned health activities. Remember to keep in mind that older persons tend to learn more effectively in small groups that foster discussion in an informal setting. Elders are also, for the most part, concrete rather than theoretical learners and learn best when the subject matter has direct practical application.

Multiple studies have touted the benefits of exercise across the life span. Exercise helps maintain fitness, stimulates and quickens the mind, helps establish social contacts, prevents and/or slows progression of some diseases, and generally improves one's quality of life.[34] Also, inactivity leads to muscle wasting and weakening of the bones. A number of chronic conditions such as heart disease, arthritis, osteoporosis, diabetes, obesity, and depression show improvement, or at least a slowing of progression, with regular physical activity.

Much has been written recently on the relationship between stress and disease. Stress can increase the risk of, or worsen, heart disease, cancer, or other chronic conditions. It can also dampen the immune response. Stress tends to originate from three sources: the environment, our bodies, and our minds.[3] Environmental stressors such as the weather, crime, and crowds are usually beyond one's control, whereas physical and mental stressors, although sometimes seemingly insurmountable, can often be controlled. There are numerous stress management techniques such as exercise, diet, muscle relaxation, meditation, deep breathing, visualization, desensitization, and biofeedback.[36] Each individual should find one that is suited to his or her lifestyle and temperament.

Substance abuse can become a major source of problems when it affects an elderly person. This is especially true with alcohol, as the elderly have a decrease in lean body mass as well as lower volume of body water. Both conditions combine to cause a higher percentage of the alcohol ingested to be absorbed by one's body. In addition to this, excessive alcohol use increases the risk of injuries and/or accidents in elderly individuals. Alcohol and other drugs can have an adverse effect on sleep and can sometimes mask the symptoms of underlying diseases. Let us not forget that nicotine is also a drug, and that smoking cessation can lead to a healthier life.

Once substance abuse has been identified in an older individual, a plan of management control must be established. This must first involve an initial screening to assess the impact of alcohol or drug abuse both physically and psychologically. Then a treatment plan, which includes education and promotes self-responsibility, must be established. Drug use and abuse are covered in depth in Chapter 6.

HEALTH CARE FINANCES

The elderly spend more money on long-term care than on any other type of health care. Most elders, however, cannot meet these overwhelming costs on their own, and Medicare coverage is limited. At an average cost of $30,000 per year, and double or triple that in some urban areas, many elders in nursing homes watch their lifetime savings evaporate within a few years.[37]

Long-term private insurance may be the answer to this dilemma, at least for those who can afford it. This form of insurance has become the fastest growing type of health insurance sold in recent years, and it promises to continue its upward growth spiral over the coming years. The industry sold 24 million policies between 1987 and 1993 and estimates that 5 percent of the elderly, and 1 percent of the general population, now have long-term insurance.[37] This, however, still leaves 30 million persons without this kind of coverage.[7]

The increased cost of health care and the aging population go hand and hand and have assumed a position on the central stage of the national policy debate. The cost of health care programs such as Medicare and **Medicaid** has risen to staggering levels. Spending on these programs as a proportion of overall spending on the elderly has increased from 6 percent in 1960 to approximately 32 percent in 1991. To give this a dollar figure, $150 billion of the $450 billion for total health care spending goes to the 12 percent of the population older than 65.[8] Individuals older than 65 with no provisions for this type of coverage are at the mercy of Medicaid after their assets have been consumed.

SUMMARY

Many factors determine how we age; not least among them are social aspects affecting aging. Each ethnic group has its own unique way of approaching aging and treatment of the elderly. Sometimes economic and educational backgrounds factor into a particular ethnic cohort's attitude toward aging.

Ageism, a systematic stereotyping of and discrimination against people who are old, fosters the notion of a gender gap. It is fueled by numerous myths regarding aging and the elderly as well as by language that conjures negative images of old persons. In its worst form, it leads to work discrimination and unequal employment opportunities. The media, through portrayal of the elderly in commercials and various screen and television productions, also play a role in perpetrating negative age stereotyping.

Many elderly persons are involved politically. Organizations such as the American Association of Retired Persons (AARP) and Gray Panthers provide opportunities for varying degrees of involvement. The ballot power of the elderly is often effective in passing legislation favorable to them.

Attitudes toward retirement vary greatly, as do lifestyles of the elderly. For some, it heralds the chance to pursue a special interest or hobby they never had time to do while working. Others see it as an opportunity to travel or return to school in order to pursue a second career. Others view it with a bit of disappointment, especially if they previously held an influential position. For most people, however, retirement is a time of relaxation to be spent with spouse, children, grandchildren, and/or friends.

Family and social roles also vary greatly among older people. For those couples whose marriage has weathered many storms, it is often a time of extreme closeness. Others approach old age alone, having lost a spouse through death or divorce. Relationships between aging parents and adult children tend to be as varied and challenging as spousal relationships. So too do relationships with brothers and sisters vary, although studies have shown that siblings generally become closer with age. Research has also pointed out that friendships are often more important to one's psychological well-being than relationships with family members. Grandparenting has been, and remains, one of the most rewarding and fulfilling experiences of later life.

Financial security is extremely important to most elderly individuals. Social Security was the major source of an elder's income in 1994. Many elderly (3.7 million) live at or below the poverty level.

As a result of improvements in health care, better diet, and more emphasis on exercise, Americans are entering their "sunset" years healthier than ever before. This trend is likely to continue with the aging of the baby boom generation. One of the greatest problems facing an aging society is health care finances. Because of the staggering costs of health care, elderly are increasingly at the mercy of government-sponsored programs such as Medicare and Medicaid.

It is important for all working with the elderly to understand the various social factors discussed in the chapter that affect ageism and the elderly. Through an appreciation of the diverse backgrounds of the elderly patients/clients, we can better serve their needs. This should also help us in our personal approach in dealing with elderly parents and our own aging process.

▧ REVIEW QUESTIONS

1. Which of the following is the fastest growing ethnic group?

   A. Hispanic
   B. African-American
   C. Vietnamese
   D. Native American

2. _____ elderly fall into the lowest socioeconomic category.

   A. African-American
   B. Native American
   C. Hispanic
   D. Chinese

3. Work discrimination against elders is a form of:

   A. Bigotry
   B. Ageism
   C. Socialism
   D. None of the above

4. The largest organization of elderly individuals is the:

   A. Gray Panthers
   B. National Council of Senior Citizens
   C. National Association on Aging
   D. American Association of Retired Persons

5. The average retirement age in most Western countries is:

   A. 55
   B. 65
   C. 70
   D. 75

6. Today the average retiree spends what percentage of life in retirement?

   A. 10%–15%
   B. 15%–20%
   C. 25%–30%
   D. 40%–50%

7. Which aged cohort copes *least well* with retirement?

   A. Black men
   B. White men
   C. White women
   D. Hispanic men

8. Which of the following holds the greatest degree of importance to the psychological well-being of the elderly?
   A. Spouse
   B. Children
   C. Siblings
   D. Friends

9. The major source of income (in 1994) for individuals older than 65 was:
   A. Social Security
   B. Private income
   C. Asset income
   D. Private pensions

10. The major cause of malnutrition in the elderly is:
    A. Depression
    B. Poverty
    C. Chronic illness
    D. Appetite-suppressing medications
    E. None of the above

11. The diet consisting of olive oil, whole-grain breads, soups, beans, vegetables, and fruits is called the:
    A. Scarsdale Diet
    B. High-protein diet
    C. LA Diet
    D. Mediterranean Diet

12. A number of studies have shown that exercise does which of the following:
    A. Increases aerobic capacity
    B. Increases mental speed
    C. Increases sleep
    D. Increases appetite
    E. A and B

13. Healthy People 2000 focuses on which of the following goals?
    A. Increase the span of a healthy life
    B. Reduce health disparities
    C. Achieve access to preventive services
    D. Universal health care coverage for all

14. An answer to the problem of providing coverage for astronomical nursing home fees is:
    A. Medicare
    B. Medicaid
    C. Long-term care insurance
    D. None of the above

LEARNING ACTIVITIES

1. Act out (role play) with a partner various examples of ageism—in work, in social situations, and in the family.

2. Videotape at least five commercials with elderly individuals (older than 65) in them. Review the tape, then play it in class, soliciting comments.

3. Establish a "mock" elder, political organization. Develop a vision statement as well as goals and objectives. Develop and describe various approaches you might use to "win over" politicians opposing elder issues or bills.

4. Develop a clearinghouse that markets and packages "lifestyles" for elderly individuals. (Example: Elder community that caters to those with computer/high tech interests).

5. Design a health promotion/disease prevention course or workshop for elderly persons.

REFERENCES

1. Maddox G (ed): Encyclopedia of Aging. Springer Publishing Company, New York, 1987.
2. Bonder, B, and Wagner, M: Functional Performance in Older Adults. FA Davis, Philadelphia, 1994.
3. Butler, RM: Ageism: Another form of bigotry. Gerontologist 9:243–246, 1969.
4. Palmore, EB: Ageism: Negative and Positive. Springer, New York, 1990, pp 183–184.
5. Aiken L: Aging: An Introduction to Gerontology. Sage, Thousand Oaks, CA, 1995.
6. Tagliareni, E, and Waters V: The Aging Experience. In Anderson, MA, and Braun, JV (eds): Caring for the Elderly Client. F.A. Davis, Philadelphia, 1995.
7. U.S. Senate Special Committee on Aging, American Association of Retired Persons, Federal Council on the Aging, and U.S. Administration on Aging: Aging America, Trends and Projections, 1991 ed. U.S. Department of Health and Human Services, Washington, DC, 1991.
8. Dychtwald, K: Age Wave. Bantam Books, New York, 1990.
9. Friedan, B: The Fountain of Age. Simon and Schuster, New York, 1993.
10. Burke, M, and Walsh, M: Gerontologic Nursing: Holistic Care of the Older Adult. Mosby, St. Louis, 1997.
11. Mulley, GP: Preparing for the late years. Lancet 34:1409–1412, 1994.
12. Riley, M, and Riley, J: Age integration and the lives of older people. Gerontologist, 34: 110–115, 1994.
13. Tournier, P: Learn to Grow Old. Harper and Row, New York, 1972.
14. The Hen Co-op: Growing Old Disgracefully. The Crossing Press, Freedom, CA, 1994.
15. Peterson, D, and Wendt, P: Training and education: Imperative for retirees. In Peterson, D, and Wendt, P: Older and Active: How Americans Over 55 are Contributing to Society. Yale University Press, New Haven, CT, 1995.
16. Menkler, M: Research on the health effects of retirement: An uncertain legacy. J Health Soc Behav 22:117–130, 1981.

17. Allison, R: Easy steps to tone up retirement. Advertising Age 67(45):32, November, 1996.

18. Kanes, C: The Rileys work to reshape attitudes about aging. The Times Record, Brunswick, ME, pp 13 and 21, October 1, 1993.

19. Bennett, D: Great grandmother goes solo. Cruising World 19(12):8–9, December, 1994.

20. Clements, M: What we say about aging. Parade magazine pp 4–5, December 12, 1993.

21. Uncle Sam wants you to volunteer. New Choices 34(2):82, March, 1994.

22. Silverstone, B, and Hyman, H: Growing Older Together. Pantheon Books, New York, 1992.

23. Adams, R, and Blieszner, R: Aging well with friends and family. American Behavioral Scientist 39(2):109–221, November/December, 1995.

24. Atchley, R: Aging: Continuity and Change. Wadsworth, Belmont, CA, 1983.

25. Goodman, S: MM interview with Arthur Kornhaber. Modern Maturity 40(1):52–56 and 68–71, January/February, 1997.

26. A Profile of Older Americans, 1995. American Association of Retired Persons, Washington, DC, 1995.

27. Koellin, K, et al: Vulnerable elderly households: Expenditures on necessities by older Americans. Social Science Quarterly 76(3):619–632, September, 1995.

28. Ozawa, M: The economic status of vulnerable older women. Social Work 40(3):323–331, May, 1995.

29. Burrell, C: Malnutrition is common among older americans. Maine Sunday Telegram, Health Resources Guide, October 13, 1996.

30. Ahmed, F: Effect of nutrition on the health of the elderly. J Am Diet Assoc 92:1102–1108, 1992.

31. Blumberg, J: Changing nutrient requirements in older adults. Nutrition Today 27(5):15–20, September/October, 1992.

32. Mediterranean diet associated with longer life for elderly. Harvard Heart Letter, Heart Line Section, April, 1996.

33. Jaret, P: Think fast. Health 10(2):44–46, March/April, 1996.

34. Anderson, M, and Braun, J: Caring for the Elderly Client. FA Davis, Philadelphia, 1995.

35. Healthy People 2000. Public Health Service, Washington, DC, 1990.

36. Huber, D: Health Promotion and Aging. Springer, New York, 1994.

37. Randall, T: Insurance—private and public: A payment puzzle. JAMA 269:2344–2346, 1993.

It is frustrating that in a time when humans have gone into and returned from outer space and can manipulate DNA, they have not conquered death. Death, indeed, remains the last 'sacred' enemy.[1]

Much of the continuing massive destruction of this planet and the consequent ills that this destruction produces for humans can be traced to overpopulation, a phenomenon that appears to show no sign of abating. Extending the life of a population that already strains global resources is, in the view of many, unconscionable.[2]

The Physiology and Pathology of Aging

David A. Sandmire

CHAPTER OUTLINE

BEHAVIORAL OBJECTIVES

Upon completion of this chapter, the reader will be able to:

1. Compare and contrast the concepts of aging as a "disease" and aging as a "process."
2. Compare and contrast preventive medicine and curative medicine.
3. Explain the difference between average life expectancy and maximum life span potential and describe the determinants of each.
4. Describe both molecular and evolutionary theories of aging.
5. Describe the cellular theories of aging and explain the possible role of free radical formation in the aging process.
6. Describe the cross-linking and glycosylation theories of aging.
7. Explain the effects of aging on the various organ systems of the body.
8. Understand the concept of homeostasis, or the maintenance of a stable internal environment in the body in the face of an ever-changing external environment.
9. Appreciate the interdependence among the body's organ systems and the ways in which these systems compensate for disturburbances in homeostasis.
10. Describe how the compensatory capabilities of the body change with advancing age.
11. Understand the concept of "illness" as an inability of the body to adequately compensate for disturbances in homeostasis.

KEY TERMS

Anemia
Aneurysm
Atherosclerosis
Autoimmune disease
Average life expectancy
Benign prostatic hypertrophy
  (BPH)
Cataract
Chronic bronchitis
Chronic obstructive pulmonary
  disease (COPD)
Dementia
Diabetes mellitus
Diverticulosis
Dysphagia

Embolism
Emphysema
Fecal incontinence
Free radical
Gastritis
Heat stroke
Hyposmia
Lipofuscin
Maximum life span potential (MLP)
Myocardial infarction
Osteoarthritis
Osteoporosis
Peptic ulcer
Postural hypotension
Presbycusis

Presbyopia   Thrombus
Senescence   Urinary incontinence
Stroke   Xerostomia

INTRODUCTION

If death is our last sacred enemy, how can efforts to extend our life span be considered unconscionable? Perhaps the view of death as an enemy to be conquered emanates from one's personal perspective, whereas considering a timely death as a necessity to conserve our earth's resources reflects a more global perspective. Indeed, it is entirely possible for an individual to share both sentiments. What is certain is that death remains one of the great mysteries of our existence. Thus, how we deal with death, and the aging process that leads to it, is in large part dictated by our religious, cultural, and philosophical upbringing. Native American cultures consider the elderly the most valuable members of society for the wisdom of their years. In a small Italian village, one finds three generations living under one roof, the younger generations taking to heart a sense of obligation to the older members of the family. Contrast these examples with the fast-paced, highly mobile society that is the United States, where the elderly are frequently placed in nursing homes in the charge of health care professionals.[3]

Culture not only influences personal perspectives and family living arrangements but also the way that scientists approach aging (often called **senescence**) and death. Scientific enterprise is a mirror of culture, and vice versa. If society views the physiological changes associated with aging as "diseases," researchers will do likewise. Indeed, Western medicine, with its greater emphasis on curative rather than preventive medicine, seems to favor the disease model of aging. We expend more time and resources curing cancer and treating heart attack victims than we do promoting healthful living. Curative medicine and the disease model of aging, in turn, help us rationalize the placement of our elderly in nursing homes and other extended-care settings. If, instead, we accept senescence as a process that can be attenuated, we are likely to focus more strongly on healthful living and preventive medicine throughout life than on a "quick fix" at the end of life.

From a strictly scientific standpoint, however, the distinction between aging and disease is, at best, a blurry one. Consider atherosclerosis, a pervasive affliction of our elderly that predisposes one to hypertension, heart attacks, and strokes. Do the fatty plaques that develop in arteries result from degenerative changes that are inevitable with the passage of time or from specific injuries to the blood vessels, perhaps due to turbulent bloodflow or microbial infection? Do low-fat diets and exercise regimens merely slow down this unavoidable "phenomenon of aging"? Or is it more accurate to view healthy lifestyle habits as measures that prevent the "disease" atherosclerosis? Paola S. Timiras suggested the following distinctions between aging and disease:[4]

- Aging is a universal process, shared by all living organisms, whereas disease is a selective process, varying with species, tissue, organ, cell, and molecule.
- Aging is intrinsic, dependent on genetic factors, whereas disease is intrinsic and extrinsic, dependent on both genetic and environmental factors.
- Aging is always progressive, whereas disease may be discontinuous and may progress, regress, or be arrested entirely
- Aging is always deleterious and likely to reduce functional competence, whereas disease is occasionally deleterious, often causing damage that is reversible
- Aging is irreversible, whereas disease may be treatable and often has a known cause.

Whether one agrees with these above descriptors or not, there is good reason to continue refining our definitions and conceptions of aging. Consider the following statistic: the **average life expectancy** in the United States has risen from about 45 years in 1900 to 76 years in 1990, an increase largely attributed to improvements in sanitation, food, and water supply and to the advent of antibiotics and vaccinations.[3,5] But during this period, there has been no change in the **maximum life span potential** (i.e., the oldest age reached by an individual in a population) of Americans, estimated to be about 115 (Fig. 3–1).[6,7] Thus, while improvements in our standard of living have helped spare us from several causes of premature death, such as cholera, tuberculosis, and influenza, they have done nothing to slow down the inherent aging process. In fact, any medical intervention that claims to slow down human aging must be shown to increase the maximum life span potential, and, to date, none have done so.

Our unchanging maximum life span potential in the face of an ever-increasing life expectancy suggests two things to those who ponder growing old. First, it supports the notion of distinguishing disease from aging. One of the most important chapters in the history of medicine has been the eradication of smallpox from the face of the earth with vaccines. But while the child who is immunized to smallpox has been spared a devastating infectious disease, he or she is not likely to age more slowly than an unimmunized child. Second, a maximum life span potential that has not budged in centuries suggests that there exists some "biological clock" that predetermines our length of existence on this planet. No such "clock" has been discovered, and it is perhaps an oversimplification of human physiology to suggest that one single mechanism in the body is responsible for aging. Nonetheless, it certainly appears that there are relatively fixed limits on how long our bodies last.

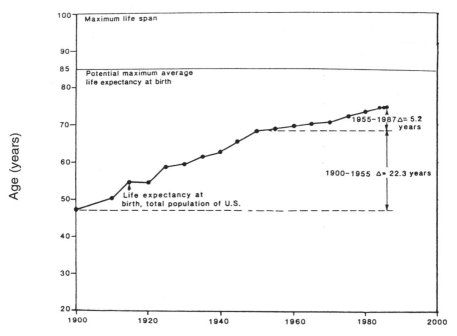

FIG. 3–1. Average life expectancy at birth and estimated maximum lifespan potential in the U.S. since 1900. (Adapted from Harman, D: The aging process: Major risk factor for disease and death. Proc Natl Acad Sci USA 88:5362, 1991, with permission.)

A fixed life span, however, does not necessarily sentence us to pain and suffering in our twilight years. Many of the physiological changes associated with aging can be slowed to some extent with a healthy diet and consistent regimen of moderate exercise, and many of the chronic diseases prevalent in the elderly are either preventable or modifiable with healthy lifestyle habits (Table 3–1). Reduction of dietary fat (especially saturated fats and cholesterol) lowers one's risk of coronary artery disease and stroke as well as breast and colon cancer.[8,9] A program of increased physical activity increases one's resting and maximum cardiac output (the amount of blood pumped out of the heart per minute) while decreasing one's chance of developing hypertension.[4,10] To the extent that exercise helps prevent obesity, it also decreases the likelihood that one will develop osteoarthritis and non-insulin-dependent diabetes mellitus or suffer from a heart attack.[8] Regular exercise, coupled with sufficient dietary calcium intake, lowers one's risk of osteoporosis and its complications, such as broken hips and slipped intervertebral disks.[3] Along with these physical benefits, exercise appears to have psychological benefits as well, lifting one's spirits and alleviating loneliness and depression.[11] On the other hand, sedentary lifestyles and, in particular, extended bedrest increase

TABLE 3–1. Common Chronic Diseases of Aging Potentially Modifiable in Middle Age Through Personal Changes in Lifestyle

Disorder	Preventive Strategy
Hypertension	Reduction of dietary sodium Reduction of body weight
Atherosclerotic cardiovascular disease	Treatment of hypertension Cessation of cigarette smoking Reduction of excess body weight Reduction of dietary saturated fat and cholesterol Increased aerobic exercise
Cancers	Cessation of cigarette smoking Reduction of dietary fat Reduction of salt- or smoke-cured food intake Minimization of radiation exposure Minimization of sun exposure
Chronic obstructive pulmonary disease	Cessation of cigarette smoking
Diabetes mellitus (Type II)	Reduction of excess body weight Diet consistent with atherosclerosis prevention
Osteoporosis	Maintenance of dietary calcium Regular exercise Cessation of cigarette smoking Avoidance of alcohol excess
Osteoarthritis	Reduction of body weight
Cholelithiasis (i.e., gallstones)	Reduction of body weight

Source: Bierman, EL, and Hazzard, WR: Preventive Gerontology: Strategies for attentuation of the chronic diseases of aging. In Hazzard, WR, et al (eds): Principles of Geriatric Medicine and Gerontology, ed 3. McGraw-Hill, New York, p 188, with permission.

the chance of thromboembolic disease, respiratory infection and decubitus ulcers (bed sores). Perhaps the most important lifestyle choice one can make is to not smoke cigarettes. Indeed, cigarette smoking is the most common preventable cause of disease and death in the United States. It leads to chronic obstructive pulmonary disease (i.e., emphysema and chronic bronchitis) and lung cancer and is a major cause of other cancers of the upper respiratory and digestive tracts.[8,12] In addition, cigarette smoking enhances one's chance of developing atherosclerosis and its complications—heart attacks and strokes.

Clearly there are many ways to enhance our health as we age, but such modifications to lifestyle, activity level, and diet must occur in early or middle life to have the maximum effect. One of the difficulties in convincing young people to adopt these measures is that, generally speaking, they already feel healthy. Persuading a teenager to quit smoking or a forty-year-old business executive to take her blood pressure medication is difficult when doing so offers them no immediate reward—delayed gratification is not something our society seems to value highly. But the tide appears to be turning, at least on some fronts, as evidenced by the growing popularity of aerobic exercise over the past three decades and the legislative effort to limit the public areas where smoking is allowed. With such societal changes, perhaps we will accomplish what gerontologists call the compression of morbidity—i.e., decreasing the period and severity of illness experienced toward the end of life.

It seems most appropriate to describe human aging as a process that runs a fairly predictable course from infancy to senescence. Superimposed on that developmental sequence, however, are lifestyle choices and environmental insults that influence how far we are able to travel along life's course and how well we feel along the journey. While we may not be able to extend our maximum life span potential, we can certainly reduce the morbidity associated with aging on our way to the 115th year. In addition, healthy lifestyles may help us accomplish what epidemiologists call a rectangularization of the survival curve—a condition where nearly everyone in a population reaches the maximum life span potential (Fig. 3–2). Perhaps there is some truth to

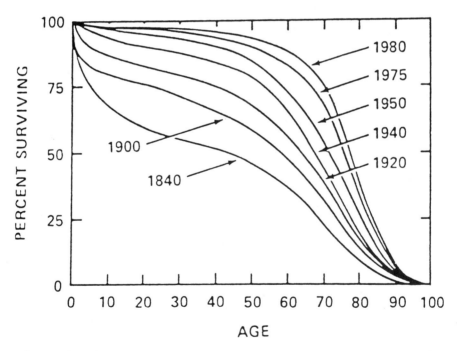

FIG. 3–2. Specific mortality survival curve, illustrating the "rectangularization" that has taken place over the past 150 years as a growing percentage of the population approaches the maximum lifespan potential. (From Cassel, CK, and Brody, JA: Demography, epidemiology, and aging. In Cassel, CK, et al [eds]: Geriatric Medicine, ed 2. Springer-Verlag, New York, 1990, p 17, with permission.)

the observation by comedian George Burns that you can never live to be 100 if you stop living at 65.[3] Burns lived to enjoy his 100th birthday.

THEORIES OF BIOLOGICAL AGING

While research on the aging process has proceeded for decades, we now seem as far away from the "fountain of youth" as we ever were. One of the stumbling blocks in senescence research is the lack of a true biological marker of aging (with the arguable exception of lipofuscin accumulation in cells, discussed later). There is, as yet, no single identifiable molecular, cellular, tissue, or organ change in the body that correlates closely with age.[13,14] Senescence appears to be a multifactorial process whose rate depends on both genetic and environmental phenomena. The following sections briefly review some theories of aging that have been proposed over the past 45 years. It is not the author's intent to suggest that any single theory explains the aging process, but rather to recognize that aging is a complex phenomenon orchestrated by events at several organizational levels in the body.

MOLECULAR AND EVOLUTIONARY THEORIES OF AGING

Because the stages of cellular, tissue, organ, and body development are, for the most part, controlled by our genetic machinery, many theories of aging have focused on the role of DNA (deoxyribonucleic acid), RNA (ribonucleic acid), and the proteins made from these nucleic acid "blueprints" (Table 3–2).

One such theory is that senescence results from the gradual accumulation of random mutations (alterations in the DNA) in somatic cells of the body.[15] According to this *somatic mutation theory,* radiation and other environmental mutagens alter the structure of the genetic code and thus change the sequence of amino acids found in enzymes and other proteins. Such minor alterations could, in turn, have damaging effects on protein function and thus on body functions. Differences in longevity among individuals might result from varying rates of mutagenesis and varying proficiencies of DNA repair. But while studies have shown that the number of DNA mutations increases with age,[16,17] proving that such changes are the cause, rather than the result, of aging has been more difficult.

The *error catastrophe theory* attributes aging to problems in the transfer of information from DNA to proteins.[18] A gradual decline in the precision of DNA transcription and RNA translation would cause the accumulation of abnormal enzymes in aging cells. If such malformed enzymes themselves were unable to play proper roles in transcription or translation, their production would, in positive feedback fashion, exacerbate the errors in transcription and translation, resulting in catastrophic changes in cellular physiology.[3,19] However, if errors in fact occurred in these critical processes, one would expect all cellular enzymes to be affected equally, and studies do not bear this out.[20–23]

TABLE 3–2. *Theories of Biological Aging*

Somatic mutation theory	Gradually accumulating random mutations of the DNA alter gene structure and function.
Error catastrophe theory	Loss of precision in the translation of the genetic code from DNA to proteins
Gene regulation theory	Changes in the expression of certain genes orchestrate the changes of aging.
Evolutionary theory	Aging is an inevitable by-product of evolution because of less intense selection against deleterious genes in the elderly.
Antagonistic pleiotropy theory	Evolutionary selection of genes that are favorable for younger individuals despite their harmful effect in older individuals
Disposable soma theory	Aging is an inevitable result of the compromise that a species reaches between diverting all of its energy to reproduction and diverting all of its energy to body maintenance and repair.
Wear-and-tear theory	Cells and thus individuals wear out from continued use.
Rate-of-living theory	Version of the wear-and-tear theory that suggests that a species' average life span is inversely proportional to its basal metabolic rate per gram of metabolizing tissue
Free-radical theory	Aging results from the random damage to macromolecules by highly reactive molecules called free radicals.
Cross-linking theory	Aging results from the accumulation of cross-linkages between macromolecules.
Glycosylation theory	Aging is attributed to the accumulation of cross-linkages between macromolecules as a result of the initial attachment of glucose molecules to those macromolecules.

In contrast to the preceding concepts of aging as something that results from molecular "mistakes," the *gene regulation theory* suggests that aging occurs along an intentional timeline that is primarily determined by changes in the regulation of gene expression.[24] If earlier stages of human development are orchestrated by the precise "turning on" and "turning off" of certain genes, then age-related changes might be as well. But studies designed to look specifically for such changes in gene expression have not been fruitful.[25,26] This may be because whole organisms or tissues were studied rather than individual cell types or because the changes in gene expression are undetectable by current research techniques.

If the characteristics of growing old are indeed due to the expression of certain genes that cause age-related changes in cells, why would such preprogrammed mortality have evolved in the first place? Some intriguing answers to this question come from evolutionary biologists. The *evolutionary theory* of aging portrays senescence as a by-product, rather than a driving force, of evolution.[27] Even if a species did not age, accidental mortality occurring at a fixed rate (e.g., due to predation) would cause the number of individuals reaching successively older ages to decline. Therefore, any DNA mutation that selectively affected an older individual's reproductive capability or survival in an adverse way would be less detrimental to the species as a whole than a mutation that selectively altered a younger individual's reproductive ability. There would be less intense selection pressure against "bad genes" programmed to affect older members of a species than against "bad genes" that preferentially affect its younger members. Those individuals lucky enough to escape accidental death earlier in life would eventually succumb to the effects of detrimental genes that have remained in the species' genetic pool.

But if the evolutionary theory's starting conditions dictate that aging did not exist initially and was instead an end-result of the course of evolution, how could certain genes initially have had age-specific effects in a species that did not age? One possibility is that while there would be little natural selection *against* genes that adversely affected aged individuals, there would be a strong selection *for* genes that benefitted younger individuals, even if such genes had adverse side effects for older members of the species.[28] These individual genes that are beneficial early in life but detrimental late in life are said to exhibit *antagonistic pleiotropy.* For example, a gene that stimulates the deposition of calcium in the bone of young individuals (a favorable effect) may also cause calcification of arteries and other soft tissues later in life (an unfavorable effect). Similarly, a gene that promotes rapid cell division during embryonic development (favorable) may predispose an elderly individual to uncontrolled cell division, or cancer (unfavorable).[29]

Another evolutionary explanation for aging, the *disposable soma theory,* proposes that a species strikes a compromise between expending all of its energy on reproduction and spending all of its energy on maintenance and repair of the body, or *soma.*[30] Members of a species that hypothetically devote all of their available energy toward reproduction without providing the necessary nutrients for feeding, growth, and tissue repair will likely die before they are able to reproduce. Conversely, organisms that devote all of their resources to maintenance of the soma would still not be able to escape the accidental mortality that all species face. In this regard, it would be wasteful to allocate too much energy to a soma that will eventually die anyway. Optimal species survival would be attained by reducing the amount of energy required for perpetual maintenance of the soma (i.e., immortality) and diverting the remaining energy to more rapid growth or greater reproductive output. Said another way, the longevity of a species would represent a balance between the natural selection for a longer reproductive period and the limits placed on the life span by environmental hazards. The soma is in this sense "disposable" as long as a species can survive to reproduce. A species such as the tree shrew that is relatively low on the food chain and therefore subjected to high rates of accidental death does better to focus more of its resources on rapid development and increased reproductive capability than on maintaining a viable soma. Its life span is thus relatively short. In contrast, an organism with virtually no natural predators, such as the African elephant, has a much longer life span because of its proportionately greater investment in somatic maintenance and repair. As a result, it has smaller numbers of progeny and longer gestational periods. Similarly, it is perhaps not surprising that human beings, who for all practical purposes have no natural predators, are the longest lived of all mammals.

CELLULAR THEORIES OF AGING

While the evolutionary theories of aging provide explanations for the origin of senescence, they do not predict the specific events in the process of cellular aging. In this section, some theories of aging are reviewed that either directly or indirectly relate to actual changes in cell structure and function.

The *wear-and-tear theory* of aging proposes that aging is inevitable as cells, much like machines, gradually wear out from continued use. The machine analogy is not a perfect one because cells, unlike machines, have several mechanisms to repair their injuries. But with the passage of time, the intracellular damage due to wear and tear might accumulate to a point at which it overcomes a cell's capacity for maintenance and repair. Cells (and therefore organisms) with higher rates of metabolism might "wear out" more quickly than those with lower metabolic rates, thus aging more quickly and dying sooner.

The inverse correlation between basal metabolic rate and longevity across a wide number of species has led some experimental gerontologists to reformulate the wear-and-tear hypothesis into a *rate-of-living theory* of aging, which attributes interspecies variation in life span to varying metabolic rates per gram of metabolizing tissue.[31] Every organism, then, is endowed with the ability to burn up a fixed number of calories in its lifetime, after which the accumulation of wear and tear results in the organism's death. Members of a species with a higher metabolic rate would burn up their fixed number of total calories more quickly, suffer from accumulated wear and tear more rapidly, and die sooner than those of a species with a lower metabolic rate.

The well-documented effect of *caloric restriction* (i.e., limiting food intake) to increase average life expectancy[32,33] seems on the surface to support the rate-of-living theory of aging. Furthermore, a multitude of studies have shown that caloric restriction not only increases average life span but also dampens many of the physiological changes associated with increasing age, such as rising serum cholesterol levels,[34] decreasing bone mass,[35] and deteriorating immune system function.[36] Nonetheless, it does not appear that caloric restriction has a significant effect on an organism's specific basal metabolic rate.[37,38] The basis for its effect must therefore lie elsewhere. Furthermore, the rate-of-living theory itself has been called into question by studies that have found exceptions to the generalization that animals with lower metabolic rates live longer than those with higher metabolic rates.[39]

But while the rate-of-living theory of aging has not panned out, it nonetheless has helped focus experimental gerontology on another promising theory, the free-radical theory of aging.

FREE-RADICAL THEORY OF AGING

The *free-radical theory* of aging is a specific version of the wear-and-tear theory that attributes cellular (and therefore organismal) aging to random accumulating damage of macromolecules by the highly reactive by-products of oxidative metabolism known as **free radicals**.[40–42] Free radicals are molecules that contain at least one unpaired electron in their outer valence shells. Free radicals most notably form in the mitochondria of cells, the site of aerobic respiration (the "burning up of food" for energy), where electrons are "stripped" from temporary carrier molecules and passed down a chain of membrane-bound protein carriers to be "accepted" by oxygen.[43,44] Free radicals are relatively rare in nature because they are chemically unstable. When formed, they usually bind with other free radicals to create more stable molecules. However, when free radicals form in cells, they can initiate chain reactions that consume oxygen and randomly damage lipid molecules, enzymes, and nucleic acids.

One part of a cell's structure that is particularly vulnerable to chemical attack by free radicals is the lipid membrane, which bounds the cell and many of its internal organelles, such as the mitochondria, endoplasmic reticulum, and Golgi apparatus. The polyunsaturated fatty acids embedded in these membranes are major targets. But cells have specific defenses against this lipid peroxidation, such as *vitamin E* (alpha-tocopherol), *vitamin C* (ascorbic acid), and several enzymes that arrest free radical chain reactions.[45]

If the levels of free radical "scavengers" such as vitamins E and C are depleted, however, damage to lipid membranes can be more permanent. Repeated peroxidation of unsaturated lipids can cause inappropriate cross-linking of lipids to proteins and nucleic acids.[46] The cross-linking of lipids with proteins leads to the formation of **lipofuscin** (or "age pigment"). Granules of this yellowish-brown pigment are found in the cytoplasm of aged cells (Fig. 3–3). Interestingly, the slow, predictable accumulation of lipofuscin is considered to be the most reliable marker of chronological age in cells, and it has been found in nearly every eukaryotic organism studied thus far.[47]

But while evidence for the age-related accumulation of lipofuscin and

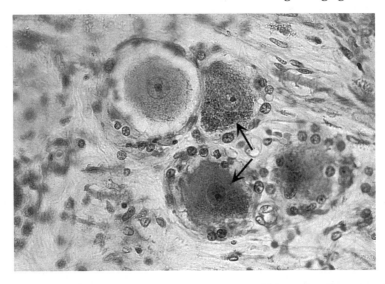

FIG. 3–3. Light micrograph of a dorsal root ganglion cell illustrating the accumulation of lipofuscin. (Courtesy of Allen Bell, University of New England.)

other types of free radical-mediated cell damage is widespread, proving that free radical damage is the primary determinant of aging has been more difficult; lipofuscin accumulation, it appears, is a result, rather than a cause, of aging.[48] Recall that any intervention that truly slows down the aging process must be shown to increase the maximum life span potential of a species. And while studies in which organisms were given supplements of vitamin E throughout life revealed that the rate of lipofuscin accumulation decreased and the average life expectancy often increased, none showed a change in the maximum life span potential.[49-54]

Nonetheless, the potential importance of free radical-mediated destruction in aging cells should not be ignored, especially when one considers its role in disease. Consider cigarette smoking, the most common preventable cause of disease and death in the United States. The smoke from cigarettes contains free radicals whose presence can alter or destroy important biological molecules such as DNA and enzymes.[55,56] Damage to DNA, in turn, may play a role in the etiology of lung cancer, while damage to enzymes, such as alpha-1 antitrypsin, may cause the progressive and irreversible destruction of lung tissue in patients with emphysema (see Respiratory System). Thus, smoking may accelerate the aging process by enhancing the free radical mechanism, a process that some researchers claim is at the heart of the natural aging process.[40] One can see how the distinction between "disease" and "pure aging" becomes less clear at the cellular level.

CROSS-LINKING AND GLYCOSYLATION THEORIES OF AGING

The *cross-linking theory* of aging attributes aging to the gradual accumulation of cross-linkages between organic macromolecules, particularly those that are closely packed together under normal circumstances, such as collagen and phospholipids.[57,58] Such binding together of large biological molecules might significantly alter their structure and function.

Intracellular macromolecules, such as enzymes and DNA, seem vulnerable to cross-linking as well.[59] The nonenzymatic attachment of glucose molecules to some proteins and DNA is an important preliminary step to their cross-linking. The extent of this glucose attachment increases with age, and long-term chemical modification of these glycosylated (i.e., "glucose-attached") macromolecules can lead to the formation of advanced glycosylation end products (AGEs), which are prone to further cross-linking.[60] The *glycosylation theory* of aging, really a subset of the cross-linking theory, implicates the accumulation of glycosylation-induced cross-links in the gradual aging of cells.[61]

Much of the impetus to study nonenzymatic glycosylation of proteins and DNA has come from its relevance to diabetes mellitus (DM), a disease marked by an elevated blood glucose level (hyperglycemia). Individuals with DM have glycosylated protein levels that are two to four times higher than those seen in nondiabetics.[62] Glycosylation of macromolecules might explain some of the long-term complications of DM, many of which are identical to the diseases commonly seen in aging individuals.[63] At the tissue level, long-term effects of DM include a loss of elasticity of arteries and joints, conditions that may help explain the accelerated hypertension and osteoarthritis, respectively, often suffered by diabetics.[64] In addition, excessive glycosylation and subsequent cross-linking of lens crystalline protein may contribute to the formation of cataracts, another diabetic complication that is also common in the nondiabetic elderly.[65,66] Finally, DM predisposes individuals to accelerated forms of atherosclerosis, emphysema, and immunosuppression—other conditions most prevalent in the aging population.[60] While these considerations certainly do not prove that glycosylation accounts for all of the age-related changes in tissues, they are nonetheless provocative—particularly since caloric restriction in rats has been shown to decrease levels of protein glycosylation and blood glucose while at the same time increasing life expectancy.[32,62]

The proposed connections between the glycosylation process, the long-term complications of DM, and the pathological conditions common to the elderly provide but one more example of the unclear boundary between aging as a *process* and aging as a *disease*. The next section focuses on the actual physiological and pathological changes that occur in the organ systems as we grow older.

AGE-RELATED CHANGES OF THE ORGAN SYSTEMS

INTEGUMENTARY SYSTEM

The integumentary system consists of the skin and all of its accessory structures, such as hair, nails, sebaceous (oil) glands, and eccrine (sweat) glands. From outermost in, skin consists of three major layers: the epidermis, dermis, and subcutaneous layers. Because it is the skin that covers our bodies, changes in its appearance are the most noticeable of all aging phenomena. We will focus here on the particular changes that occur in the epidermis, dermis and subcutaneous layers with age and the consequences of those changes for the structure and function of the integumentary system (Fig. 3–4).

The *epidermis* is a multilayered sheet of epithelial cells called keratinocytes, which are named for their production of keratin, a fibrous protein that gives this layer its strength. Interspersed among the keratinocytes are smaller numbers of melanocytes, which produce the melanin pigment that browns the skin, and Langerhans cells, which may play a role in cell-mediated immunity. The epidermal cells rest on a thin layer of tissue called the basement membrane, which separates the epidermis from the underlying dermis. This membrane is normally undulated, which helps hold the two layers together. However, with age it flattens out, making the skin more vulnerable to shearing forces, abra-

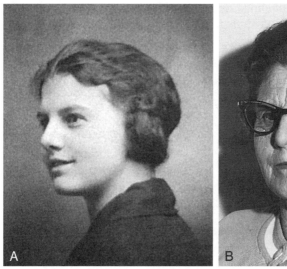
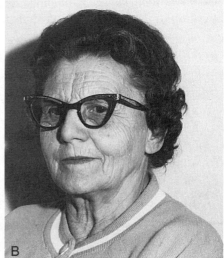

FIG. 3–4. Change in the appearance of the skin with aging. The same woman is shown at (*A*) age 19 and (*B*) age 70.

sion, and blister formation[67] (Fig. 3–5). Because of the everyday wear and tear on the skin, the epidermal cells must be continuously replaced with new cells that divide by mitosis in the lowest layers. The new cells slowly get "pushed up" through the epidermis and ultimately are shed from the skin, a process that takes about 28 days. Thus, our epidermis is completely replaced every month. The turnover rate, however, decreases by 30 to 50 percent between ages 20 and 70, which increases the time during which individual epidermal cells are exposed to carcinogens (i.e., cancer-causing agents) such as ultraviolet light from the sun.[68,69] Furthermore, the number of melanocytes, and therefore the amount of protective melanin pigment, decreases with age, making ultraviolet light more dangerous. When one couples these considerations with the fact that the number of macrophage-like Langerhans cells also declines with age, it becomes clear why the elderly are particularly prone to develop *skin cancer*.

The *dermis* is a thick layer of loose connective tissue that is well supplied with blood vessels, lymphatic vessels, nerves, and accessory organs such as sweat glands, sebaceous glands, and hair follicles. The predominant cells found in the dermis are fibroblasts, mast cells, and macrophages. Fibroblasts produce and release collagen and elastin into the extracellular matrix, which give skin its strength and elasticity, respectively. Mast cells release substances that mediate the inflammatory response following injury to the skin. The rich supply of blood vessels in the dermis provides oxygen and nutrients as well as an efficient mechanism for regulation of body temperature. When the body is overheated, blood flow to the dermis increases so that heat can be released through the skin. This, together with the action of sweat glands, allows for the release of large amounts of heat in a short period of time.

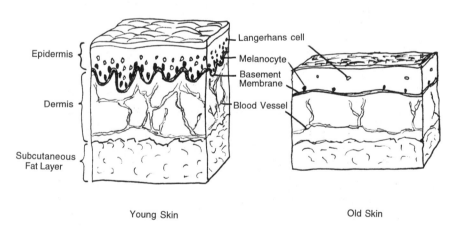

Young Skin   Old Skin

FIG. 3–5. Changes in the structure of skin with aging. Note that older skin has a thinner epidermis, a flatter basement membrane, fewer melanocytes and Langerhans cells, a diminished dermal blood supply, and a thinner subcutaneous fat layer.

The amount of collagen and elastin in the dermis decreases as we age, accounting for the thinning and wrinkling of the skin in the elderly. Loss of collagen makes the skin more susceptible to wear and tear, while loss of elastin causes skin to lose its resiliency over time. The density of the dermal blood supply also decreases with age, blunting the outward signs of inflammation in elderly skin. This is particularly important to realize, because the elderly often lack some of the early warning signs of tissue injury (e.g., redness and swelling) from, for example, sunburn, bacterial infection, or skin cancer. The diminished blood flow to the dermis also impairs wound healing and, together with the gradual loss of functioning sweat glands, makes the elderly especially vulnerable to overheating syndromes such as **heat stroke.** The dermis contains sensory receptors called pacinian and Meissner's corpuscles, which make the skin sensitive to vibration, pressure, and light touch. The gradual loss of these receptors with age decreases the *tactile sensitivity* of the skin and probably increases the threshold for pain stimuli.

The *subcutaneous layer* of the skin is largely adipose (i.e. fat) and loose connective tissue. This fat layer provides cushioning and thus protection to the underlying tissues. It also serves to insulate the body from rapid heat loss or gain. With age comes a thinning (or atrophy) of this layer, particularly in the face, backs of the hands, and soles of the feet. Loss of this "fat pad" on the soles can increase the physical trauma of walking and thus exacerbate other foot conditions in the elderly.

Perhaps the most striking age-related changes to the integumentary system are the graying, thinning, and loss of the hair. Hair follicles are specialized epidermal cells packed into cylinders rooted in the dermis. Hair growth is made possible by mitotic cell divisions at the base of the follicle, and hair color is dependent on varying amounts of melanin pigment within the specialized cells. Blonde, brown, and black hair have successively higher concentrations of melanin. With advancing years, the number of hair follicles decreases, and those follicles that remain grow at slower rates and have smaller concentrations of melanin (due to declining numbers of melanocytes at the base of the hair follicles), causing the hair to become thin and white. Such changes over the scalp hamper hair's ability to screen the skin on the scalp from the damaging effects of sunlight.

Chronic exposure to sunlight, in fact, is the biggest scourge of aging skin. It is to the skin what cigarette smoking is to the internal organs and is largely responsible for the wrinkling, yellowing, coarseness, and irregular pigmentation of the skin with advancing years. It is also implicated in the development of several benign dermatological lesions, such as skin tags, seborrheic keratoses, and sebaceous nevi. More importantly, the ultraviolet component of sunlight predisposes one to the three major forms of skin cancer: *malignant melanoma, basal cell carcinoma,* and *squamous cell carcinoma.* The latter two comprise more than 50 percent of all malignancies in the United States.[70] Yet, despite all of the damaging effects of "photoaging," the vanity of our youth often directs us to cultivate the "great tan" rather than to protect our skin. Again, the rewards of a great tan are immediate, whereas the benefits of skin protection come decades later. Nonetheless, if one still wants to look great at 80, the use of protective hats and clothing, along with sunscreens of sun protection factor 15 (SPF-15) strength or higher, is in order.

NERVOUS SYSTEM

The nervous system is the principal regulatory system of the body. An intact nervous system, therefore, is requisite to the proper functioning of all the other systems. The central nervous system, consisting of the brain, brain stem, and spinal cord, regulates and monitors peripheral activities via the nerves, the communication networks that form the peripheral nervous system. The *neuron* is the functional unit of the nervous system, capable of transmitting electrochemical impulses (or "messages") over its cell body and cell extensions (the axon and dendrites) (Fig. 3–6). Neurons form functional boundaries, or *synapses*, with other neurons and with target structures such as muscles and glands. In response to electrochemical impulses, signaling chemicals called *neurotransmitters* are released from neurons at these synapses to bind with and activate (or inhibit) the next cell in the sequence. The number of neurons in the

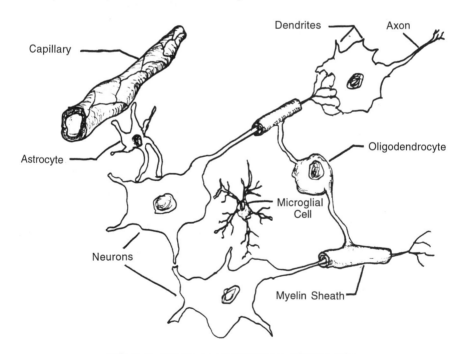

FIG. 3–6. Neurons and related neurologlial cells.

nervous system is relatively fixed early in life because mature neurons lack the ability to divide. The continued development of the nervous system throughout life (to make possible learning and memory formation, for example) is thus not attributed to an increase in the number of cells, but most likely to an increase in the complexity of neuronal circuits (due to axonal sprouting) and to intracellular modifications. More than 100 billion neurons are distributed throughout the nervous system, and any single neuron can synapse with several thousand other neurons. The neurons are supported by an even larger number of *neuroglial cells* (e.g., astrocytes, microglial cells, and oligodendrocytes) which help nourish, protect, and myelinate the neurons. Given these considerations, one can understand the claim that the human nervous system is the most complex functioning system in nature.

Because of its complexity and relative inaccessibility to study, the nervous system is probably the least understood of all body systems. Thus, we know relatively little about the effects of aging on the central nervous system. Furthermore, the age-related microscopic structural alterations to this system are unobservable until autopsy. And even at autopsy, it is often difficult to distinguish disease-related changes from changes due to normal aging. Our meager progress in understanding the brain is reflected in the fact that central nervous system disorders remain one of the most common causes of disability in the elderly, accounting for almost 50 percent of disability in those older than 65.[71] Nonetheless, some generalizations can be made concerning the appearance of the aged brain. Overall, the number of neurons does not change significantly during healthy aging, although certain parts of the nervous system show significant decreases in neuron density in individuals with Parkinson's disease (in the substantia nigra) and Alzheimer's disease (in the locus ceruleus and nucleus basalis of Meynert).

While the number of neurons changes little throughout life, there are nonetheless important structural and functional alterations in these cells as one ages. *Axons* in some parts of the nervous system lose moderate amounts of myelin (a lipid "wrapping" around the axon that increases the speed of the nerve impulse) or become swollen with age. These changes may contribute to the 10 percent decrease in nerve impulse conduction velocity noted with aging, a phenomenon that is partly responsible for the slowed reaction time in the elderly.[72] The number of *dendrites,* and therefore synapses, decreases along with a declining function of the neurotransmitter signaling mechanisms. These changes impair communication throughout the nervous system.

The nervous system utilizes several different neurotransmitters, some of which are excitatory and some of which are inhibitory. The more well characterized neurotransmitters include acetylcholine, dopamine, gamma-aminobutryic acid (GABA), serotonin, and glycine. Individual neurons may store and release more than one type of neurotransmitter. The smooth functioning of the nervous system appears to rely on the appropriate balance in

activity among the various neurotransmitters. The neurotransmitter dysfunction that occurs with aging has more to do with a loss of this balance
than with an absolute loss of any one particular neurotransmitter.

Like any other organ system, the nervous system is vulnerable to the effects
of atherosclerosis with advancing age. As fatty plaques narrow cerebral arteries, blood flow to the brain diminishes. Blood clots (thrombi) developing in
these narrowed arteries can block off the blood supply completely. Within
minutes, brain tissue deprived of oxygen can be irreversibly damaged, resulting in infarction of tissue. The symptoms from this particular type of stroke depend on which area of the brain has been damaged. Repeated episodes of cerebral infarction can lead to multi-infarct dementia, which accounts for 8 to 29
percent of all cases of dementia in the elderly, surpassed in frequency only by
Alzheimer's disease, which accounts for about 50 percent of the total.[73]

Dementia should be distinguished from the memory loss that occurs normally with age. Although most mental functions do not decline with age, mild
loss of memory for recent events is quite common, while long-term memory
remains intact in most cases. Dementia, on the other hand, is less common.
Defined as generalized mental deterioration in orientation, memory, intellect,
judgment, and emotional status despite clear consciousness, dementia in its
severe form affects only 5 percent of individuals older than 65, and in the
mild-to-moderate forms affects only 10 percent. However, two thirds of all
nursing home patients have dementia, and as the elderly segment of our population becomes proportionately larger, we can expect the care of those with
dementia to account for a large proportion of health care costs.[71]

Gradual impairment of *locomotor function* is another important contributor
to disability in the elderly. Chief among these symptoms are a slowing of fine
motor tasks, diminished postural reflexes, and alteration of the gait, or pattern of walking. The confident, long stride of our youth changes to a more
hesitant, broad-based gait as we age. Such deficiencies in motor skills have
been attributed primarily to an overall decrease in function of motor control
centers in the brain, such as the basal nuclei, cerebellum, and cerebral cortex. However, they result in part from diminished sensory input to these areas as well—diminished *proprioception* (sense of body position), *vestibular sensation* (sense of head movement), and *kinesthetic sensation* (sense of body
movement). Interestingly, many of the characteristics of the elderly stride,
such as the tentative, shuffling steps and stooped posture, are identical to
those seen in the early stages of Parkinson's disease. These changes in balance and movement place the elderly at risk for falls.

Finally, the aging process brings about notable changes in the pattern and
quality of *sleep* one gets. The total amount of time spent sleeping changes little over the course of a lifetime, but as one ages, episodes of sleep are shorter
and more frequent. Thus, a single 8-hour interval of sleep at night might be
replaced by 6 hours of sleep a night supplemented by two or three daily naps.

In addition, the proportion of stages 3 and 4 sleep decreases with advancing years. These are the deepest levels of sleep and are thought to be, physiologically speaking, the most rejuvenating forms of slumber. Their diminished presence might account for the observation that the elderly are "light sleepers." Conversely, the increased period of time spent in stage 1 corresponds to the common complaint that it takes longer to fall asleep as one ages. Indeed, about one third of the elderly population suffers from insomnia.[74] The difficulties with sleep are exacerbated by the anxiety, stress, and depression that can affect the elderly population.

SPECIAL SENSES

Vision

All of the special sensory systems undergo changes with aging. The changes in vision result from alterations in the structure of a number of the components of the visual system (Fig. 3–7). The cornea and the lens are the principal focusing structures in the eye; they refract (or bend) incoming light rays so that

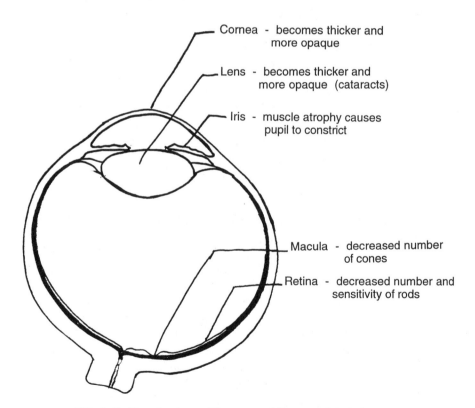

FIG. 3–7. The structure of the eye and its age-related changes.

images can be brought into focus on the retina in the back of the eye. Both the cornea and lens undergo predictable changes. The convex *cornea* is the thin and transparent anterior border of the eye. With advancing years, it becomes thicker and more opaque. The biconvex *lens* is largely acellular and transparent, consisting of several layers of crystallin lens protein. Its attachment to the surrounding sphincter-shaped ciliary muscle allows us to regulate its curvature. To focus on near objects, the ciliary muscle contracts, causing the lens to become rounder (a process called *accommodation*). Conversely, to focus on distant objects, the lens flattens out. With age, the lens increases in anterior-posterior diameter as successive layers of crystallin protein are laid down. It also becomes more opaque as its proteins become increasingly oxidized, glycosylated, and cross-linked (see earlier theories of aging)—severe degrees of which cause **cataracts.** These molecular changes render the lens less elastic and more rigid, which significantly impairs accommodation and thus the ability to focus on near objects, a condition called **presbyopia.** This change is so universal that nearly everyone older than 55 needs corrective convex lenses to read.

The *iris* is a pigmented ring of tissue whose opening, or pupil, regulates the amount of light entering the eye. Two sets of smooth muscle, the dilator and constrictor muscles, regulate the diameter of the pupil. Over time, the dilator muscle atrophies to a greater extent than the constrictor muscle, causing the average diameter of the pupil to decrease. The *retina* is the photoreceptive surface in the back of the eye. It is covered with highly sensitive *rods* (which detect white light) and less sensitive *cones* (which detect colored light). Both the number and photosensitivity of the rods decrease with age, which, coupled with the inability to completely dilate the pupils, makes night vision more difficult for the elderly. There is also a gradual loss of cones, which are normally densely packed in the *macula* of the retina. This may contribute to the decreased visual acuity common with aging.

Hearing

As with vision, impairment of *hearing* is very common in the elderly, affecting about 40 percent of those older than 63 years old.[75] We normally hear and interpret sounds through a multi-stepped process that converts sound waves (air pressure) into nerve impulses (Fig. 3–8). The sound waves travel through the external auditory canal and set the *tympanic membrane* (eardrum) into vibration, which in turn causes the lever-like *ossicles* (middle ear bones) to vibrate, all at the same frequency as the original sound. The smallest ossicle "taps" on the oval window, which creates a fluid pressure wave that travels through the *cochlea* of the inner ear. Specialized cochlear *hair cells* sense this wave and generate nerve impulses that travel via the auditory nerve to the brain stem and brain. Hair cells at the base of the spiral-shaped cochlea are sensitive to high-pitched sounds, whereas hair cells at the apex are sensitive to low-pitched sounds.

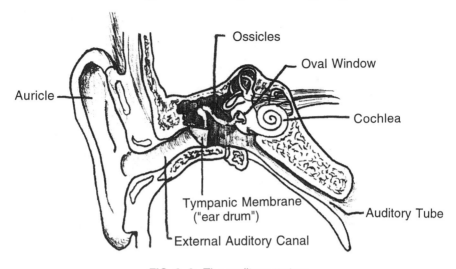

FIG. 3–8. The auditory system.

With aging comes a gradual, progressive hearing loss called **presbycusis.** Men are affected more than women, and urban dwellers suffer greater losses than those living in rural areas (suggesting a role played by chronic exposure to environmental noise). The degree of loss is more severe for high-frequency sounds than for low-frequency sounds. This selectivity suggests that the origin of the problem is in the inner ear and/or the nerve pathways to and through the brain. Cochlear hair cells near the base of the cochlea, for example, accumulate lipofuscin in proportion to the degree of high-frequency loss. Other likely mechanisms for age-related damage include altered mechanical function of the basilar membrane (on which the hair cells sit), damage to the neurons in the auditory nerve, and diminished blood flow to the cochlea. The selective loss of high-frequency hearing makes it especially difficult for the elderly to hear consonants. Vowel sounds, on the other hand, are lower pitched and can still be heard fairly well. Overall, these changes cause speech to sound muffled. Many elderly compensate for this loss by lip-reading, which is easier to do for consonant sounds than for vowel sounds. Hearing conversations in a crowded room can be very difficult for an elderly person, not only because of the presbycusis, but also because the elderly have a diminished ability to localize sound and to mask those sounds that are deemed less important.

Taste

There appears to be a decline in sensitivity to *taste* with age as well. Our ability to taste results from the activation of taste cells, which are clustered together in the taste buds on our tongue and other regions of the oral cavity.

Nerves transmit this information to the brain stem and on to higher centers in the brain. Taste buds have been classically described as being of four types—sweet, sour, bitter, and salty—which are regionally distributed over the tongue. The degree of taste impairment seems to vary from taste to taste, being least profound for sweet and most profound for salt. The decline in taste is consistent with the age-related loss in the number of taste buds on the tongue but may also be due to the decreased production of saliva and resultant dry mouth one experiences with aging. The elderly also have more difficulty gauging the intensities of tastes and identifying individual tastes, like salty, in a mixture of flavors. This impairment may cause older individuals to add excessive amounts of salt to foods, which could be detrimental, particularly if they have hypertension or congestive heart failure.

Smell

Another functional decline with important ramifications is the impairment of the ability to *smell*, a condition known as **hyposmia.** Similar to taste, the degree of impairment varies with the particular odor, and the ability to identify individual odors in a mixture is gradually lost with age. Interestingly, men are more profoundly affected than women. Smell is made possible by the activation of sensory cells in the upper mucosal surface of the nasal cavity, which pass the sensory information through the bony roof into the *olfactory bulb* at the base of the frontal lobe. From there, the information is processed and relayed through the *olfactory tract* to higher brain centers. As one might expect, there is an age-related decline in the numbers of mucosal sensory cells and olfactory bulb relay cells, accounting for the decreased sensitivity to smell. Because of the crucial role played by smell in distinguishing the tastes of different foods, hyposmia makes foods less desirable, causing a decreased appetite and irregular eating habits with subsequent weight loss and malnutrition in the elderly. In addition, the inability to smell can have dire consequences if a person fails to notice a poison gas leak or other toxic inhalant. The elderly, for example, have a 10 times higher threshold than younger individuals for the smell of ethyl mercaptan, an odiferous substance added to propane gas to warn individuals of gas leakage.[76] Clearly, the sense of smell has protective value.

MUSCULOSKELETAL SYSTEM

Musculoskeletal dysfunction is a major cause of disability in the elderly, altering mobility, fine motor control, and the mechanics of respiration. As a result, the elderly are more prone to falls (and thus fractures), respiratory infections, and the general physiological decline that accompanies an increasingly sedentary lifestyle. One of the most significant changes in the aging skeleton is **osteoporosis.** Defined as a reduction in bone mass and bone density, this condition predisposes an individual to fractures, especially in the vertebrae, proximal femur, and distal radius. In the United States, an estimated 1.5 million fractures per year result from osteoporosis, the morbidity of which accounts for about $10 billion in health care costs annually.[77] Important risk factors for osteoporosis include estrogen depletion (in postmenopausal women), calcium deficiency (exacerbated in the elderly because of decreased intestinal absorption of calcium), decreased bone mass at the end of development, physical inactivity, testosterone depletion (in males), alcoholism, and cigarette smoking. The loss of bone mass in the vertebrae and the thinning of the intervertebral disks account for a gradual decrease in height of about 2 inches between ages 20 and 70.[78] Collapse or severe wedging of the vertebrae cause the characteristic appearance of kyphosis, an exaggerated convex curvature of the upper spine leading to a "hunch-backed" posture. Concomitant deformity of the rib cage can alter the normal mechanics of breathing. At about age 40, the rate of bone resorption surpasses the rate of new bone formation, with a subsequent loss of about 40 percent of total bone mass in women and 30 percent in men over the course of the lifespan.[79] Bone resorption is most extreme in the inner spongy bone at the enlarged ends (epiphyses) and along the inside rim of long bones, making older bones more vulnerable to fractures from both compression and lateral impact.

Osteoarthritis, also called degenerative joint disease, is the second most common cause of disability in this country, affecting more than 50 million Americans.[80] Its incidence increases with age, affecting 85 percent of persons aged 70 to 79.[81] So common is this disease in the elderly that, for many years, it was believed to be a normal aspect of aging. More recent histological studies, however, have revealed clear differences in joint and cartilage structure between the healthy aged and those with osteoarthritis. Osteoarthritis is marked by ulceration and destruction of joint cartilage, leading eventually to exposure and destruction of underlying bone. The normal cushioning effect of cartilage is lost, causing bone to rub on bone. As one might guess, the weight-bearing joints are the most commonly affected (e.g., knee and hip joints), and obesity is a major risk factor. But other highly used, freely movable joints, such as the proximal and distal interphalangeal joints of the fingers, are also commonly affected. Inflamed joints are marked by pain, swelling, and decreased range of motion. Other less common forms of arthritis that increase in incidence with age include rheumatoid arthritis, gout, pseudogout, and polymyalgia rheumatica.

Skeletal muscle undergoes changes with aging as well. Overall, the number of skeletal muscle fibers (cells) decreases with age, although the rate of decline varies from muscle to muscle. For example, little change is noted in the diaphragm, the primary breathing muscle which never relaxes for more than a few seconds; muscles used less frequently, such as those of the extremities, exhibit greater rates of muscle cell loss. Other microscopic changes in aging skeletal muscle include a variable decrease in muscle fiber size (atrophy) and capillary supply, an increase in deposition of lipofuscin and adipose (fat) cells, and a spotty loss of the motor neuron innervation. These microscopic changes result in a gradual decline in muscle strength and efficiency over time, although this too varies from one muscle group to the next. It cannot be overemphasized, however, that regular physical training can improve muscle strength and endurance, even in the very old. This fact, coupled with the benefits of exercise in maintaining bone strength and cardiovascular fitness, argues for a cautioned exercise regimen for almost everyone.

CARDIOVASCULAR SYSTEM

The cardiovascular system consists of the *heart* and *blood vessels.* It is responsible for the circulation of the blood which allows for the delivery of oxygen and nutrients to and removal of waste products from all parts of the body. Damage to this system, therefore, can have negative implications for the entire body. The *ventricles* of the heart generate the pressure that propels the blood through the arteries, arterioles, capillaries (the site of nutrient and waste exchange), venules, and finally the veins, the blood vessels that return the blood back to the *atria* of the heart. The left ventricle has the thickest muscular wall and pumps blood out to the systems of the body (via the higher pressure *systemic circulation*), while the right ventricle pumps blood to the lungs (via the lower pressure *pulmonic circulation*) (Fig. 3–9).

The significance of cardiovascular disease in the middle-aged and elderly cannot be overemphasized. It is the most common cause of death worldwide. While mortality due to cardiovascular disease has been decreasing in the United States since the late 1960s, probably as a result of healthier diets, increased exercise, less smoking, and better control of hypertension (high blood pressure), it is nonetheless still a major killer.

Although the heart may increase in size considerably as a result of chronic congestive heart failure, its size and weight change very little with age in healthy individuals. Nevertheless, the heart exhibits several structural alterations with advancing years. Lipofuscin is deposited at a regular rate and mitochondrial DNA is damaged in cardiac muscle cells. Adipose tissue accumulates in and around the heart. The inner lining, or endocardium, undergoes fibrosis (i.e. scarring), and there is a gradual loss of the specialized conduction cells (autorhythmic cells) that coordinate the events of the cardiac contraction cycle.

Coinciding with these changes are important functional alterations. The resting *cardiac output,* defined as the total volume of blood pumped out of the heart in 1 minute while at rest, decreases by 1 percent per year after age 30.[78] To understand the reasons for this, one must be familiar with the determinants of cardiac output, which is computed by multiplying the *heart rate* (in beats per minute) by the *stroke volume* (the volume of blood pumped out of

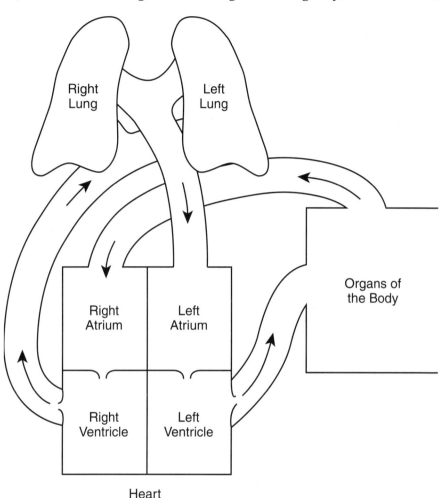

FIG. 3–9. The cardiovascular system. The arrows indicate the direction of blood flow.

the ventricle in one contraction). A decline in the resting cardiac output with age is primarily due to a decrease in stroke volume, which in turn is caused in part by a decreased efficiency of cardiac muscle as well as a decreased responsiveness of the heart to the sympathetic nervous system, the branch of the nervous system whose effect is normally to increase the strength of the heart's contraction, or *contractility.*

Other factors influencing stroke volume, and therefore the cardiac output, are the preload and afterload work requirements placed on the heart. *Preload* is a measure of the amount of blood filling the ventricles just prior to contraction. When the volume of blood filling the ventricles increases, the heart responds by contracting more strongly, pumping out more blood to keep pace. Conversely, a decreased preload causes a weaker contraction. This phenomenon, known as *Starling's law of the heart,* ensures that blood does not get "backed up" in the venous circulation. However, with aging comes changes in the elasticity and smooth muscle of the venous walls and subsequent dilations, or varicosities, of the veins. This increases the capacity of the veins to hold blood and decreases the rate of venous return to the heart, ultimately causing a decreased preload and cardiac output. Afterload is a measure of the pressure against which the ventricles must pump to force blood out into the arteries. All other things being equal, the greater the afterload, the smaller the stroke volume, and therefore cardiac output. Systemic hypertension, which is more prevalent in the aged population, increases afterload and thus reduces cardiac output. Successful treatment of high blood pressure, therefore, reduces the workload placed on the heart.

Despite these changes, the cardiac output generally remains sufficient for the body's resting needs well into old age. It is during physical exertion that the decreased work capacity of the heart becomes more evident. During exercise, heart rate and stroke volume normally rise to meet the body's increased metabolic needs. These changes, which are part of the so-called *fight-or-flight response* to stress, occur largely under the direction of the sympathetic nervous system. At the same time that the heart is working harder, the sympathetic nervous system preferentially redirects blood flow to skeletal muscles, the brain, and heart muscle while limiting blood flow to the "less vital" organs of the digestive, reproductive, and urinary systems. But these normal responses to exercise are dampened as we age, largely because of decreased sympathetic nervous system activity. The maximum heart rate during exercise, calculated roughly as 220 minus one's age, decreases with advancing years. Thus, the elderly become short of breath (*dyspnea*) and tire more quickly than younger individuals during exercise. A related problem, probably also due in part to insufficient sympathetic nervous system activity, is **postural hypotension,** which is a fall in systemic blood pressure upon rising from a supine to a standing position. It can cause lightheadedness when a person stands up and can thus increase the risk of falling. It is difficult to tell whether these age-related changes in heart structure and function are due to aging per se or to an increasingly sedentary lifestyle. However, since regular exercise improves cardiac functioning in the young and middle-aged, it is likely to have similar benefits in the elderly, provided that regimen is safe and commensurate with the abilities of the individual. In fact, one study found that healthy 60- to 71-year-old subjects improved their maximal oxygen consumption (a measure of physical fitness) in response to regular exercise to the same relative extent as younger individuals, independent of initial level of fitness.[82]

The predominant change that occurs in the blood vessels with age is **atherosclerosis,** defined as the development of fatty plaques and the proliferation of connective tissue in the walls of arteries. The slow destruction of the arterial wall can lead to blockage of the artery, particularly when a blood clot develops on its damaged surface. So prevalent is this condition that one may argue that it is an inevitable phenomenon of aging. And while the clinical consequences of atherosclerosis are often sudden and life-threatening (e.g., heart attacks and strokes) and come toward the end of life, it has become clear in recent years that the earliest evidence of fatty accumulation is detectable in the first decade of life, and that the lesions progress throughout life.

Knowledge of the normal structure of the artery wall is necessary to understand the changes of atherosclerosis. The three major layers of arteries, from the innermost out, are the intima, media, and adventitia (Fig. 3–10A). The *intima* is a thin layer of connective tissue covered on the inner surface by endothelial cells. The *media* is primarily smooth muscle, bounded on its inner and outer surfaces by elastic connective tissue. The *adventitia* is a connective tissue layer that contains the tiny blood vessels (vasa vasorum) that nourish the outer half of the arterial wall. The inner half of the artery wall receives its nutrients by direct diffusion from the blood in the lumen of the artery.

According to one widely held theory of atherogenesis (fatty plaque formation), white blood cells called monocytes adhere to the surface of the intima in areas where microscopic damage has occurred (e.g., because of turbulent blood flow). These cells transform into macrophages and begin to ingest lipids from the bloodstream. Lipids and proteins from the blood begin to accumulate in the intra- and extracellular spaces of the intima and media as endothelial, smooth muscle, and macrophage cells begin to proliferate. As the lipid deposits enlarge, they become visible as *fatty streaks,* which form as early as the first decade of life (Fig. 3–10B). As the fatty deposits grow and the arterial wall thickens, cells of the intima and media are forced farther away from their nutrient supplies and ultimately die and disintegrate, leaving behind a fatty paste, or *atheroma.* In an effort to contain the damage, fibroblasts form a fibrous connective tissue capsule around the atheroma. The encapsulated lesion, referred to as a *fibrous (or fatty) plaque,* appears as early as the second decade of life (Fig. 3–10C).

Fatty plaques create several problems for us as we age. Firstly, enlargement of the fatty deposits may partially or completely block blood flow through the artery. Secondly, the thickening of artery walls makes them more rigid, which in turn can raise systolic blood pressure and increase the afterload work requirement of the heart. Thirdly, destruction of the inner layers of the artery wall can weaken it and cause it to balloon out under the force of the blood pressure. These dilations, called **aneurysms,** are prone to rupturing and causing severe internal bleeding. Finally, breaks in the fibrous capsule of fatty plaques can cause ulcerations, leaving the underlying fat deposits exposed to the bloodstream. This is ominous because such ulcerations attract platelets from the bloodstream, which clump and release substances that stimulate the formation of a blood clot, or **thrombus** (Fig. 3–10D). Enlarging thrombi can

(A)

(B)

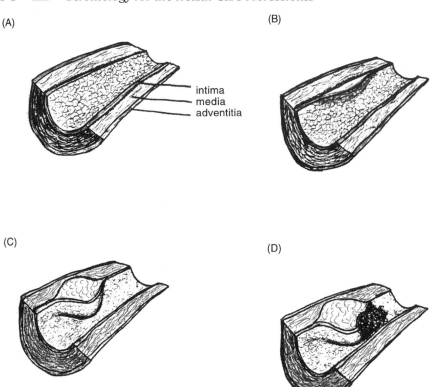

intima
media
adventitia

(C)

(D)

FIG. 3–10. The progressive changes in arteries due to atherosclerosis. (*A*) Normal structure. (*B*) Fatty streak formation. (*C*) Fatty plaque formation. (*D*) Ulcerated fatty plaque with overlying thrombus blocking the artery lumen.

very quickly occlude arteries, or break off and travel farther down the bloodstream to lodge in a smaller vessel, a phenomenon known as **embolism.**

The complications of atherosclerosis begin as early as the fourth decade of life and increase in frequency with each succeeding decade. The particular consequences of the disease depend on the artery or arteries involved. Blockage of the coronary arteries can cause **myocardial infarction** (heart attack), while occlusion or rupture of a cerebral artery can result in a **stroke.** The development of fatty plaques in the renal arteries can cause hypertension and kidney failure, while blockage of an artery in the leg can cause severe pain (called claudication) and ulcerations of the skin. While nearly everyone is prone to some degree of atherosclerosis, there are several risk factors that seem to accelerate the disease process. They include age, genetic predisposition, hypertension, diabetes mellitus, high blood-cholesterol level, cigarette smoking, obesity, poor physical fitness, and "type A" personality. While there is nothing one can do about some of these factors, many are in fact modifiable. Thus, it makes good sense to "eat right," exercise, keep trim, avoid cigarettes, and comply with any prescribed high blood pressure medications. But as is true of most preventive health measures, these interventions are more effective if initiated early in life.

RESPIRATORY SYSTEM

The function of the respiratory system is to transport oxygen to and remove carbon dioxide from the bloodstream. The air breathed in is warmed, humidified, and cleansed as it passes successively through the mouth and/or nasal cavity, pharynx, larynx, trachea, and bronchi to reach the lungs (Fig. 3–11). In the lungs, the inhaled air continues through smaller bronchi, bronchioles, and alveolar ducts to finally reach the **alveoli,** the tiny, thin-walled air sacs covered by capillaries that are the major site of gas exchange between the air and the bloodstream. The 300 million alveoli in the lungs account for most of the lung volume and provide about 75 m^2 of surface area available for gas transport to and from the blood. The lungs, located in the thoracic cavity (or thorax), are enclosed from the sides and top by the thoracic vertebrae and rib cage and from below by the **diaphragm,** a dome-shaped skeletal muscle. During inhalation, the diaphragm contracts, lowering the floor of the thorax while the external intercostal muscles between the ribs contract to swing the ribs forward and upward. Both of these actions help expand the thorax, creating a vacuum-like effect that draws air into the respiratory tract and lungs. The lungs expand passively during this process because of their adherence to the inner wall of the thorax. Exhalation is normally a passive process whereby the relaxation of the breathing muscles causes the thorax to contract down to a smaller volume, largely by elastic recoiling of the rib cage and lungs. The elastic recoiling (and lowering of volume) of the lungs during exhalation is due to two factors (Fig. 3–12A):

- The tendency of individual alveoli to become smaller at lower air pressures because of the surface tension generated by the watery inner alveolar lining
- The recoiling of elastic tissue around the respiratory airways that was stretched out during inhalation

The elastic tissue in the lungs is tethered between alveoli and bronchioles in such a way that actually prevents the bronchioles from completely collapsing during exhalation. Elastic recoiling of the rib cage and lungs decreases the thoracic volume, thus increasing air pressure in the thorax and creating the necessary pressure gradient to force much of the air back out of the respiratory system.

A major indicator of pulmonary fitness is the *forced vital capacity* (FVC), defined as the maximal volume of air breathed out during one forced exhala-

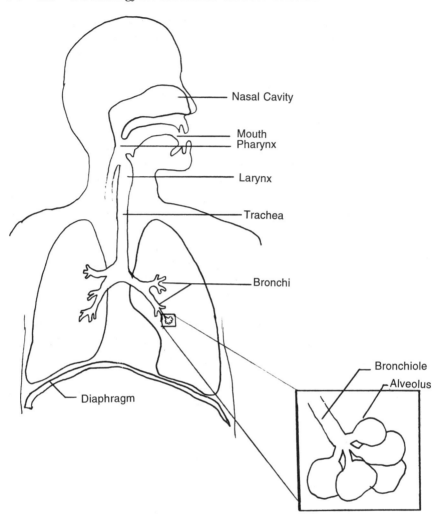

FIG. 3–11. The respiratory system.

tion after maximal inhalation. The normal FVC in adults is 3 to 4 L in women and 4.5 to 5.5 L in men. FVC increases with growth of the body during childhood, adolescence, and early adulthood, reaching a peak at about age 25. Thereafter, FVC declines at a steady rate of about 21 ml/year, primarily because of changes in the soft tissue of the lungs.[83] As we age, the elastin fibers in the lungs are altered, probably by both excessive cross-linking between fibers and breakage of individual fibers. As a result, the lungs, as a whole, lose some of their elastic recoil, and the small bronchioles tend to partially or completely collapse during exhalation, causing obstruction of air flow and trapping of air in the alveoli (Fig. 3–12B). Air-trapping decreases the rate of oxygen delivery to and carbon dioxide extraction from the bloodstream. In addition, air-trapping in the alveoli increases the *residual volume,* which is the volume of air remaining in the lungs after a forced exhalation. Because the *total lung capacity* (or maximum volume of air that the lungs can hold) changes very little in a healthy aging person, any increase in the residual volume comes at the expense of decreasing the FVC (Fig. 3–13). Further hampering of gas exchange occurs with age as a result of a gradual loss of alveolar wall surface area, estimated to be a 4 percent decline per decade after age 30.[84] These changes in lung elasticity and alveolar surface area are similar to, but smaller in scale than, the changes that occur in emphysema.

Coupled with the changes in the lung tissue are changes in the mechanical properties of the wall of the thorax. As we grow older, the rib cage stiffens, largely because of the calcification of the cartilage between the ribs and the vertebrae and to the exaggerated curvature of the thoracic spine (kyphosis). These skeletal changes limit the mobility of the rib cage, making it difficult for the external intercostal muscles (as well as the accessory muscles of inhalation, such as the sternocleidomastoid and pectoralis minor) to expand the rib cage. While a healthy elderly person might breathe adequately to meet the body's needs at rest, the previously described changes may limit his or her tolerance for exercise, especially when coupled with the age-related

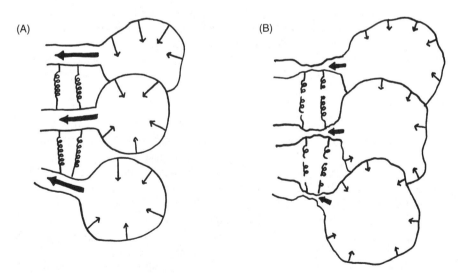

FIG. 3–12. (*A*) Normal elastic recoil of alveoli and unobstructed bronchiolar airflow in healthy lungs. (*B*) Decreased elastic recoil of alveoli and obstructed bronchiolar airflow noted with emphysema.

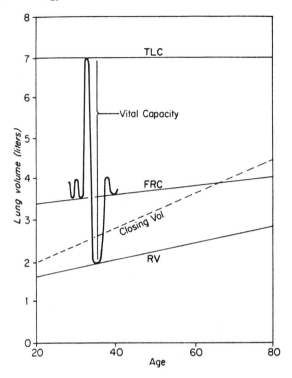

FIG. 3–13. The effect of age on subdivisions of lung volume. TLC = total lung capacity, FRC = functional residual capacity, RV = residual volume. Values shown are for men of average height; the changes with age are similar for women. (Adapted from Tockman, MS: Aging of the respiratory system. In Hazzard, WR, et al (eds): Principles of Geriatric Medicine and Gerontology. McGraw-Hill, New York, 1994, p 557, with permission.)

decrease in cardiac output described earlier in this chapter. Thus, it is not surprising that the elderly, in general, experience shortness of breath (dyspnea) more quickly during exercise than do younger individuals.

Superimposed on the normal age-related changes to the respiratory system are certain diseases that increase in frequency from the fifth decade of life onward. They include emphysema, chronic bronchitis, pneumonia, and lung cancer. The first two are referred to together as **chronic obstructive pulmonary disease (COPD),** and along with lung cancer, are caused primarily by cigarette smoking. The steps leading to **emphysema** begin when cigarette smoke irritates the respiratory tract, stimulating proliferation of white blood cells called macrophages. These macrophages release chemicals that attract large numbers of another type of white blood cell, the neutrophil, to the inflamed area. Neutrophils, in turn, release protease enzymes, one of which called elastase can damage the elastin protein found in elastic tissue of the lungs. The effects of elastase are limited by a protective enzyme called alpha-1 antitrypsin, which inactivates elastase. However, alpha-1 antitrypsin is damaged by the free radicals produced from cigarette smoke. Thus, elastase is free to destroy lung tissue. The stage is then set for the slow, irreversible loss of functional elastic tissue in the lungs, resulting in the loss of alveolar wall surface area and the premature collapsing of small bronchioles during exhalation (hence, the "obstructive" in chronic obstructive pulmonary disease).[85–89] As more air gets "trapped" distal to the bronchiolar obstruction, the lung volume increases, creating the classic "barrel chest" appearance. In the end stages of emphysema, destruction of alveolar walls can be so extreme that large, visible air pockets form in the lungs. Collapsed bronchiolar airways are more difficult to reopen on inhalation. Thus, emphysema increases the work of breathing so that an individual must use the accessory muscles of inhalation to supplement the activity of the diaphragm and external intercostal muscles. This exaggerated use of the accessory muscles gives rise to the "barrel-shaped" chest noted in emphysema. Because of the diminished rate of gas transport and the increased work of breathing, the sufferer of emphysema is short of breath and cannot tolerate rigorous exercise well.

Chronic bronchitis, like emphysema, is more common in the elderly, especially in those with a long history of cigarette smoking. It is clinically defined as a chronic cough ("smoker's cough") productive of sputum, occurring on most days for at least 3 months' duration over at least 2 consecutive years. Whereas emphysema primarily affects the smallest airways, chronic bronchitis is an inflammation of the larger bronchi, brought about by the irritating effects of cigarette smoke or other environmental inhalants. The inflammatory process causes excessive mucus production, which is difficult to clear from the lungs, not only because of its abundance, but also because the tiny, beating cilia covering the bronchi that normally help move the mucus upward are damaged by smoking. The pooling of excessive mucus can block the bronchi (hence, the "obstructive" in chronic obstructive pulmonary disease) and provide a nutrient-rich environment for bacterial infection. When one considers that the elderly immune system is not as efficient, nor is the cough reflex that helps clear excess mucus and aspirated food from the respiratory tract, it is easy to understand why an older smoker with chronic bronchitis is at increased risk for the spreading of the inflammation and infection to the bronchioles and alveoli—the development of *pneumonia.*

HEMATOLOGICAL SYSTEM

The hematological system consists of those organs and tissues in the body that contribute red blood cells (RBCs), white blood cells (WBCs), and platelets to the bloodstream. Production of these cells from precursor stem cells, a process called *hematopoiesis,* occurs primarily in the bone marrow. The WBCs, or *leuko-*

cytes, protect the body from infectious organisms and cancer cells, coordinate the events of the inflammatory and allergic responses, and participate in tissue and organ transplant rejection. Following their production in the bone marrow, WBCs travel through blood and lymphatic vessels to "seed" other organs, such as the spleen, tonsils, and lymph nodes, where they provide a continuous supply for life. Their role in aging is discussed in the next section. Platelets, or *thrombocytes*, are really cell fragments produced by the disintegration of large megakaryocyte cells in the bone marrow. They play a role in hemostasis (i.e. the stoppage of bleeding) by clumping together and releasing chemicals that stimulate blood clot formation in damaged blood vessels.

This section focuses on RBCs, called *erythrocytes*, which are flexible, disk-shaped cells filled with hemoglobin, an iron-containing protein that reversibly binds to and helps transport oxygen and carbon dioxide through the bloodstream. The life span of a RBC is relatively short, lasting only about 120 days. This is because RBCs undergo significant wear and tear as they are repeatedly squeezed through the small capillaries of the circulation. In addition, mature RBCs lack a nucleus (it is extruded from the RBCs during their final stage of development) and thus cannot repair themselves when damaged. For these reasons, RBCs must be produced at the astonishing rate of more than 2 million per second in healthy bone marrow (a process called *erythropoiesis*). They are broken down by macrophages at the same rate in the spleen. When the rate of erythropoiesis is equal to the rate of RBC destruction, there is no net change in the oxygen-carrying capacity of the blood over time. This capacity is often gauged by measuring the *hematocrit*, defined as the percentage of total blood volume taken up by red blood cells. The normal range for hematocrit is 42 to 52 percent and 37 to 47 percent in healthy men and women, respectively.

A major hematological concern in geriatric medicine is the high prevalence of **anemia** (defined as a lower than normal oxygen-carrying capacity of the blood) in the elderly, particularly those older individuals in acute and long-term care settings. It is important to understand that anemia is not a single disease, but rather a syndrome that has several different causes. Individuals with anemia often have pale skin, shortness of breath, and fatigue as a result of the subnormal hematocrit. The majority of the blood's oxygen is carried in RBCs, and anemias are caused by inadequate production or premature destruction of these RBCs. It has become clear in recent years that the high incidence of anemia in the elderly is not due to aging per se, but rather to the high frequency of other age-related illnesses that can cause anemia. In healthy elderly individuals, there is no significant decline in the rate of erythropoiesis under normal conditions. However, when the body is stressed in ways that require an increase in erythropoiesis (e.g., chronic bleeding), aged bone marrow has a more difficult time "keeping up" than does young bone marrow.

The most common category of anemia diagnosed in the elderly is *hypopro-*

liferative anemia, defined as anemia due to a lower rate of RBC production than would be expected for the degree of hematocrit decline. The most common cause of hypoproliferative anemia in the aged is an inadequate supply of iron to make the hemoglobin in RBCs. However, the problem in most cases is not insufficient iron in the diet, but rather excessive loss of iron and/or the inability to recycle the iron that collects in macrophages from broken-down RBCs. Excessive loss of iron is caused by acute or chronic bleeding, which in the elderly occurs most frequently in the digestive tract (e.g., due to ulcers, diverticulitis, or colon cancer). Another type of hypoproliferative anemia, the anemia of inflammation, affects those individuals undergoing inflammatory responses as a result of conditions such as infection, tissue damage, or cancer. Extensive inflammation hampers the recycling of iron from macrophages in the spleen and liver. Thus, as older RBCs are continuously broken down, the supply of iron available for erythropoiesis in the bone marrow is inadequate. Chronic diseases such as rheumatoid arthritis and inflammatory bowel disease (e.g. ulcerative colitis and Crohn's disease) have a similar effect. These anemias can be exacerbated by protein and caloric malnutrition, which appears to decrease levels of the protein erythropoietin, a hormone produced by the kidneys, whose normal effect is to stimulate erythropoiesis in the bone marrow.

Other types of anemia that can afflict the elderly fall under the category of *ineffective erythropoiesis,* defined as a group of anemias that result from destruction of developing RBCs while still in the bone marrow or immediately after they are released into the circulation. Anemia due to vitamin B_{12} deficiency is an example of ineffective erythropoiesis often diagnosed in the elderly. Vitamin B_{12} is a coenzyme required for DNA production. When levels of this vitamin are deficient, RBCs develop abnormally in the bone marrow. Specifically, the cells cannot divide efficiently, and maturation of the cell nucleus lags behind maturation of the cytoplasm. The large, nucleated RBC precursors called megaloblasts (hence, the alternative name, megaloblastic anemia) that form are often destroyed in the bone marrow before they can be released into the bloodstream. The cause of the vitamin B_{12} deficiency may be any of the following:

- Insufficient dietary intake (particularly in those who suffer from alcoholism)
- Inflammation or destruction of the ileum, the terminal portion of the small intestine, where vitamin B_{12} is absorbed
- Inflammation or destruction of the stomach lining (e.g., due to an autoimmune disorder called pernicious anemia), and thus the cells that produce intrinsic factor, a glycoprotein required for successful vitamin B_{12} absorption in the ileum

Having just reviewed the cardiovascular, respiratory, and hematological systems, it becomes clear that all three of these systems are required to ensure adequate delivery of oxygen to the tissues. An age-related decline in the function of one or two of these systems will exacerbate any physiological dysfunction present in the others. The presence of anemia in someone with congestive heart failure would be much more detrimental than it would be in an otherwise healthy individual. If that person with anemia and congestive heart failure also had emphysema, the disruption to the body would be still more extreme. It is this interdependence of our organ systems that, on the one hand, allows for appropriate compensatory adjustments to homeostatic disturbances in younger, healthy individuals but, on the other hand, can create a "chain reaction" of dysfunction in older, less healthy persons with decreased functional reserve.

IMMUNE SYSTEM

The ability of our bodies to remain free of infections and cancer requires that the WBCs of our immune system are able to distinguish "self" (i.e., our own healthy cells) from "non-self" (i.e., invading microorganisms and parasites or structurally altered cancer cells). To appreciate the enormity of this task, one need only think about the thousands of different types of organisms that can invade the body, each of which must be specifically recognized by the immune system as "foreign" and destroyed without damaging the integrity of our own tissues in the process. Similarly, imagine the countless number of precancerous cell types, each of which may differ from normal cells in only very subtle ways, that are recognized and destroyed by the immune system on a regular basis. Indeed, in its prime, the immune system is to be marvelled for its fidelity. But, as is true of most systems, age takes its toll on this system. A discussion of the most important aspects of the immune response is followed by a review of those age-related changes in immunity that have implications for our health and well-being.

To be "immune" to an infection implies being protected from it. The development of immunity to a particular infectious organism, however, usually requires initial exposure to it, which in turn often causes mild illness. Nonetheless, on recovery from the sickness, the individual is immune to subsequent infection and illness from that organism; the body has developed an "immunological memory" so that it can act more swiftly and effectively the next time it is exposed to the same invader. The development of this immunological memory occurs by one of two general processes, called the humoral-mediated and cell-mediated immune responses. The former process produces proteins called antibodies, which circulate through the blood (or "humor") and specifically bind to the foreign organism; the latter process activates white blood cells called killer T-lymphocyte cells, which directly destroy the invading organism.

In the *humoral-mediated immune response,* the invading organism, for example a streptococcal bacterium, is initially "trapped" and ingested by scavenger *macrophage* cells "hiding out" in the lymph nodes (Fig. 3–14A). The macrophage digests the bacterium but re-presents some of the bacterial molecules (or antigens) on its own cell surface. This antigen presentation signals a helper T-lymphocyte (or *T-helper cell*) to bind to the macrophage. There are several distinct populations of T-helper cells available in our body for this purpose, but the beauty of our immune system is that only the T-helper cell with the appropriate receptor for that particular presented streptococcal antigen will bind to the macrophage. Other T-helper cells will not bind because their receptors do not make a nice "hand-in-glove" fit with that specific antigen. The macrophage, once bound to the appropriate T-helper cell, releases a chemical called interleukin-1, which, in turn, stimulates the T-helper cell to mature and multiply, forming a large population of clones, all bearing receptors for the streptococcal antigen. These activated T-helper cells then bind to and activate another type of white blood cell called the B-lymphocyte (or *B-cell*), which is specialized to make antibodies. But again, the correct population of B-cells is selected (clonal selection). In other words, only that particular population that makes the antibody that binds specifically to the streptococcal antigen is selected. These activated B-cells multiply, forming an entire "army" of fully developed, antibody-producing cells called *plasma cells.* The abundant supply of antistreptococcal antibodies released from the plasma cells bind to the streptococcal bacteria in the tissues, lymphatics, and bloodstream, tagging them for efficient destruction by other macrophages and by membrane-piercing chemicals called complement factors. In the process, some of the dividing B-cells are stored away as "memory B-cells," primed and ready to go for the next time the same strain of streptococcus enters the body.

While antibodies are effective in neutralizing extracellular microorganisms, another strategy must be used to destroy those microbes that "hide out" inside our cells, most notably viruses. This strategy, called the *cell-mediated immune response,* is similar in many respects to humoral-mediated immunity (Fig. 3–14B). The invading virus enters the macrophage, leaving some of its protein coat antigen on the surface. This signals the correct T-helper cell to bind, become activated, and subsequently activate the correct clone of killer T-lymphocytes (or *T-killer cells*). As a result, a growing population of T-killer cells are formed, each cell of which is specifically programmed to kill those of our body cells infected by that particular virus. In addition, some of the "primed" T-killer cells are stored away as "memory T-cells," poised for the next invasion by that same virus. The ability to detect and destroy cancer cells in the body probably also involves populations of these T-killer cells, along with another population of white blood cells called *natural killer cells.*

The age-related decline of immune system functioning gives rise to three general categories of illness that preferentially afflict the elderly:

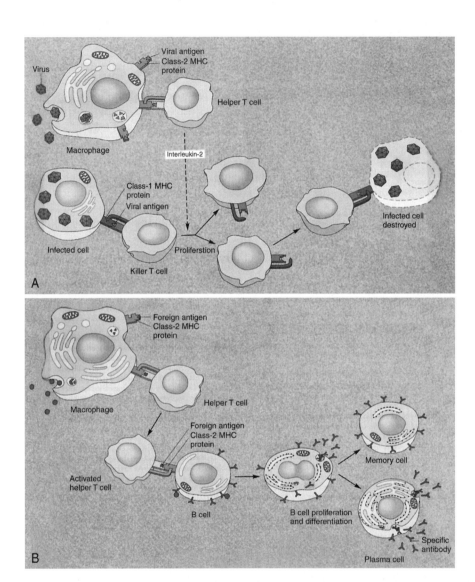

FIG. 3–14. (*A*) Humoral-mediated immune response. (*B*) Cell-mediated immune response. (From Van de Graaff, KM, and Fox, SI: Human Anatomy and Physiology, ed 4. William C. Brown Pub., Dubuque, IA, 1994, pp 672–673, with permission.)

- Infections
- Cancer
- Autoimmune disease

The overall incidence of *infectious disease* rises in late adulthood. Particularly prevalent among the aged are influenza, pneumonia, tuberculosis, meningitis, and urinary tract infections. Deficiencies in both humoral- and cell-mediated immunity have been implicated in the increased incidence of infections. The age-related decreases in the numbers and activities of various clones of T-cells may be due to the slow, postpubertal destruction of the thymus gland, an organ that stimulates the development of T-helper and T-killer cells by releasing various hormone-like chemicals. Another possible reason for diminished functioning of T-cells is the derangement of precursor stem cell development in the bone marrow. Regardless of the cause, it is important to bear in mind that any decline in T-helper cell function will have widespread repercussions for our health because this cell is the "catalyst" for both humoral- and cell-mediated immunity (it is, incidentally, the destruction of these cells by the human immunodeficiency virus [HIV] that makes acquired immunodeficiency syndrom [AIDS] such a devastating disease). There appears to be an age-related decline in the number and function of different B-cell clones as well. Thus, there is a general decline in the body's ability to generate antibody responses to certain infections.

Cancer increases in prevalence with age as well, particularly leukemia, lung, prostate, breast, stomach, and pancreatic cancer. This rise may be due in part to the altered immune surveillance of precancer and cancer cells that comes with aging. Several components of the immune system probably play roles in cancer protection, including the previously mentioned natural killer cells. Both the number and function of natural killer cells in animals decline with aging. If this is the case in humans, it may partly explain the rising incidence of cancer in the elderly.

Autoimmune diseases are also more common in the elderly. These diseases are marked by the mistaken immunological destruction of the body's own cells. In such diseases, the body loses the ability to distinguish "self" from "non-self." Prominent examples of autoimmune diseases affecting the elderly are rheumatoid arthritis, Hashimoto's thyroiditis, lupus, and chronic hepatitis. Tolerance to our own tissues develops early in life (during development of the immune system), when the thymus gland selects out and eliminates those clones of T-cells programmed to destroy our own tissues— a process called *clonal deletion*. However, with the slow, age-related destruction of the thymus gland, the body may lose the ability to detect and destroy these potentially self-harming T-cells. Indeed, with aging comes increased levels of "autoantibodies."

DIGESTIVE SYSTEM

The primary function of the digestive system is to process incoming food so that nutrients can be absorbed into the body. The primary structural feature of this system is the digestive tract, made up of the mouth, pharynx, stomach, small intestine, large intestine (or colon), rectum, and anus (Fig. 3–15). This canal works like an assembly line, with each part having a specialized function in digestion. Attached to the digestive tract along the way are exocrine glands, such as the salivary glands, pancreas, and liver, which secrete substances to aid in digestion and absorption. While aging in an otherwise healthy individual has minimal effects on the digestive system, many specific diseases of this system increase in frequency with advancing years. The age-related alterations in structure and function are discussed in descending order, starting with the mouth and proceeding to the rectum.

Food entering the *mouth* undergoes the initial stages of mechanical digestion (via chewing) and chemical digestion (via release of salivary amylase en-

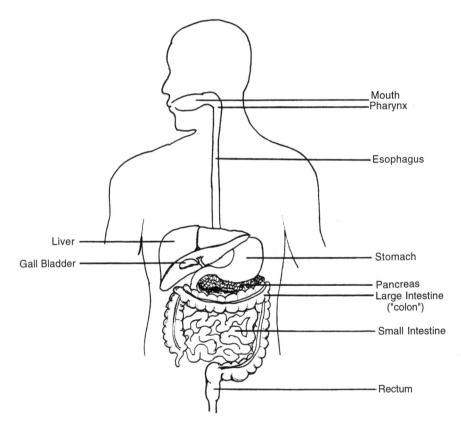

FIG. 3–15. The digestive system.

zyme). In the mouth, the teeth undergo perhaps the most visible changes with age, becoming yellowish-brown (because of exposure to coffee, cigarette smoke, and other staining agents) and worn on the surface (because of years of chewing, night-grinding, and jaw-clenching). Osteoporotic changes of the jaw bones (maxilla and mandible) can cause teeth to loosen from their sockets. This change, coupled with the recession of the gums (*periodontal disease*), can cause loss of teeth in the elderly. Indeed, about half of U.S. citizens have lost the majority of their teeth by age 65.[90] While dental caries (cavities) are not an inevitable result of aging, the diminished strength and dexterity of the elderly can make teeth-brushing difficult, thus increasing the likelihood of dental caries. **Xerostomia,** or dry mouth, is another problem of aging and has several causes, including decreased saliva production, cigarette smoking, and medication side effects (e.g., from certain blood pressure medications).

Once sufficiently chewed, the food is swallowed by the complex coordination of several muscles of the tongue, palate, pharynx, and esophagus. In this regard, a common problem in the elderly is **dysphagia,** or difficulty swallowing. This may be due to weakness of the tongue muscles, improper nervous system control of the swallowing reflex, or uncoordinated muscular action of the pharynx or esophagus. Severe dysphagia can cause aspiration of food into the larynx and farther down the respiratory tract, which in turn puts one at risk for aspiration pneumonia. Treatment of more severe cases of dysphagia may require the expertise of a speech and language pathologist.

In the *stomach,* the swallowed food is chemically digested by virtue of hydrochloric acid (gastric acid) and pepsin enzyme secretion and is mechanically digested by the stomach's muscular churning action. The rate of gastric acid secretion decreases with age, while the incidence of **peptic ulcer** and **gastritis** (i.e., inflammation of the stomach lining) increases. The latter two phenomena may be due to an increased incidence of *Helicobacter pylori* bacterial infection in the elderly, drug ingestion (e.g., aspirin, caffeine, alcohol), or genetically programmed changes with age. Chronic bleeding from a peptic ulcer or gastritis can result in iron-deficiency anemia, while acute bleeding can place severe stress on the elderly individual's cardiovascular system. *Carcinoma* (or cancer) of the stomach is most common in the very old, and carries a poor prognosis for survival.

The initial section of the *small intestine,* called the *duodenum,* receives the partially digested food (or chyme) from the stomach and continues the process of digestion with the help of secretions from the liver and gallbladder (the bile) and from the pancreas (digestive enzymes and bicarbonate-rich fluid). As the chyme is further digested, nutrient molecules become small enough to be absorbed through the small intestinal wall, a process that occurs primarily in the more distal parts of the small intestine (the *jejunum* and *ileum*). Movement of the chyme through the small intestine by peristaltic contractions of the muscular wall is fairly slow to allow sufficient time for nutrient absorption. Aging has surprisingly little effect on the small intestine's digestive function and smooth muscle contractility. In addition, with the possible exceptions of calcium, vitamin D, and iron, most nutrients are absorbed efficiently in the small intestine in the healthy elderly. The decreased calcium and vitamin D absorption may contribute to the increased incidence of osteoporosis in the elderly.

The *liver* has several functions, some related to digestion and others not. It produces the bile that is stored below in the gallbladder until its release into the duodenum. Bile is required for the emulsification of fats in the chyme. Without bile, fats would pass through the digestive tract without being absorbed, a condition called *steatorrhea*. The storage of bile in the gall bladder can lead to its precipitation into solid stones, or *gallstones,* a phenomenon that is increasingly likely as we age. Gallstones, in turn, can get lodged in the ducts that normally convey the bile to the duodenum, resulting at times in obstructive jaundice, inflammation of the gallbladder (*cholecystitis*) or pancreas (*pancreatitis*), and steatorrhea (Fig. 3–16).

The liver also detoxifies many of the foreign and potentially damaging chemicals that enter, or are produced within, the body. Indeed, many of the medications given for disease and illness are broken down by the liver and are either released through the bile or into the bloodstream to be eliminated

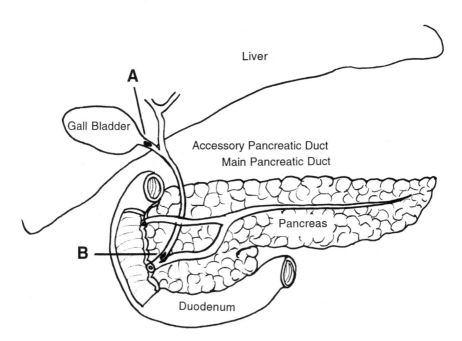

FIG. 3–16. Hepatobiliary tree with gallstone lodged in (*A*) the cystic duct and (*B*) the common bile duct.

by the kidneys into the urine. But with age, this detoxifying ability is diminished. This is particularly important to realize, because it means that many drugs given to the elderly remain in the body for longer periods of time. Thus, recommended dosages of many drugs for the elderly are smaller than they would be for younger individuals. Failure to consider this leads to the dangerous overdosing of medications for the elderly (see Chapter 6).

The remainder of the small intestinal contents (largely water and undigestible fiber) enters the *large intestine* (or *colon*), an area of the digestive tract that is heavily colonized by a normal flora of bacteria. The large intestine reabsorbs much of the remaining water and stores the feces until defecation. One common problem in the elderly is **diverticulosis,** which is the development of small sacs where the large intestinal lining has herniated through the muscular wall. These herniations usually result from the muscular spasms and increased intracolonic pressure associated with diets low in fiber. These pockets, or diverticuli, can become impacted with feces, resulting in ulceration and inflammation of the mucosal lining (*diverticulitis*). Also with age comes decreased motility of the smooth muscle in the large intestinal wall, prolonging the time that feces are stored in the colon and rectum. This, in turn, causes excessive water reabsorption and hardening of the feces, leading to *constipation* and, in extreme cases, intestinal obstruction. On the other end of the spectrum, the elderly may suffer from **fecal incontinence** (the inability to voluntarily control defecation), largely because of the weakening of the external anal sphincter muscle. This can be exacerbated when there is a simultaneous increase in intrarectal pressure caused by episodes of *diarrhea.*

The small and large intestine, like most other parts of the body, are vulnerable to the ravages of atherosclerosis. Blockage of the mesenteric arteries supplying the intestines can result in *ischemia* (reversible tissue damage due to oxygen depletion) and, ultimately, *infarction* (tissue death and breakdown). In the latter case, perforations can develop in the intestinal wall, allowing the bacteria-laden feces to spill out into the normally sterile peritoneal cavity, causing severe inflammation (*peritonitis*), a life-threatening condition. Finally, the large intestine is susceptible to cancer as well. In fact, in those people 70 and older, *colon cancer* is the second most common malignancy (behind lung cancer).[91]

GENITOURINARY SYSTEM

The paired *kidneys* serve two principal, somewhat overlapping, functions:

- Excretion of certain waste products from the body
- Maintenance of homeostasis (stability) in the fluid compartments of the body, such as the plasma and the interstitial fluid

The fact that these two fairly small organs (each weighing only 5 ounces) receive about 20 percent of the cardiac output illustrates their importance in carrying out these tasks. Failure to perform these functions can result in the build-up of nitrogenous waste products (e.g., urea) in the bloodstream and in the imbalanced levels of water, electrolytes, or acids in the body, any of which can in turn alter normal physiological processes. One would expect organs of such importance to have considerable functional reserve so that they could make the necessary compensations when damaged in any way. For the most part, this is true. Consider the *nephrons,* the microscopically sized functional units of the kidneys that filter the blood and then "choose" which substances of the filtered fluid to excrete and which substances to place back in the bloodstream. At age 25, there are approximately 1 million nephrons in each kidney. By age 85, 30 to 40 percent of them have been lost, yet an otherwise healthy 85-year old can still maintain homeostasis under normal circumstances.[78]

Nonetheless, because of the loss of nephrons and the less efficient functioning of those that remain, the kidneys of the elderly have a more difficult time responding to any added metabolic stressor on the body. Thus, as is true of the other organs we have discussed, older kidneys work well under normal conditions but have reduced tolerance for disease processes, whether originating from the kidneys themselves or from other organs. This is why, compared with younger individuals, the elderly more commonly suffer from *acute* and *chronic renal failure,* conditions in which toxic metabolites build up in the body because of the inability of the kidneys to remove them at a sufficient rate. It is also important for the health care provider to understand that the kidneys, like the liver, help eliminate drugs and their breakdown products from the body. The decreased functional reserve capacity that comes with age makes it more likely that the kidneys will not be able to efficiently excrete drugs. Thus, to prevent overdosing of medications, the elderly typically require smaller drug dosages than do younger individuals (see Chapter 6).

One of the major roles of the kidneys is to maintain water balance in the body. Indeed, the amount of water in fluid compartments such as the blood, interstitial fluid, and intracellular fluid is a major determinant of the concentrations of all the substances dissolved in those fluid compartments. Therefore, to maintain levels of sodium, potassium, calcium, and other vital components within the appropriate narrow concentration ranges, the kidneys must regulate the rate of water removal from the body. Severe dehydration (e.g., due to excessive sweating or inadequate fluid intake) might increase the concentration of dissolved substances in the body to dangerously high levels, if not for the ability of the kidneys to respond by producing smaller volumes of very highly concentrated urine, thus minimizing the amount of water lost. On the other hand, when someone is overhydrated, the kidneys respond by producing large volumes of very dilute urine. But this ability to regulate the concentration according to the body's needs diminishes with age. For this reason, the elderly are more likely to become dehydrated, especially when confusion, immobility, or fear of urinary incontinence (discussed later) prevents them from drinking adequate amounts of liquids. This dehydration may be exacerbated by the overdosing of diuretics, medications used for congestive heart failure and hypertension, whose effect is to increase urinary output.

Other age-related changes in the genitourinary system pertain to the structures required for urinary collection and removal—i.e. the *ureters, urinary bladder,* and *urethra* (Fig. 3–17). Normally, urine produced by the kidneys flows continuously through the ureters to be temporarily stored in the bladder. As the bladder fills with urine, its walls stretch out, initiating a reflexive contraction of the bladder wall. The expanding bladder compresses the

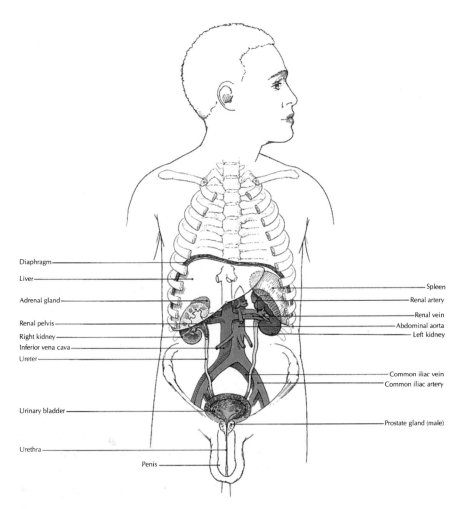

FIG. 3–17. The urinary system. (From Van Wynsberghe, D, et al: Human Anatomy and Physiology, ed 3. McGraw-Hill, New York, 1995, p 889, with permission.)

ureteral openings, preventing the reflux of urine in the bladder back into the ureters. In addition, the smooth muscle sphincter at the urethral opening (internal urethral sphincter) prevents urine in the bladder from entering the urethra. Nonetheless, as the fluid pressure in the bladder rises, the internal urethral sphincter opens up and urine enters the proximal urethra. However, a more distal, voluntary, skeletal muscle sphincter (the external urethral sphincter, located in the pelvic floor) must relax before urine can exit through the urethra. Thus, while the release of urine, called micturition, is made possible by an involuntary reflex, we nonetheless have voluntary control over it under normal conditions.

The loss of this voluntary control of micturition, called **urinary incontinence,** is a common problem in the elderly population. Indeed, 50 to 60 percent of those living in institutions suffer from this embarrassing and distressing condition.[92] Post-menopausal women are prone to this problem because lowered estrogen levels cause the skeletal muscles of the pelvic floor and the smooth muscle of the urethra to weaken. Women who have had multiple pregnancies are particularly susceptible and may involuntarily urinate whenever intraabdominal pressure rises, for example when coughing, sneezing, or laughing. This is called stress incontinence. In elderly men, urinary incontinence is often caused by an enlarged *prostate gland.* The prostate gland, which produces some components of the semen, is "wrapped around" the beginning of the urethra. It undergoes enlargement as one ages, which can partially or completely obstruct the urethra. This enlargement is either benign (**benign prostatic hypertrophy [BPH]**) or malignant (*prostate cancer*). In either case, the bladder must contract more forcefully to eliminate the urine. Over time, the bladder can become very distended (a condition called *urinary retention*) and its muscular wall can weaken, leading to a lack of coordination of micturition and, in turn, incontinence. Urinary retention, in turn, increases the chance of *urinary tract infection* and kidney damage (due to the build-up of fluid pressure). To avoid these complications, surgery is often performed to remove that part of the prostate gland blocking the urethra (a procedure called transurethral resection of the prostate, or TURP).

ENDOCRINE SYSTEM

Like the nervous system, the endocrine system is a principal regulatory system in the body. It helps control several aspects of our physiology, such as body temperature; basal metabolic rate; growth rate; carbohydrate, lipid, and protein metabolism; stress responses; and reproductive events. Clearly, dysfunction of this system could have widespread ramifications for one's health and well-being. Only a few of the many age-related changes to this system are highlighted here.

The endocrine system is a collection of glands that produce and secrete into the bloodstream chemical messengers called *hormones* that have physiological effects on various *target organs* throughout the body. The cells of target organs have protein *receptors* that specifically bind to the hormone in question. This binding initiates a cascade of metabolic events within the target cell that mediate the effects of the hormone.

While the endocrine glands are spread throughout the body, there is a hierarchical control of the release of most hormones, which begins in the central nervous system (CNS) (Fig. 3–18). Neural activity from higher centers in

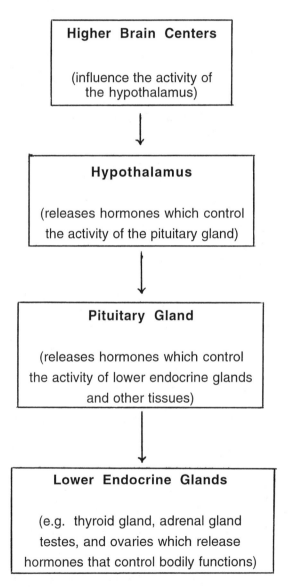

FIG. 3–18. The hierarchy of control over the endocrine system.

the CNS is relayed to the **hypothalamus,** a small but extremely important structure that, in turn, controls the activity of the **pituitary gland** by releasing hormones that stimulate or inhibit its hormonal production and release. The pituitary gland, under the influence from these higher control centers, releases a battery of tropic hormones that have selective stimulatory effects on glands such as the thyroid, adrenal, and gonadal glands (ovaries and testes). It should be emphasized, however, that even the structures at the top of this endocrine hierarchy are influenced by "lower" events. For example, the thyroid gland is stimulated to release thyroid hormone in response to the sequential release of thyrotropin-releasing hormone (TRH) from the hypothalamus and thyroid-stimulating hormone (TSH) from the pituitary gland. But as its level in the blood rises, thyroid hormone "turns off" further production of TRH and TSH in the higher centers in a negative feedback fashion—in effect, the endocrine system operates under a system of checks and balances, so that under normal conditions the appropriate levels of all hormones are maintained.

The *thyroid hormone* released from the *thyroid gland* has many physiological effects, such as regulation of tissue growth and development (particularly of the skeletal and nervous systems), stimulation of the basal metabolic rate (BMR) by promoting oxygen consumption and heat production in most tissues (i.e. a calorigenic effect), enhancement of the effects of the sympathetic nervous system (or fight-or-flight response), increased mental alertness, and possibly regulation of cholesterol metabolism. As one ages, the level of thyroid hormone secretion declines, but this is matched by a decrease in its rate of removal from the bloodstream, so that, overall, levels change very little over the years. Furthermore, aging per se does not appreciably affect the increased release of TRH, TSH, or thyroid hormone in times of greater need. However, several characteristics of the elderly, such as a reduced metabolic rate, suboptimal regulation of body temperature, decreased effectiveness of the fight-or-flight response, reduced mental alertness, and increased incidence of cholesterol-related atherosclerosis, are also symptoms of reduced thyroid activity (hypothyroidism). Thus, it is likely that the age-related changes in thyroid function result from inadequate responses of target cells to thyroid hormone, rather than from direct damage to the thyroid gland.

The paired *adrenal glands* consist of an outer layer called the adrenal cortex and an inner section called the adrenal medulla (which, from a functional standpoint, is more aptly considered part of the sympathetic nervous system, and thus is not discussed here). The *adrenal cortex* produces a number of corticosteroid hormones, such as cortisol, which helps the body adapt to stress; aldosterone, which helps the body conserve sodium and thus water; androgens, which have masculinizing effects; and estrogens, which have feminizing effects. The latter two hormones, whose levels decline with age, supplement the action of the testosterone and estrogen released from the testes and ovaries, respectively. The loss of estrogen production from post-menopausal ovaries appears to upset the androgen-estrogen balance in favor of the androgens produced in the adrenal gland. This might explain the mild masculinization of a woman's physique as she ages.

Aldosterone levels also fall as one ages, impairing an important component of blood pressure regulation. Normally, this hormone stimulates the reabsorption of sodium ions from the renal tubules back into the bloodstream, which osmotically draws water back in as well, thus increasing blood volume and therefore blood pressure when needed. While the aldosterone mechanism is just one of many ways to increase blood pressure, its loss may bring the body one step closer to disruption of homeostasis.

Cortisol is the quintessential "stress hormone," released into the bloodstream during prolonged periods of physical or psychological stress. It is a catabolic hormone whose function is to mobilize the body's energy reserves, increasing blood levels of glucose, fats, and amino acids during times of illness, physical injury, or emotional distress. In addition, baseline cortisol release (in conjunction with release of the hormone glucagon from the pancreas) in the absence of stress helps prevent blood glucose levels from falling dangerously low during sleep and in between meals.

As was true of thyroid hormone, cortisol levels remain normal well into old age because of a balance between the hormone's decreased production and its decreased excretion. In addition, stress-induced increases in cortisol release are not affected by aging. However, it appears to take the elderly longer to reestablish normal blood-cortisol levels following the stressful event, possibly as a result of a faulty negative feedback system in which the hypothalamus and pituitary gland fail to slow down the release of corticotropin-releasing hormone (CRH) and adrenocorticotropic hormone (ACTH), respectively, when cortisol levels are increased. The persistently elevated cortisol level may actually have a negative impact on the health of the elderly. Some of the well-documented effects of chronically high blood-cortisol levels include hyperglycemia (excessively high blood glucose level), hypertension (high blood pressure, due to the aldosterone-like effects of cortisol), and immunosuppression (increased susceptibility to infection and cancer). It is plausible then that elevated cortisol responses to stress might exacerbate concomitant diabetes mellitus, hypertension, and infectious disease in the elderly.

Unlike in the thyroid gland, adrenal cortex, and gonads, control of hormone release from the endocrine cells of the *pancreas* is not primarily controlled by the hypothalamus and pituitary gland. Instead, the two major hormones produced by the pancreas, *insulin* (which decreases the blood-glucose level) and *glucagon* (which increases the blood-glucose level), are released at various rates based primarily on blood glucose levels. Deficient insulin action causes **diabetes mellitus** (DM), a condition marked by hyperglycemia and long-term complications such as blindness (due to cataracts and retinal damage), renal failure, nerve damage, atherosclerosis, and gangrenous infection often necessitating amputation of all or part of the leg. Non-insulin-dependent diabetes mellitus (NIDDM) is a type of diabetes mellitus that increases in frequency with age and accounts for about 90 percent of all cases. It appears to be caused by deficient target organ responses to the effects of insulin—the level of insulin itself is actually normal or increased. Because it is so common in the elderly, affecting more than 15 percent of those aged 65 and older, non-insulin-dependent diabetes mellitus is of great interest to geriatric medicine.[93]

SUMMARY

It is clear that our health and well-being depend on the degree to which our organ systems can successfully work together to maintain homeostasis, or internal stability, in the body. Diminished function in one organ system is minimized by appropriate compensatory mechanisms in other systems. An elderly individual with emphysema, and therefore less efficient ventilation of the lungs, often has an elevated hematocrit (i.e., a greater proportion of RBCs in the blood) to maintain adequate oxygen delivery to the bloodstream and tissues. An individual with systemic hypertension will have enlargement of the muscle in the heart's left ventricle, generating a greater force of contraction to maintain adequate cardiac output in the face of the increased afterload. A person's excessive exposure to sunlight not only stimulates increased production of the protective melanin pigment in the skin but may also heighten immune surveillance for precancerous epidermal cells.

However, also apparent is the gradual impairment of these homeostatic mechanisms with age, most likely as a result of the linear decline that seems to characterize many physiological functions, such as cardiac output, forced vital capacity, the number of functioning nephrons, bone mass, and epidermal melanocyte density. What is gradually lost with age is the functional reserve capacity of our organ systems. A physiological disturbance that is easily correctable at age 30 may cause significant illness at age 60 or death at age 90. Perhaps it should not be surprising that coinciding with the linear decline in physiological functioning is a logarithmic increase in mortality.[4] It is as though our bodies function well during the younger years despite the accumulation of environmental and genetic insults. However, at some stage in life, we reach a "critical mass" of impairment, a point beyond which our homeostatic correction mechanisms are no longer able to keep pace. When this point is reached, the likelihood of illness, disease, and death rises exponentially.

Nevertheless, we may take comfort in the fact that much of the illness and suffering that comes with old age can be delayed or at least modified by taking care of ourselves. And it must be remembered that the hallmarks of preventive medicine, such as eating right, exercising, and avoiding cigarettes, are most effective when initiated early in life. While there may be wisdom in the adage, "live for the day," it is equally wise, from a health perspective, to "live for tomorrow."

REVIEW QUESTIONS

Multiple Choice/Matching:

1. Which of the following statements is correct?
   A. Improvements in sanitation have helped to increase the maximum life span potential of U.S. citizens over the past 100 years.
   B. Most of the increase in average life expectancy over the past 100 years can be attributed to advances in medical technology.
   C. The percentage of U.S. citizens nearing the maximum life span potential is higher today than it was 100 years ago.
   D. In the effort to increase the average life expectancy, curative medicine is more cost-effective than preventive medicine.
   E. Dietary practices such as vitamin intake and caloric restriction can prevent aging.

2. Match the following theories of aging with their most appropriate descriptions:
   _____ Rate of living theory
   _____ Free-radical theory
   _____ Error catastrophe theory
   _____ Disposable soma theory
   _____ Gene regulation theory
   _____ Somatic mutation theory
   _____ Evolutionary theory
   _____ Glycosylation theory
   A. Aging results from the compromise that a species reaches between devoting all of its energy to reproduction and devoting all of its energy to body maintenance and repair.
   B. Aging results from accumulating damage to cells caused by molecules that have unpaired electrons in their outermost valence shells.
   C. Certain species live longer because they have lower metabolic rates.
   D. Aging is an inevitable result in a species that faces the possibility of accidental death (e.g. due to predation).
   E. The random accumulation of DNA mutations and subsequent errors in protein production cause aging.
   F. Aging results from a gradual decline in the precision of DNA transcription and RNA translation.
   G. The aging process begins with the attachment of glucose to important molecules such as proteins and DNA.
   H. Aging occurs along an intentional timeline dictated by the sequential expression of particular genes in cells.

3. The skin gradually loses its brown tone with age as a result of a decrease in the number of _____ in the skin.

   A. Melanocytes
   B. Keratinocytes
   C. Fibroblasts
   D. Mast cells
   E. Langerhans cells

4. Which of the following is *not* a characteristic change in the nervous system as one ages?

   A. A decrease in the nerve conduction velocity
   B. A loss of moderate amounts of myelin around some axons
   C. A generalized and substantial decrease in the number of neurons
   D. A decrease in the number of dendrites
   E. An increase in the size of fatty plaques in the cerebral arteries

5. Which of the following is not a risk factor for osteoporosis?

   A. cigarette smoking
   B. sedentary lifestyle
   C. depletion of estrogen levels following menopause
   D. high blood pressure
   E. calcium deficiency

6. Which of the following statements regarding the cardiovascular system is false?

   A. With aging comes a gradual decline in the maximal heart rate during exercise.
   B. Insufficient activity of the sympathetic nervous system can cause postural hypotension in the elderly.
   C. The cardiac output is obtained by multiplying the heart rate by the stroke volume.
   D. The walls of arteries become more rigid with age, increasing the likelihood that an older individual will develop hypertension.
   E. The first changes of atherosclerosis are not detectable in arteries until middle age.

7. Occasionally a blood clot can dislodge from its area of formation and travel farther down the bloodstream to block a more distal artery. This is called a(n):

   A. Thrombus
   B. Embolism
   C. Aneurysm
   D. Infarction
   E. Atheroma

8. Which of the following statements about chronic bronchitis is false?

   A. It is marked by excessive production of mucus in the bronchi.
   B. It is a condition that typically lasts only a week to 10 days.
   C. Cigarette smoke can play a key role in its development by irritating the respiratory lining.

D. It is more likely to cause pneumonia in the very old because of the diminished effectiveness of their immune system.

    E. It can lead to blockage of the bronchi.

9. An elderly woman complains of bruising and bleeding easily. A deficiency of which of the following types of cells might cause these symptoms?

    A. Erythrocytes

    B. Thrombocytes

    C. Macrophages

    D. Fibroblasts

    E. Leukocytes

10. A decline in the functioning of the immune system in the elderly population may help directly explain the increased prevalence of all of the following categories of illness except:

    A. Cancer

    B. Renal failure

    C. Viral infection

    D. Autoimmune disease

    E. Bacterial infection

11. The elderly are at increased risk of developing small, sac-like herniations through the wall of the large intestine. This condition is called:

    A. Cholecystitis

    B. Peritonitis

    C. Fecal incontinence

    D. Steatorrhea

    E. Diverticulosis

12. Which of the following statements about non-insulin-dependent diabetes mellitus (NIDDM) is false?

    A. Poorly treated NIDDM results in elevated blood-glucose levels.

    B. Individuals with NIDDM are at increased risk for cataracts.

    C. One's risk of developing NIDDM increases with age.

    D. NIDDM is caused by the inability of the pancreas to secrete insulin.

    E. Sufferers of NIDDM are more likely to develop hypertension than are healthy individuals.

13. The clouding of the lens of the eye is called:

    A. Presbyopia

    B. Cataract

    C. Dyspnea

    D. Presbycusis

    E. Hyposmia

14. Elderly individuals commonly experience an inability to focus on near objects due to the inelasticity of the lens of the eye. This is called:

    A. Presbyopia

    B. Cataract

    C. Dyspnea
    D. Presbycusis
    E. Hyposmia

15. Older individuals who have lost the coordination of their tongue, palatal, and pharyngeal muscles find it difficult to swallow food. This phenomenon is called:
    A. Dyspnea
    B. Dysphagia
    C. Xerostomia
    D. Emphysema
    E. Dementia

Short Answer Essay Questions:

1. Distinguish between preventive and curative medicine, and describe five things a young adult can do to help stay healthy into old age.

2. How might aging be a by-product of evolution?

3. For a drug or other medical intervention to truly slow down aging, what must it be shown to do?

4. List five changes that occur in the skin as one ages. Describe a clinical consequence of each change you listed.

5. Define the term *presbyopia* and describe its effect on an individual.

6. Why might hyposmia, the impairment of one's ability to smell, be a life-threatening condition?

7. Why does the successful treatment of hypertension (high blood pressure) reduce the workload placed on the heart?

8. List seven risk factors for the development of atherosclerosis.

9. What is emphysema, and how does cigarette smoking increase one's risk of developing it?

10. List three causes of anemia that fall under the category of ineffective erythropoiesis.

11. Explain why the elderly are at increased risk of overdosing their medications.

12. List seven reasons why elderly individuals are more prone to becoming dehydrated than are younger individuals.

LEARNING ACTIVITIES

1. Compare and contrast aging and disease. How do the effects of cigarette smoking on the body illustrate the difficulty of distinguishing aging from disease?

2. A 76-year-old man with a long history of peptic ulcer disease has become increasingly fatigued and short of breath over the past 3 weeks. He complains of a dull pain below his sternum that is worse following meals. On physical examination, he looks pale and has a slightly elevated heart rate.
   A. What might be this man's diagnosis?
   B. Suggest some possible explanations for his:
      i. shortness of breath
      ii. elevated heart rate
   C. From a physiological standpoint, why might it be more difficult for this man to compensate for his current problem than it would be for a 30-year old man? In your answer, explore possibilities from at least three different organ systems.

REFERENCES

1. Timiras, PS: Introduction: Aging as a stage in the life cycle. In Timiras, PS (ed): Physiological Basis of Aging and Geriatrics, ed 2. CRC Press, Boca Raton, FL, 1994, p 1.

2. Hayflick, L: Myths of aging. Sci Am 276:110, 1997.

3. Schneider, EL: Aging research: Challenge of the twenty-first century. In Woodhead, AD, et al (eds): Molecular Biology of Aging. Plenum Press, New York, 1985, p 1.

4. Timiras, PS: Aging and disease. In Timiras, PS (ed): Physiological Basis of Aging and Geriatrics, ed 2. CRC Press, Boca Raton, FL, 1994, p 23.

5. National Center for Health Statistics: Vital Statistics of the United States 1985. PHS Publ No 88–1104, Life Tables, Vol 2, Sect 6. US Department of Health and Human Services, Hyattsville, MD, 1988, p 9.

6. Comfort, A: The Biology of Senescence, ed 3. Elsevier, New York, 1979, p 81.

7. Finch, CE: Longevity, Senescence, and the Genome. University of Chicago Press, Chicago, 1990.

8. Bierman, EL, and Hazzard, WR: Preventive gerontology: Strategies for attenuation of the chronic diseases of aging. In Hazzard, WR, et al (eds): Principles of Geriatric Medicine and Gerontology, ed 3. McGraw-Hill, New York, 1994, p 187.

9. Committee on Diet and Health, Food, and Nutrition Board, Commission on Life Sciences, National Research Council: Diet and Health. National Academy Press, Washington, DC, 1989.

10. Evans, W, and Rosenberg, I: Biomarkers. Simon & Schuster, New York, 1991.

11. Ruuskanen, JM, and Ruoppila, I: Physical activity and psychological well-being among people aged 65 to 84 years. Age and Ageing 24:292–296, 1995.

12. Wynder, EL: Etiology of lung cancer: Reflections on two decades of research. Cancer 30:1332, 1972.

13. Timiras, PS: Demographic, comparative, and differential aging. In Timiras, PS (ed): Physiological Basis of Aging and Geriatrics, ed 2. CRC Press, Boca Raton, FL, 1994, p 7.

14. Martin, GM: Interactions of aging and environmental agents: The gerontological perspec-

tive. In Baker, SR, and Rogul, M (eds): Environmental Toxicity and the Aging Process. Alan R Liss, New York, 1987, p 25.

15. Szilard, L: On the nature of the aging process. Proc Natl Acad Sci USA 45:30, 1959.

16. Martin, GM, et al: Increased chromosomal aberrations in first metaphases of cells isolated from the kidneys of aged mice. Israel Journal of Medical Sciences 21:296, 1985.

17. Curtis, HJ: Cellular processes involved in aging. Fed Proc 23:662, 1964.

18. Orgel, LE: The maintenance of the accuracy of protein synthesis and its relevance to aging. Proc Natl Acad Sci USA 49:517, 1963.

19. Medvedev, ZA: The nucleic acids in development and aging. In Strehler, BL (ed): Advances in Gerontological Research, Vol 1. Academic Press, New York, 1964.

20. Holliday, R and Tarrant, GM: Altered enzymes in aging human fibroblasts. Nature 238:26, 1972.

21. Lamb, MJ: Biology of Aging. John Wiley & Sons, New York, 1977.

22. Reiss, V, and Gershon, D: Comparison of cytoplasmic superoxide dismutase in liver, heart, and brain of aging rats and mice. Biochem Biophys Res Commun 73:255, 1976.

23. Kanungo, MS, and Gandhi, BS: Induction of malate dehydrogensae isoenzymes in livers of young and old rats. Proc Natl Acad Sci USA 69:2035, 1972.

24. Kanungo, MS: A model for ageing. J Theor Biol 53:253, 1975.

25. Sierra, F, et al: T-kininogen gene expression is induced during aging. Mol Cell Biol 9:5610, 1989.

26. Friedman, V, et al: Isolation and identification of aging-related cDNAs in the mouse. Mech Ageing Dev 52:27, 1990.

27. Medawar, PB: An Unsolved Problem in Biology. HK Lewis, London, 1952.

28. Williams, GC: Pleiotropy, natural selection and the evolution of senescence. Evolution 11:398, 1957.

29. Miller, RA: The biology of aging and longevity. In Hazzard, WR, et al (eds): Principles of Geriatric Medicine and Gerontology, ed 3. McGraw-Hill, New York, 1994, p 3.

30. Kirkwood, TBL: Evolution of ageing. Nature 270:301, 1977.

31. Pearl, R: The Rate of Living. University of London Press, London, 1928.

32. McCay, CM, and Crowell, MF: Prolonging the life span. The Scientific Monthly 39:405, 1934.

33. Barrows, CH, and Kokkonen, GC: Relationship between nutrition and aging. Adv Nutr Res 1:253, 1977.

34. Masoro, EJ, et al: Temporal and compositional dietary restrictions modulate age-related changes in serum lipids. J Nutr 113:880, 1983.

35. Kalu, DN, et al: Life-long food restriction prevents senile osteopenia and hyperparathyroidism in F344 rats. Mech Ageing Dev 26:103, 1984.

36. Weindruch, R, et al: Influence of controlled dietary restriction on immunologic function. Fed Proc 38:2007, 1979.

37. Masoro, EJ, et al: Action of food restriction in delaying the aging process. Proc Natl Acad Sci USA 79:4239, 1982.

38. McCarter R, et al: Does food restriction retard aging by reducing the metabolic rate? Am J Physiol 248:E488, 1985.

39. Austad, SN, and Fischer, KE: Mammalian aging, metabolism, and ecology: Evidence from the bats and marsupials. J Gerontol 46:B47, 1991.

40. Harman, D: The aging process: Major risk factor for disease and death. Proc Natl Acad Sci USA 88:5360, 1991.

41. Harman D: Aging: A theory based on free radical and radiation chemistry. J Gerontol 11:298, 1956.

42. Chance, B, et al: Hydrogen peroxide metabolism in mammalian organs. Physiol Rev 59:527, 1979.

43. Nohl, H, and Hegner, D: Do mitochondria produce oxygen radicals in vivo? Eur J Biochem 82:563, 1978.

44. Lippman, RD: The prolongation of life: A comparison of antioxidants and geroprotectors versus superoxide in human mitochondria. J Gerontol 36:550, 1981.

45. Leibovitz, BE, and Siegel, BV: Aspects of free radical reactions in biological systems: Aging. J Gerontol 35:45, 1980.

46. Pryor, WA: The formation of free radicals and the consequences of their reactions in vivo. Photochem Photobiol 28:787, 1978.

47. Sohal, RS (ed): Age Pigments. Elsevier/North-Holland, Amsterdam, 1981.

48. Timiras, PS: Degenerative changes in cells and cell death. In Timiras, PS (ed): Physiological Basis of Aging and Geriatrics, ed 2. CRC Press, Boca Raton, FL, 1994, p 47.

49. Berg, BN: Study of vitamin E supplements in relation to muscular dystrophy and other diseases in aging rats. J Gerontol 14:174, 1959.

50. Porta, EA, et al: Effects of the type of dietary fat at two levels of vitamin E in Wistar male rats during development and aging. I. Life span, serum biochemical parameters and pathological changes. Mech Ageing Dev 13:1, 1980.

51. Blackett, AD, and Hall, DA: Vitamin E: Its significance in mouse ageing. Age Ageing 10:191, 1981.

52. Ledvina, M, and Hodanova, M: The effect of simultaneous administration of tocopherol and sunflower oil on the life-span of female mice. Exp Gerontol 15:67, 1980.

53. Tappel, AL: Lipid peroxidation damage to cell components. Fed Proc 32:1870, 1973.

54. Packer, L, and Smith JR: Extension of the lifespan of cultured normal human diploid cells by vitamin E: A reevaluation. Proc Natl Acad Sci USA 74:1640, 1977.

55. Nakayama, T, et al: Generation of hydrogen peroxide and superoxide anion radical from cigarette smoke. Gann 75:95, 1984.

56. Church, DF, and Pryor, WA: Free radical chemistry of cigarette smoke and its toxicological implications. Environ Health Perspect 64:111, 1985.

57. Nagy, I: Memorial lecture: Verzar's ideas on the age-dependent protein cross-linking in the light of the present knowledge. Arch Gerontol Geriatr 5:267, 1986.

58. Bjorksten, J: The crosslinkage theory of aging. J Am Geriatr Soc 16:408, 1968.

59. Kohn, RR: Principles of Mammalian Aging, ed 2. Prentice Hall, Englewood Cliffs, NJ, 1978.

60. Monnier, VM: Nonenzymatic glycosylation, the Maillard reaction and the aging process. J Gerontol 45:B105, 1990.

61. Cerami, A: Hypothesis: Glucose as a mediator of aging. J Am Geriatr Soc 33:626, 1985.

62. Masoro, EJ, et al: Evidence for the glycation hypothesis of aging from the food-restricted rodent model. J Gerontol Biol Sci 44:B20, 1989.

63. Cerami, A, et al: Role of nonenzymatic glycosylation in the development of the sequelae of diabetes. Metabolism 28:431, 1979.

64. Kohn, RR, and Schneider, SL: Glycosylation of human collagen. Diabetes (suppl)31:47, 1981.

65. Araki, N, et al: Immunochemical evidence for the presence of advanced glycation end products in human lens proteins and its positive correlation with aging. J Biol Chem 267:10211, 1992.

66. Monnier, VM, and Cerami, A: Nonenzymatic browning in vivo: Possible process for aging of long-lived proteins. Science 211:491, 1981.

67. Montagna, W, and Carlisle K: Structural changes in aging human skin. J Invest Dermatol 73:47, 1979.

68. Grove, GL, and Kligman, AM: Age-associated changes in human epidermal cell renewal. J Gerontol 38:137, 1983.

69. Leyden, JJ, et al: Age-related differences in the rate of desquamation of skin surface cells. In Adelman, RD, et al (eds): Pharmacological Intervention of the Aging Process. Plenum Press, New York, p 297.

70. Kaminer, MS, and Gilchrest, BA: Aging of the skin. In Hazzard, WR, et al. (eds): Principles of Geriatric Medicine and Gerontology, ed 3. McGraw-Hill, New York, 1994, p 414.

71. Timiras, PS: Aging of the nervous system: Functional changes. In Timiras, PS (ed): Physiological Basis of Aging and Geriatrics, ed 2. CRC Press, Boca Raton, FL, 1994, p 103.

72. Shock, NW: The physiology of aging. Sci Am 206:100, 1962.

73. Jarvik, LF, et al: Dementia and delirium in old age. In Brocklehurst, JC, et al (eds): Textbook of Geriatric Medicine and Gerontology, ed 4. London, Churchill Livingstone, 1992, pp 332, 338.

74. Morgan, K: Sleep in normal and pathological aging. In Brocklehurst, JC, et al (eds): Textbook of Geriatric Medicine and Gerontology, ed 4. London, Churchill Livingstone, 1992, p 122.

75. Gates, GA, et al: Hearing in the elderly: The Framingham cohort, 1983–1985. Ear Hear 11:247, 1990.

76. Stevens, JC, et al: Aging impairs the ability to detect gas odor. Fire Technology 23:198, 1987.

77. Berg, RL, and Cassells, JS: The Second Fifty Years: Promoting Health and Preventing Disability. National Academy Press, Washington, DC, 1990, p 76.

78. Kallenberg, GA, and Beck, JC: Care of the geriatric patient. In Rakel, RE (ed): Textbook of Family Practice, ed 3. W. B. Saunders, Philadelphia, 1984, p 249.

79. Mazess, RB: On aging bone loss. Clin Orthop 165:239–252, 1982.

80. Sorensen, LB: Rheumatology. In Cassel, CK, et al (eds): Geriatric Medicine, ed 2. Springer-Verlag, New York, 1990, p 185.

81. Timiras, PS: Aging of the skeleton, joints, and muscles. In Timiras, PS (ed): Physiological Basis of Aging and Geriatrics, ed 2. CRC Press, Boca Raton, FL, 1994, p 259.

82. Kohrt, WM, et al: Effects of gender, age, and fitness level on response of VO_2 max to training in 60–71-year-olds. J Appl Physiol 71:2004, 1991.

83. Crapo, RO, et al: Reference spirometric values using techniques and equipment that meet ATS recommendations. Am Rev Respir Dis 123:659, 1981.

84. Timiras, PS: Aging of respiration: Erythrocytes, and the hematopoietic system. In Timiras, PS (ed): Physiological Basis of Aging and Geriatrics, ed 2. CRC Press, Boca Raton, FL, 1994, p 226.

85. Pryor, WA, et al: The inactivation of alpha-1-proteinase inhibitor by gas-phase cigarette smoke: Protection by antioxidants and reducing species. Chem Biol Interact 57:271, 1986.

86. Weiss, SJ: Tissue destruction by neutrophils. N Engl J Med 320:365, 1989.

87. Travis, J, and Salvesen, JS: Human plasma protease inhibitors. Annu Rev Biochem 52:655, 1983.

88. Janoff, A: Elastase in tissue injury. Annu Rev Med 36:207, 1985.

89. Boross, M, et al: Effect of smoking on different biological parameters in aging mice. Z Gerontol 24:76, 1991.

90. Timiras, PS: Aging of the gastrointestinal tract and liver. In Timiras, PS (ed): Physiological Basis of Aging and Geriatrics, ed 2. CRC Press, Boca Raton, FL 1994, p 248.

91. Nelson, JB, and Castell, DO: Gastroenterology. In Cassel, CK, et al (eds): Geriatric Medicine, ed 2. Springer-Verlag, New York, 1990, p 356.

92. Herzog, AR, and Fultz, NH: Prevalence and incidence of urinary incontinence in community dwelling populations. J Am Geriatr Soc 38:273, 1990.

93. Goldberg, AP, and Coon, PJ: Diabetes mellitus and glucose metabolism in the elderly. In Hazzard, WR, et al (eds): Principles of Geriatric Medicine and Gerontology, ed 3. McGraw-Hill, Inc, New York, 1994, p 826.

So we always keep the same hearts,
though the outer framework fails and
shows the touch of time.
Sarah Orne Jewett
(The Country of the Pointed Firs)

The Psychological, Behavioral, and Cognitive Aspects of Aging

Regula H. Robnett

CHAPTER OUTLINE

BEHAVIORAL OBJECTIVES

Upon completion of this chapter, the reader will be able to:

1. Differentiate aspects of personality that may tend to change over time from those that may not, based on current research.
2. Describe the five-factor (trait theory) model of personality.
3. List the three basic factors that cause cognitive impairments in the elderly.
4. Define and provide examples of sustained attention, divided attention, alternating attention, and selective attention, and relate how these may change with the aging process.
5. Define orientation and give examples of A&O×1, A&O×2, and A&O×3.
6. Define four different types of memory and explain how these may change over time.
7. List six recommendations to stimulate remembering that may be used by elderly people to compensate for decreased memory skills.
8. Define the seven types of intelligences described by Gardner and describe how each of these may change with the aging process, according to current research findings.
9. Compare and contrast fluid and crystallized intelligence.
10. Describe how vision may change with age, and list compensatory measures for the primary impairments.
11. Define perception and describe how perceptual skills may change as one ages.
12. Describe how hearing changes with age, and list four recommendations for health care professionals who work with people who are hard of hearing.
13. Define hyposmia and describe the impact of this impairment.
14. Define praxis and describe the features of praxis that are likely to change with the aging process.
15. Describe the core principles of quality of life, and relate the five factors believed to contribute to increased quality of life in elderly people.
16. List the symptoms of clinical depression and potential suicide, and know when to refer a client for additional help in these areas.
17. Describe the bereavement process, and state recommendations for health care professionals who are working with bereaved individuals.
18. Define dementia (including Alzheimer's disease), and list the signs and symptoms associated with it.
19. List the general rules for working with people who have dementia.
20. List the disorders that can be confused with the onset of dementia or clinical depression.

KEY TERMS

Age-associated memory impairment (AAMI)

Aging-associated cognitive decline (AACD)

Alternating attention

Alzheimer's disease (AD)

Attention

Bereavement

Bodily-kinesthetic intelligence

Cerebrovascular accident (CVA)

Cognition

Crystallized intelligence

Dementia

Depression

Divided attention

Endurance

Executive functioning

Failure to thrive (FTT)

Fluid intelligence

Hypothyroidism

Integrity versus despair

Intelligence

Interpersonal intelligence

Intrapersonal intelligence

Learned helplessness

Linguistic intelligence

Logical-mathematical intelligence

Long-term memory

Malnutrition

Memory

Musical intelligence

Orientation

Perception

Personality development

Physical performance

Praxis

Primary memory

Quality of life (QOL)

Reaction time

Remote memory

Secondary memory

Selective attention

Self-efficacy

Senescence

Sensation

Short-term memory

Spatial intelligence

Sustained attention

Tertiary memory

Trait theory

Working memory

 INTRODUCTION

Change is a constant in our lives. Our bodies undergo change second by second, cells constantly being renewed or sloughed off. Intangibly, thoughts and opinions evolve and can as easily dissolve. Most of the time these changes escape our conscious attention unless they are brought on by sudden or dramatic physical, psychological, or cognitive events. For example, falling in love, the onset of pain or illness, accidents, and the mastering of a new skill all can significantly affect our emotional or physical state. While the living, and thus aging, process inevitably entails change, not all changes are negative, and not every aspect of our humanness experiences change.

In the previous chapter, focus was on many of the physical changes that take place within the aging body. **Senescence,** or the process of physical decline, does occur, but perhaps at a slower or more variable rate than originally believed. This chapter discusses the concurrent psychological, behavioral, and cognitive changes that are associated with the structural changes previously described. The reader will discover that not all behaviors undergo transformation from middle age into old age. This chapter also explores those aspects of cognition and psychological makeup that remain more consistent.

▦ PERSONALITY DEVELOPMENT

Personality is what makes a person a unique individual. Each one of us has a set of character traits, attitudes, habits, and emotional tendencies that distinguish us from everyone else. These dispositions can be intimated by our appearance (e.g., blue spiked hair or conservative clothing) but are essentially inner characteristics that cause us to behave as we do. Many studies have looked at the development of personality in youth and into young adulthood, while fewer studies have concentrated on personality evolvement during older adulthood. The question is whether or not significant personality change takes place during old age (in both healthy adults and those afflicted with disease).

There are many theories on personality. One that may already be familiar to many readers is the eight stages of psychosocial development described by Erik Erikson.[1] He and his colleagues present a view on the changing personality of elders to include the final era of life: **integrity versus despair.** Erikson contends that during old age, those who successfully transcend this stage are able to develop a sense of pride in their past accomplishments and present lives. They judge their own lives as being worthwhile. Others, who do not successfully complete this stage, experience instead a feeling of despair, not only about the course of their lives thus far but also because they do not believe that they have enough time left to improve their sense of life satisfaction. Overall, Erikson views this last stage of life as a time that can be positive and integrating for the well elderly.[2]

While several well-known theorists (Maslow, Piaget, Freud) devote little attention to the personality of elders per se, many social scientists are completing contemporary research in this field. One project of particular interest is the **trait theory** espoused by McCrae and Costa.[3] Their five-factor model includes the following:

1. Neuroticism
2. Extraversion
3. Openness to experience
4. Agreeableness
5. Conscientiousness

They found that these traits have the greatest instability between the ages of 17 and 35 and then tend to become more fixed. When these traits were studied in elderly people over 3- and 6-year intervals, they found strong stability of all five traits using both self and spousal reports. Even when the intervals between testing increased to as much as 50 years, stability coefficients still remained statistically significant, with the strongest stability measures in the traits of neuroticism and extraversion.

Other evidence in support of the permanence of personality traits in healthy, older adults is presented by Mitchell and Helson[4] and others. They have found that people who are optimistic and managed their lives well at one stage of life tend to feel more positive about their lives at other times as well. Hayflick,[5] in citing the results of the Baltimore Longitudinal Study of Aging (BLSA), maintains that when elders are well, personality traits remain essentially the same throughout the life span, although he states that most people older than 50 do begin to prefer slower-paced activities. This is a valuable piece of information for health care professionals who work with the elderly. Pacing health care intervention for the convenience of the client, rather than the provider, is essential for good care.

The evidence for personality change is also abundant. Research shows that men, as they age, often become more nurturing and open about their feelings, while women become more assertive, confident, and comfortable with themselves. Social scientists believe these changes could be influenced by hormonal fluctuations that may cause a diminution of the character distinctions between the genders.[4]

Representations of the self such as goals, values, coping styles, and control beliefs are likely to change over the course of a lifetime. The elders in a study done by Erikson and colleagues[1] described themselves as more tolerant, patient, open-minded, understanding, compassionate, and less critical than when they were younger. However, many participants viewed both themselves and other elders as more set in their ways. Erikson discusses this seeming contradiction by explaining that because people are increasingly integrating their own style as they age, they perhaps can also gain a new understanding and tolerance of others' personal styles of behavior.

Labouvie-Vief and colleagues[6] make a further assertion that the thinking patterns of mature adults differ from those of youth. While young adults and adolescents tend to think of themselves (and others) in static contrasts (black/white, self/other, right/wrong), mature adults are better able to envision dynamic possibilities and have an increased tolerance for ambiguity. While these researchers found evidence to indicate that this type of self-representation peaks in middle age, other researchers have found elders to be more tolerant, patient, and open-minded.[1]

Self-efficacy is a construct that was introduced by Bandura[7] in the 1970s. It relates to the beliefs that each of us hold about the level of control we have over our future. Those who have strong self-efficacy, or internal locus of control, feel empowered to shape the future for themselves. On the other hand, those with low self-efficacy or related external locus of control, believe that the course of their lives is determined by the whims of the world and that they, personally, can have little influence over their own future.

The tendency has been to attribute to the elderly a more external locus of control, perhaps because of the various situations, such as medical emergencies and living on fixed incomes, that occur more frequently as one grows older. Older people may have fewer choices about their personal living arrangements as well. However, Rhee and Gatz[8] drew a different conclusion. Older adults in their study showed a higher level of self-perceived internal control as compared with college students. Additionally, the college students actually had lower self-perceived locus of control than attributed to them by the elders.

The strength of one's sense of self-efficacy may be variable across time and across different domains of life and may be a factor in the initiation of behaviors in these realms.[9] For example, people may feel empowered about financial matters yet feel that their health is beyond their personal control. Other domains besides health and finances include productivity, transportation, family, friends, safety, and living arrangements. McAvay and her colleagues[9] were interested in the perception that elderly people (age 62 and older) had of their own self-efficacy in the different domains mentioned and the factors that could influence these perceptions over time. They found that the trait of self-efficacy in any domain was quite stable over the course of 2 months. For each domain listed, a majority of respondents (65% to 95%) reported a high degree of self-efficacy, indicating that at least these older people believed that they have a high level of control over many aspects of their lives. The only domain in which less than half of the respondents reported a high level of self-efficacy was finances. This finding is logical; many elderly people may feel a lack of control over finances because they are on fixed incomes and no longer a part of the paid work force.

A decline in health (as evidenced by an increase in number of medical conditions) was significantly correlated to decreased self-efficacy in the domains of productivity, family, friends, and living arrangements. Perhaps not surprisingly, prior depression was the one factor that corresponded most closely with the decline in self-efficacy across all domains. Elderly people who feel depressed have a tendency to feel powerless about the course of their lives, which subsequently leads to even further social withdrawal. The downward spiral of depressed mood and withdrawal emphasizes the need for medical intervention. Depression in the elderly is not likely to simply go away unaddressed. McAvay and her colleagues[9] also pointed out the importance of developing and maintaining social support systems and learning coping strategies to effectively deal with daily problems.

A significant correlation has been found between a high level of self-perceived self-efficacy and positive health behaviors such as healthy diet, exercise, and non-smoking. On the other hand, chronic illnesses may lower the level of perceived control,[10] and this in turn may decrease one's motivation to maintain a healthy lifestyle.

Overall, in the realm of personality, we can see that there are no definitive answers in regard to aging. People adhere to their personhood throughout life: they remain unique individuals with distinct features. Extreme diversity is found even within a set population. While we can use stereotypes to explain and explore the personality of the aging individual, these theories will never adequately illuminate any one person.

🔀 COGNITION

Cognition is a multifaceted construct. Our brains control everything we do intentionally. It is a well-known assertion that cognition declines with advancing age. However, this premise is only partially true. Several aspects of cognition, and how the aging process differentially affects these, are explored in this chapter (Table 4–1).

Zec[11] asserts that cognitive impairments in the elderly are primarily caused by three factors:

1. Disease
2. Aging
3. Disuse

It is beyond the scope of this text to examine the effects of disease processes beyond an introduction to the effects of Alzheimer's disease, which is the most common disabling condition of aging. The most significant focus is on the cognitive correlates of normal aging, but there is also discussion of disuse, since this is a truly preventable aspect of intellectual decline and one that can be positively influenced by front-line health care professionals. To simplify the presentation, cognition is divided into several domains. However, it is important to keep in mind that these domains often do not have distinct boundaries and that they have an impact on one another regularly throughout performance of our daily tasks.

ATTENTION

Attention can be defined as being tuned in to the task which is being completed over a set period of time. This is the simplest kind of attention—**sustained attention** or vigilance. More complex kinds of attention include

- **Divided attention**—Paying attention to two or more tasks simultaneously. An example of divided attention would be driving a car and listening to an audiotape (perhaps a foreign language tape that requires concentration as well). It is easiest to sustain divided attention on tasks that are routine or overlearned.

TABLE 4–1. *Effects of Aging on Components of Cognition*

Cognitive Function	Significant Aging Effects	Mild or Insignificant Effects of Aging
Attention	−Complex attention tasks −Auditory alternating attention tasks	+Sustained attention to task +Visual alternating attention tasks
Orientation	−Possibly orientation to time due to lifestyle changes	+Most aspects of orientation (self, situation, location)
Memory	−Short-term and working memory −Newly learned information	+Long-term or remote memory +Procedural memory +Overlearned information
Intelligence	−Fluid intelligence −Mechanics of intelligence	+Crystallized intelligence +Pragmatics of intelligence
Learning	−Timed learning tasks −Nonverbal, novel situations −Understanding new concepts/methods/situations	+Intellectual attainments +Verbal tasks +Recalling acquired information, past experience
Problem Solving	−Immediate problem solving ability −Ability to solve novel problems −Flexibility in problem solving −Abstract reasoning	+Previously accumulated experience +Drawing on acquired knowledge/wisdom +Routine problem solving +Overlearned, well-practiced abilities
Performance	−Psychomotor skills −Speed of performance −Unfamiliar and difficult tasks −Spatial abilities	+Verbal abilities and performance +Familiar and/or easy tasks +Routine habits

This table is based on information referenced in text and adapted from table in Salthouse, TA: Theoretical Perspectives on Cognitive Aging. Lawrence Erlbaum Associates, Hillsdale, NJ, 1991, pp 11–13.

- **Alternating attention**—Quickly alternating concentration between two or more tasks. An example could be alternating attention between cooking dinner and a craft project.
- **Selective attention**—Paying attention to relevant stimuli while filtering out the noise or unimportant data. An example of this becomes evident in city driving tasks, which demand that the driver pay attention to pertinent stimuli while ignoring the constant barrage of irrelevant input (e.g., horns honking, people on the sidewalk, road conditions, landmarks).

All types of attention can involve various means of sensory stimulation, most often including at least visual and/or auditory input. The studies concerning attention levels in the elderly have demonstrated generally consistent results.

Investigations of sustained attention over an extended performance of a task do not yield reliable age differences, although age-related differences may occur in the accuracy of detection of stimuli.[11] Divided attention skills do seem to decrease with advancing age, but only when completing two or more complex tasks. When the test tasks were simple (such as visual search tasks between a pair of displays), no significant age-related differences were found.[12] In a study by Tun and Wingfield,[13] older adults were questioned about their perceptions of their own abilities to complete 16 different divided-attention tasks, such as walking and talking, or driving and planning a schedule. The researchers found that routine tasks and those involving speech processing were not deemed as becoming more difficult over time. Relative to younger adults, however, the elderly reported that dual task performance on more demanding tasks (such as driving and planning) was becoming increasingly problematic for them.

An age-related decline in alternating attention from one task to another (also called attentional switching) does seem evident from both anecdotal and empirical inquiries. An often stated concern that seems to occur more frequently with advancing age is the problem mentioned by McDowd and Birren[12]: one enters a room and forgets the intended reason for being there. While attending to the goal of going somewhere new, the goal of retrieving on item (or completing a task) gets misplaced. Perhaps both the slowed performance of the ability to switch tasks and the additional strain placed on short-term memory in this type of attentional task contribute to the relative decline in attentional switching over time. However, when visual switching of tasks is involved (rather than auditory attentional switching), Hartley and colleagues[14] did not find significant age differences.

Selective attention allows a person to focus only on important input, while filtering out the rest. In today's fast-paced world, this may be getting more difficult for everybody. When the selective attention task is particularly arduous (e.g., concentrating when there is a lot of excess stimulation or complex directions), the elderly do show a decline in this skill. Older adults are able to shift attention in a manner similar to young adults. However, older people may have more difficulty with inhibitory control over behavior (i.e., they may be less able to stop a task or to not respond),[11] or their decline may be attributed to a decreased ability to activate this type of attention.[15]

The health care professional must take into account the potential changes in attention when working with an elderly person. The older person is likely to be able to sustain attention as well as a younger person but may show decreased attentional skills during complex task completion. Divided or alternating attentional tasks are more demanding and therefore may be more problematic as well. For example, if an elderly person demonstrates decreased balance and must concentrate just on walking without falling, it would not be appropriate to demand that they simultaneously listen to unrelated instructions about another activity. While perhaps self-evident, a point worth emphasizing is that all people favor tasks or activities in which they have an interest. People will show increased attention in an inherently stimulating task. Additionally, other sensory losses and cognitive impairments may inhibit attentional processes in ways that we do not yet fully understand.

ORIENTATION

The **orientation** level of patients or clients is often documented in health care charts as alert and oriented (A&O): A&O×1, A&O×2 or A&O×3. The descriptor A&O×1 means that the person is alert and understands only who he or she is (i.e., he or she knows and responds to his or her name), A&O×2 means that the person also knows where he or she is, and A&O×3 means he or she knows not only who and where but also has an understanding of the concept of time. Occasionally the designation A&O×4 is used, which refers to the observation that the patient also understands his or her situation. Well elderly people are generally alert and oriented in all realms (A&O×3 or A&O×4). However, retirement—rather than a disease process—may contribute more to an apparent disorientation to exact date or time of day. Without a planned schedule or daily appointments, it is easy to lose track of days. Therefore, when determining whether someone is oriented, allow a little flexibility and consider the potential influence of an unstructured lifestyle.

A psychiatric disturbance is indicated when a person is alert but is not oriented at least to self. This is not a common occurrence in elderly people, except for those with severe dementia or another disease process, or those who are currently delirious under the influence of medication. For those who do display confusion about where they are, the time, and the situation, compensatory strategies may be helpful. One such intervention is the use of reality orientation boards often found in hospitals and long-term care facilities. These large display boards contain information about the date, day, location, and occasionally the weather. While these can be extremely useful, they do presume that the person is able to read, and they must be kept current. Inaccurate or outdated reality orientation boards (which unfortunately are spotted often in health care facilities) can lead to more rather than less confusion. Other compensatory tools that may have a positive influence on orientation level include calendars, scheduling books, clocks and watches, photograph albums, and current periodicals.

MEMORY

Betty and Joe were happily married for many years. Joe was such a devoted husband, he would do anything that Betty requested. One day Betty asked Joe to go and get her a hot fudge sundae. She said she wanted vanilla ice cream, chocolate syrup, nuts, whipped cream, and a cherry on top. She told Joe to write it down because he was likely to forget. He said no, he'd remember just fine. Ten minutes later, Joe came home with a hot dog for Betty. She saw it and stated with exasperation:

"Joe, I told you to write it down! You forgot the mustard!" *An anonymous joke about faulty (aging) memory*

Memory is not a simple construct. The story about Joe humorously describes declining short-term memory, which many people seem to experience with advancing age. On the other hand, the character Joe could instead be experiencing decreased sustained attention or alternating attention, or he could just have selective hearing, about which many wives of all ages complain. Although, generally speaking, memory does decline with age, one must qualify exactly what the construct of memory entails and explore the different aspects of memory in relation to the aging process.

There are several types of memory. A few are described here, although many different categories have been proposed.

- **Primary or short-term memory**—This type of memory has limited capacity and is used for information that will be used or forgotten in a matter of seconds or minutes. An example of normal short-term memory is being able to recall a 7-digit number (for example, a telephone number).
- **Working memory**—A newer concept similar to short-term memory; however, working memory refers to actively being able to use or manipulate the information from this (short-term) storage base. For example, it involves not only recalling the 7-digit telephone number but actually using that number to make a call.
- **Secondary or long-term memory**—Permanent or long-term storage of newly acquired information.
- **Tertiary or remote memory**—Storage of well-learned or previously experienced information.[11]

In addition to these, there are ways of classifying memory based on the type of information encoded. Examples include episodic memory (for events, dates), semantic memory (for words and symbols), procedural memory (which is performance based, such as riding a bicycle), spatial memory, prospective memory (remembering what needs to be done in the future), explicit memory (which requires an intention to remember), and implicit memory (which involves subconscious rather than conscious learning).

Not all types of memory are affected equally by the normal aging process. Critical differences have been found between memory systems. For example, explicit memory tasks that require concentration and the motivation for new learning (e.g., memorizing a poem or remembering a list of grocery items) can be profoundly affected by age, while the ability to complete implicit or subconscious memory tasks (e.g., completing stems of words that have been previously viewed) is maintained or only decreases slightly. Research in the area of episodic versus semantic memory has often demonstrated a more severe decline in memory for events while verbal memory tends to be better preserved.[18]

A great number of studies (more than 400 were received on request of the authors of the *Handbook of the Psychology of Aging*)[18] have been completed on the four initial types of memory highlighted on the previous page. Again no clear-cut assertions could be made, but general trends were noted. Secondary memory appears to be more affected by the aging process than primary memory. This seems logical, because secondary memory involves a deeper level of encoding information (in order for it to enter long-term storage). Think for example of the multitude of bits of information we take in and then discard (from short-term memory) throughout the course of a single day. If we had to place all that information into permanent (secondary) storage, our lives would be much more complicated.

Another implication of memory and aging research is that working memory declines more sharply with age than short-term or primary memory. Again this makes sense, because working memory tasks demand that the person not only recall the information but also be able to manipulate it. Most elderly people were able to retain telephone numbers as well as their younger counterparts. They were even able to use a 7-digit number almost as well while completing a functional telephoning task during the study, but when a 10-digit number was used (e.g., a long-distance telephone number), the elderly did not perform as well.[19]

In conclusion, the introductory joke does hold a grain of truth, but perhaps only that. Even though disease processes and hypoxia (insufficient oxygen to the brain) can severely impair memory functioning, the simple passing of years does not alone cause such major devastation. Indeed, Gorman and Campbell[19] maintain, and others concur, that while even well elders show a decline in their ability to recall names, dates, events, facts, and items on a list, this level of forgetfulness, although perhaps annoying, is usually not critical or disabling to the elderly persons' daily lives.

Compensatory and adaptive techniques may be necessary to maintain quality of life if memory skills start to diminish significantly. Self-help books on this subject are readily available. For the health care professional, several tactics are helpful when working with people who are forgetful:

- Make the material to be learned interesting (applicable to the client's life).
- Use multimodal sensory input.
- Use repetition, but not ad nauseam.
- Use cuing, but only as needed.

If possible, make the data that the elderly need to remember more enticing. The health care professional may more easily catch and hold the client's attention (which is an absolute prerequisite to conscious learning) if necessary information is provided through a story or anecdote. Relevant information will more likely be able to take hold in secondary memory storage. The use of more than one form of sensory input is crucial; that is, the practitioner can tell a client what he or she needs to know and write it down for him or her as well. Even demonstrating instructions to enhance remembering may be helpful. Immediately following an instruction session, it is often beneficial to have the client then show or tell what he or she has just learned, applying the adage that one learns best by teaching. Repetition is a key ingredient in facilitating the learning and remembering process. However, redundancy can easily lead to boredom, which then will decrease attention to task.

Following are some tips to stimulate remembering adapted from a list by Dr. Robert Lucci[20] of the Huffington Center on Aging at Baylor:

- *Pay attention*—Information can only be remembered if it is initially acknowledged.
- *Repeat* what you want to remember by rehearsing. If you meet someone and want to remember his or her name, be sure to use the name in conversation within the next few minutes.
- *Make lists*—Write down what you want to remember (but then practice remembering without the list).
- *Establish habits*—For example, always put your keys on the hook, or always park in the same section of the parking lot at the mall.
- *Relax*—Sometimes just taking a deep breath and relaxing will help to facilitate recall, while stress can hinder learning and memory.
- *Self and environmental cues* can be invaluable for stimulating memory skills. Environmental cues can be as diverse as a sign on the door to remind one of what is behind the door to using a kitchen timer to remember to turn off the oven.

Pure memory remediation (versus compensation for decreased memory) may be difficult if not impossible to achieve. However, there are many resources regarding this form of memory training as well.

Since some level of cognitive decline in the general population as people get older has been accepted as fact (see next section), the World Health Organization (WHO) proposed a diagnostic criteria for **aging-associated cognitive decline (AACD).** This refers to cognitive functioning below age and educational norms, but above what is expected for those with dementia. Studies comparing AACD with the onset of **age-associated memory impairment (AAMI)** have found that the prevalence of AACD was lower than that of AAMI.[21] This coincides with the previously mentioned findings in memory, which propose that although memory decline is evident, it very often does not interfere with day-to-day functioning.[19]

▦ INTELLIGENCE

According to Howard Gardner,[22] **intelligence** is not a single construct but rather one that encompasses several different types of skills, including the following:

1. **Linguistic intelligence**—excelling in language
2. **Logical-mathematical intelligence**—having logical, mathematical, and scientific ability
3. **Spatial intelligence**—having the ability to form mental models of the spatial world
4. **Musical intelligence**—being capable of understanding and composing music
5. **Bodily-kinesthetic intelligence**—being able to use the body effectively, as in sports and dance
6. **Interpersonal intelligence**—understanding and getting along well with others
7. **Intrapersonal intelligence**—having knowledge of the internal aspects of one's self to be used in guiding one's own behavior

Although numbered here, these skills do not fall into a particular order of importance. Gardner did not explore these types of intelligence over the course of the life span, although this would make fascinating study. What we do find is a variety of studies that investigate different aspects of these types. However, no universal consensus exists about the exact meaning of intelligence or how it should be measured. In this chapter, each of these aspects of intelligence is briefly discussed, although they are not necessarily referred to as intelligence. We have already examined some facets of inter- and intrapersonal intelligence (#6 and #7) when we discussed the age-related changes in personality. We will review the traditional aspects of intelligence (#1 and #2) and then explore other types (#3, #4, and #5) in other sections of this text.

Traditionally, intelligence quotient (IQ) tests have not covered all the aspects of intelligence mentioned here. The Wechsler Adult Intelligence Scale (WAIS) and other standard test batteries tend to focus more on the first and second types of intelligence: verbal, mathematical, and logical problem solving. In addition, many studies have taken a cross-sectional view of intelligence with generally comparable results. Younger people get higher scores than their older counterparts. However, this should not be taken to imply that younger people are more intelligent, because confounding factors such as cultural bias and level of formal education need to be taken into account. Younger people have tended to have more educational opportunities. Other potential confounding variables include speed as a determinant of the IQ score, decreased sensory functioning (especially eyesight), and the influence of memory skills, which may or may not be encompassed in the true measurement of intelligence (whatever that may be).

Therefore longitudinal cohort studies are more helpful in determining what is happening to intelligence over the course of peoples' lifetimes. Schaie[23] cites several studies that have taken this long-term view. Tests have typically shown more long-term stability of linguistic intelligence subtests (rather than performance-based) in elderly people (ages 60 to 81). One noteworthy longitudinal study found insignificant or only slight decrements prior to age 60, and then gradual average declines in all (five) areas studied. However, few people showed an overall global decline, and 85% of the respondents remained stable or even showed improved performance in certain areas. By the age of 81, between 30 and 40 percent of the participants showed significant decrements. While these figures may seem alarmingly high, we must keep in mind that the results describe a general population of aged persons, many of whom may be afflicted with disease processes that can significantly affect cognitive functioning. In another study mentioned by Schaie,[23] this hypothesis was explored and verified. Those who showed the greatest decline had a significantly greater number of diagnosed illnesses. The key, then, to staying intellectually fit may be to stay physically healthy, an idea that has accumulated a large measure of support in the past few years.

Other studies, including those by Baltes,[24] broadened the view of at least the two types of intelligences described here. These researchers have examined the concepts of cognitive mechanics (or **fluid intelligence**) and cognitive pragmatics (or **crystallized intelligence**). Fluid intelligence is "the hardware of the mind," including the speed and accuracy of information processing, such as discrimination, comparison, and categorization, and is understood to be largely evolutionarily and genetically based. Crystallized intelligence is "the software of the mind," and includes skills such as language comprehension, educational qualifications, and life and occupational skills. Baltes researched these two types of intelligences in young and old subjects and found that only fluid intelligence, or biologically based mechanics, showed a significant decline in the elderly. While memory-training sessions tended to improve memory scores, every member of the group older than age 70 was still functioning below the mean level of the younger group. Baltes proposed that when learning potential was no longer evident (i.e., when practice or memory training no longer had an additional effect), the participant could have been starting the process of pathological rather than normal aging. However, even though this study and others have shown that the human mind has its limitations, Baltes also pointed out that these limits often are not apparent, because the brain is generally not used to its full potential. He drew an interesting analogy of a young and an old person strolling together. Walking together works out well until the couple approaches a hill; the steeper the hill the harder it may be for the older person to keep up.

In contrast, crystallized intelligence does not tend to show a similar decline in older persons. Baltes compared this type of intelligence with what we term wisdom, or "an expert knowledge system in the fundamental pragmatics of life permitting excellent judgment and advice involving important and uncertain matters of life."[24] When presented with life scenarios, study participants' answers were judged by wisdom criteria. Several other studies have yielded similar results, showing no significant age differences between those who were 30 and those who were 70 when measuring this construct. A later study by Baltes and others[25] used as participants "wisdom nominees" from the community with an average age of 64. The findings project optimism into the outlook of cognitive aging, not only because people may be gaining wisdom as they age, but also because with practice and cognitive stimulation, elders can often improve the mechanics of cognitive functioning as well.

Another aspect of intelligence involves executive functioning. This high-level cognitive functioning is largely mediated by the frontal lobe of the brain. **Executive functioning** includes abstract reasoning, inductive and deductive (logical) reasoning, and cognitive flexibility in order to devise alternative solutions to a problem. A portion of community-living, normal individuals cannot easily complete these sorts of tasks anyway. Albert[26] found age-related differences between young and old people (she tested 30- to 85-year-olds) but also concluded that significant differences did not occur until after age 70 in healthy older adults. She also found great variability in the elderly as well as the younger subjects and noted that many elderly participants performed extremely well. These complex, high-level skills may show a decline in intelligent people without others even taking notice, because the types of executive skills mentioned generally are not used in social situations.

The fourth type of intelligence, musical intelligence, bears brief mentioning here. Little has been written on the aging of musical intelligence. However, music is an international language that can be used between people who do not speak in the same tongue. This may be true for communicating with the elderly as well. Basic musical abilities, such as singing, playing an instrument, and appreciating music, may be talents that are preserved even when dementia has robbed an elderly person of many other skills. A case example of an octogenarian in rehabilitation may illustrate the point.

> Mrs. N. was in the rehabilitation hospital because of a hip fracture. She had to learn new ways of completing daily tasks and practicing ambulating with a walker. The therapists were making little progress, because Mrs. N. had moderate dementia and often was distracted by her own thoughts and images. She showed little carry-over from one session to another. One day the occupational therapist happened to sing a little portion of an old folk song to get Mrs. N.'s attention. Mrs. N. perked up immediately and started singing the same and other familiar, old songs. For the rest of her stay Mrs. N. did make a little progress because she learned a few simple new "rules" by learning to sing them.

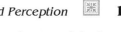

This true story suggests that musical intelligence may be one of the longest-lived types of intelligence. Sometimes music can be appreciated and enjoyed by people with cognitive impairments, even after other types of communication and entertainment are no longer meaningful.

LEARNING

Intelligence tests merely measure one's knowledge base and ability to problem-solve in a specific area. We also need to discuss the ability to learn new information as one ages. Certainly the old (and we hope, outdated) adage that "an old dog can't learn new tricks" does not apply to well elderly people. Research is beginning to support the premise that even older (middle-aged and beyond) brains can develop new interneuronal connections and "add system capacity" to enhance learning.[27] Older individuals may need more practice sessions repeated more often in order to master a task. They also may need to have the instructions presented in a variety of means (e. g. verbal, written or demonstrated) before learning can occur. Two other quotes—"use it or lose it" and "it's never too late to learn"—may be more appropriate descriptors of what happens to aging brains that are motivated to "remain open for business" (Fig. 4–1 A, B).

SENSATION AND PERCEPTION

Sensory changes occur with aging. (See Chapter 3 for the physiological details.) Some of these changes are quite familiar and arrive almost expectedly after a half-century of life. For example, visual skills are known to decrease with age, beginning in one's twenties. The good news is that the majority of elderly people are able to maintain an acuity level of 20/20 with corrective lenses well into their eighties.[5] Other visual skills are known to show a decline with advancing age:

- Visual processing speed
- Light sensitivity or ability to see well in dim light
- Near vision, especially problematic for reading small print
- Dynamic vision, which includes
     Visual tracking or saccades, needed for reading
     Visual pursuits of a moving target (such as watching the movement of a tennis ball)

Visual skills that tend to be preserved include color vision and the ability to maintain fixation on a target.[28] For the health care professional working with older persons, several simple compensatory measures can be used to mitigate the effects of decreased eyesight. Table 4–2 outlines some of these measures. If the elderly person is having difficulty with daily tasks because of impaired visual skills, a rehabilitation teacher (who works exclusively with the blind and visually impaired) or an occupational therapist can be of assistance.

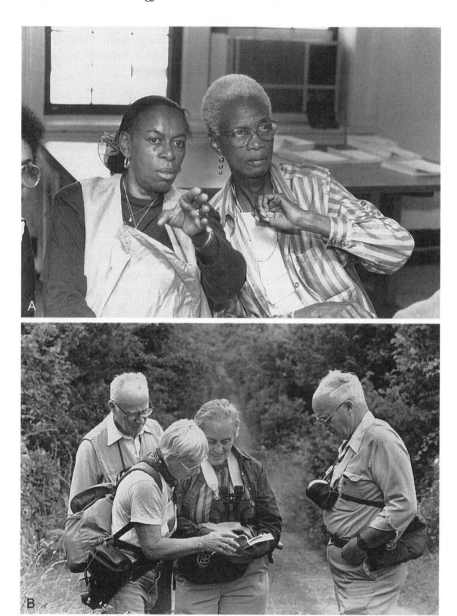

FIG. 4–1. On college campuses throughout the country, Elderhostel provides many learning opportunities for older adults. These opportunities include adult education classes (*A*) and field trips (*B*). (Photographs reprinted with permission by Jim Harrison and courtesy of Elderhostel, Inc.)

TABLE 4–2. Compensations for Specific Visual Impairments

Visual Impairment	Compensatory Measures
Decreased visual acuity	• Corrective lenses • Larger print—font size 10–12 • Larger images/signs • Closed circuit television
Increased sensitivity to light	• Use nonreflective materials on walls, floors, and ceilings • Use yellow film to reduce glare • Wear protective lenses • Shield light fixtures • Provide overhangs on windows
Decreased ability to see in dim light	• Use halogen lighting • Use night-lights • Avoid driving at night, dawn or, dusk
Decreased ability to see contrasts	• Use black with white or yellow contrasts • Highlight obstacles or changes in floor surface levels • Avoid difficult color discriminations, such as blue/green

Sources: Data from Charness, N, and Bosman, EA: Human factors design for the older adult. In Handbook of the Psychology of Aging, ed 3. Academic Press, San Diego, CA, 1990, pp. 452–453; and Zoltan, B: Vision, Perception and Cognition. Slack, Thorofare, NJ, 1996.

Perception is defined as the ability to meaningfully interpret sensory information. Usually this refers to advanced visual skills, but it can also refer to auditory, olfactory, and gustatory perception. One must have adequate vision for visual perception to be intact. Surprisingly, visual perception skills do not show a uniform decline with aging. One study by Lindfield and colleagues[29] researched the ability of people of varying ages to complete visual closure tasks (in which one must identify the figure of a given object when shown only fragments of the object). In this study the elderly were actually able to identify the fragmented pictures more accurately than their younger counterparts. When given a series of pictures, which were of the same object in ascending more complete detail, they were more accurate in identification, but they also took longer to give the correct answer. Fozard[28] presents the theory that, because of decreased sensory functioning, elderly people may become more proficient at inferring meanings from less sensory input. However, they are slower at processing the information and take in less information per unit of time.

As described in Chapter 3, hearing is another sensory modality that tends to decline with age. Men especially lose the ability to hear high frequencies, which includes consonant sounds.[5] Older people tend to have more difficulty tuning out background noise. Because of the discomfort brought on by the inability to understand others at social gatherings owing to the increased noise level, this impairment may easily lead to social isolation. Also, people in general cannot recall as much of the previous conversation if the number of words spoken per minute is increased. Both younger and older subjects were able to recall more verbal information if the words were spoken in the context of normal sentences rather than in random word strings. However, the elders' accuracy decreased more dramatically than the younger participants with unrelated words.[28] These studies and past experiences lead to the following recommendations for working with the elderly:

- Speak in a tone that can be heard. While some older people do need you to increase your volume or decibel level, do not assume this is the case. More likely the person who has difficulty hearing will need you to *lower* the pitch of your words. It is always all right to ask the person what is best for him or her.
- Make sure that your rate of speech is not too fast, but not so slow as to sound condescending.
- Whenever possible, keep background noise to a minimum.
- Do not verbally jump from one idea to the next too quickly, as older people are more likely to use the context of what is being said to understand the conversation.

As noted in Chapter 3, other perceptions that change with time include taste and smell. These closely related declines have psychological implications. The ability to detect smells in general and correctly identify differing odors decreases with age. Studies have shown a high incidence of hyposmia (decreased smell sensation) and anosmia (complete loss of smell) in participants aged 65 and older. However, in a study by Nordin and colleagues,[30] 77 percent of the elderly with smell loss (but no other apparent disease diagnoses) reported that they had a normal sense of smell. This finding corresponds with other studies that also have shown underreported olfactory deficits in the elderly. Even disregarding those who are unaware of their problem because of dementia, this sensory loss and subsequent unawareness still constitutes a serious safety issue for those wishing to remain independent to their own homes. Compensatory measures, such as natural gas/smoke detectors and having someone else with a normal sense of smell check for spoilage of food, are recommended.

Since olfaction provides a backdrop for taste sensation, decreased smell sensation can contribute to decreased pleasure in eating as well (perhaps leading to yet more social withdrawal). As people age, their ability to detect salty or bitter tastes decreases, but their capability of tasting sweet and sour foods is maintained.[5] Thirst sensation also declines, which increases the probability of dehydration in older persons.[31] Booth and colleagues[32] have suggested that inadequate dietary intake may actually cause a loss of taste perception, rather than the reverse being true. This implication points to the extreme importance of maintaining an adequate diet, especially as we age (see Chapter 5).

🔲 PRAXIS AND PERFORMANCE

Praxis is defined as the ability to carry out purposeful motor actions. Dyspraxia refers to a decreased ability to plan and/or execute purposeful movements, while apraxia refers to the total inability to carry out these motor plans. During most of our daily routines, we do not need to think about our performance; we complete many tasks (such as eating or dressing) automatically. Repetition allows us to convert novel actions into habits over time. Goal-directed actions occur throughout our self-care, work, leisure, and home management tasks. If the level of motor performance significantly decreases for any reason (e.g., injury, aging, or disease), our ability to live independently can be threatened.

When reviewing studies involving the **physical performance** of the elderly, we do find differences cross-sectionally between age groups, as well as longitudinally, but not always in the expected direction of deterioration. Age-related performance has been measured in several domains: gross motor coordination (including balance and mobility), reaction time, strength, endurance, and work-related performance (job tasks).

Perhaps the most straightforward trend when viewing performance, is an increase in both simple and complex **reaction time** over the course of years. An example of needing to take action quickly with one specific response is presented when driving a car: when one sees brake lights directly ahead, he or she perceives the need to step on the brake immediately. As people age, in general, they are not able to react as quickly. Other responses while driving (and during other activities) can be even more complex, because a person may need to decide on one or several reactions from an array of possibilities. In the Baltimore Longitudinal Study of Aging (BLSA)[33] researchers determined that slowing of behavior was a continuous process over the course of a lifetime and that increasing the complexity of task demands further increased the response time needed. Stimulus-response time tends to become about 20 percent slower between the ages of 20 and 60, and the responses made are less likely to be accurate.[5] However, the BLSA study[33] and others note that the variability within any one age group (cohort) also significantly increases with age. Therefore, at age 80, for instance, one still can be nearly as fast in responding as he ever was and still have perfectly adequate reaction time to be successful in independent living skills such as driving. (A masculine pronoun was used purposefully, because studies have tended to show that slowed reaction time is greater in older women.[33]) It is also interesting to note that when only verbal (instead of psychomotor) responses were required, the slowing has not been nearly as pronounced and may not be evident at all.[34]

Gross motor coordination is another crucial prerequisite for the completion of daily tasks without assistance. Specifically, mobility or ambulation seems to be an extremely valued skill. Falls are more prevalent in the elderly population, which would indicate a decrease in balance, coordination, and/or strength. All these areas have been studied and have generally shown age-correlated declines. Again we must point out the increasing variability among cohorts, and the fact that the vast majority of elderly people still have adequate amounts of strength and coordination to do the tasks that they want or need to do.

Endurance is defined as the ability to maintain physical involvement in an activity. It is not the same as strength, although the two are related. Several studies[34] have noted that the decrease in muscular endurance during one's lifetime is proportionately less than the decrease in muscle strength. On a hopeful and health-related note, several researchers[5] also have found that involvement in physical conditioning and exercise (doctor approved) can improve aerobic capacity, strength, and endurance, and in so doing can actually slow the course of physiological aging. (See Chapter 3 for further details.)

With the alleged, age-related deterioration of functional component skills, such as balance, reaction time, and muscle strength, one might surmise that the physical and cognitive performance of elderly workers on the job would be inferior to that of their younger counterparts. However, empirical sources and many anecdotal quips lead us to conclude that this is not the case. Many employers are beginning to realize what an asset they have in older workers.

In defense of the elderly worker, one employer speaks of their stronger work ethic,[35] while others praise the older employees' experience and sense of leadership.[36] Indeed these are subjective reports, but experimental research has supported these findings. Salthouse,[37] who completed a series of studies on the performance of older workers, states "that there is little convincing evidence that older workers are either less productive or less competent than young workers." Past relevant work experience may be a more important factor than specifically tested cognitive abilities in predicting work performance. After completing three studies, one involving architects and two involving engineers, Salthouse proposed that occupation-specific experience, while it did not seem to moderate the inverse relationship between age and basic cognitive processes, did however contribute to successful performance on the job for older workers. In yet another study, he assessed the motor functioning of older secretaries and found that, although the older secretaries had slower reaction times, they were still able to type as quickly as their younger counterparts (Fig. 4–2). This led Salthouse to surmise that years of practice helped them to more effectively scan ahead and maintain their youthful speed through a phenomenon he called "anticipatory processing."[34]

Overall, although there do seem to be age-related declines in cognition, sensation, perception, and physical performance, for most elderly people these changes do not make a substantial impact on either their comprehensive work performance or essential daily living skills.

🔲 QUALITY OF LIFE

Quality of life is an elusive construct about which a profusion of documents have been written, but that can only be truly understood on a very personal level. Each person has his or her own sense of what constitutes life quality. Health care professionals must keep in mind that stereotypical information will be helpful in understanding the elderly as a global population, but as mentioned earlier in this chapter, the older generations are an extremely diverse group of people, and therefore one description will not fit all.

According to Schalock,[38] quality of life is an overarching, multidimensional concept, which has several core principles:

- Quality of life (QOL) is best understood from the perspective of the individual.
- QOL embodies feelings of well-being.
- A high QOL is experienced when a person's basic needs are met and he or she has opportunities to pursue and meet personal goals and challenges.
- QOL can be enhanced by giving people choices and encouraging them to make decisions that affect their own lives.
- A sense of community enhances QOL.
- QOL for all persons (including those with disabilities and the elderly) is composed of the same dimensions (although the level and priority of these dimensions will differ among individuals).

These dimensions are as follows:

- Emotional well-being, including safety and spirituality
- Interpersonal relations
- Material well-being
- Personal development, including education and skills
- Physical well-being
- Self-determination, including personal control and goals/values
- Social inclusion, including roles and supports
- Rights, such as voting and accessibility

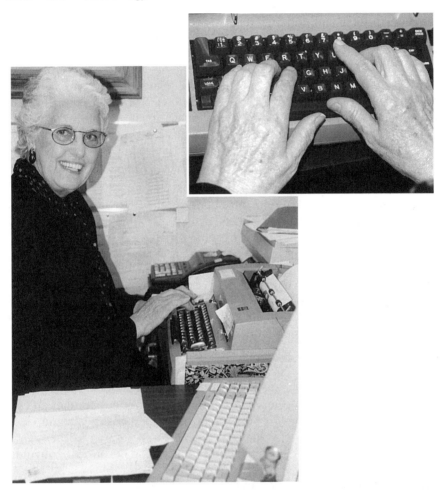

FIG. 4–2. Typing is an integral part of Connie's job at a large university. Connie is in her seventies. (Photograph reprinted with permission.)

Among the elderly population it is assumed that the degree of health or illness can have a significant impact on the level of quality of life. In a study done on life satisfaction in the elderly,[39] lack of health was listed as the biggest threat to happiness five times more frequently than any other threat, even death. These researchers concluded that health status was an excellent predictor of happiness.

In another study on robust or successful aging[40] (which could also be viewed as aging with a comparatively high quality of life), four factors were determined to promote well-being in these "successful agers" and distinguish them from those who were aging less well:

- Greater social contact
- Self-reported health satisfaction, including better vision
- Low vulnerability scores on the personality scale
- Fewer significant (stressful) life events in the past 3 years

While age did have a somewhat negative impact on robust aging, Garfein and Herzog[40] found that many members of the oldest-old group (80 and older) fit into the robust aging category. These researchers, therefore, encourage us to no longer view older age as a "phase of waning health and declining resources," but rather to put more emphasis on aging well.

From a different perspective, a research effort spearheaded by Ardelt[41] explored the impact of wisdom on life satisfaction in old age. She maintains that objective life conditions, such as health, finances, social relationships, and physical environment, can explain only a small portion of the variation of life satisfaction scores in previous studies. Her contention is that one's level of wisdom explains much of the variability of life satisfaction in the elderly. She defines wisdom as "an integration of cognitive, reflective and affective elements" including an "awareness and acceptance of human limitations" that allow us to view the human condition with humor, compassion, and detachment. This is an interesting premise because it allows those with even poor *objective* life conditions to have a great amount of *subjective* life satisfaction. It gives the level of quality of life an existential sense of personal control or insight. In fact, there may even be reason to believe that the hardships of life may challenge a person in such a way as to stimulate increased wisdom and thereby improve life satisfaction. When viewed in this light, one can more easily understand why there are many elderly people who, in spite of aging and ongoing, daily concerns, find their lives satisfying and fulfilling.

Despite a great deal of research, QOL remains a nebulous construct. We need to keep in mind that each elderly person is unique and deserving of respect for his or her own opinions. Exploring these life meanings with clients can help promote an optimal level of life satisfaction. As health care professionals, our contributions to clients' life quality may be minimal, or through the use of keen listening skills, client-centered approaches, creative problem solving, and/or by making referrals to others who may be able to provide direct assistance, our input may be invaluable and much appreciated.

🔲 DEPRESSION IN THE ELDERLY

As many as one of five people older than age 65 who live in the community show signs of clinical **depression.** This number rises sharply in long-term care facilities, where the prevalence of depression reaches up to one of every three residents.[42] In spite of this high incidence, depression in the elderly often goes unnoticed and therefore undiagnosed. This is an especially sad fact when we consider that depression is often amenable to treatment. The purpose of this section is to make the health care professional aware of the signs and symptoms of clinical depression and to offer guidelines for treatment and referral. A brief screening tool is included for the reader's use, because elderly persons may benefit from a quickly administered, routine screening for depression.[43]

A SCREENING INSTRUMENT FOR DEPRESSION IN LATE LIFE

The even Briefer Assessment Scale for Depression (EBAS DEP) is shown in (Box 4–1).

DSM-IV CRITERIA FOR DEPRESSION

According to the Diagnostic and Statistical Manual of Mental Disorders, 4th edition (DSM-IV),[44] the following are common signs and symptoms of depression:

- *Depressed mood*—the person may feel sad or appear tearful. The person may complain of feeling hopeless. (This may be the easiest symptom to recognize, but since we all have "off" days it may go unnoticed.)
- *Anhedonia*—the person has difficulty experiencing pleasure doing formerly enjoyable activities.
- Weight gain or loss of more than 5 percent of body weight within 1 month.
- Sleep disturbances—either sleeping more or less than usual.
- Psychomotor disturbances—either slowness in movements or agitated/hyperactive movements.
- Feelings of worthlessness or lowered self-esteem.
- Loss of energy nearly every day.
- Cognitive changes—such as inability to concentrate or to complete cognitive tasks that were formerly successfully completed.
- Indecisiveness nearly every day.
- Recurrent thoughts of death and/or suicide.
- While the DSM-IV also lists guilt as a symptom of depression,[44] others claim that the expression of guilt is not a common feature of depression in the elderly.[45]

BOX 4–1. EBAS DEP SCREENING INSTRUMENT

Question	Assessment	Rating	
1. Do you worry? In the past month?	Admits to worrying in the past month.	1	0
2. Have you been sad or depressed in the past month?	Has had sad or depressed mood during past month.	1	0
3. During the past month have you ever felt that life was not worth living?	Has felt that life was not worth living at some time during past month.	1	0

BOX 4–1. EBAS DEP SCREENING INSTRUMENT (*Continued*)

Question	Assessment	Rating	
4. How do you feel about your future? What are your hopes for the future?	Pessimistic about the future or has empty expectations (i.e., nothing to look forward to)	1	0
5. During the past month have you at any time felt you would rather be dead?	Has wished to be dead at any time during the past month.	1	0
6. Do you enjoy things as much as you used to—say like you did a year ago?	Less enjoyment in activities than a year previously. *(If question 6 rated 0, then rate 0 for question 7 and skip to question 8. If question 6 rated 1, ask question 7.)*	1	0
7. Is it because you are depressed or nervous that you don't enjoy things as much?	Loss of enjoyment because of depression/nervousness.	1	0
8. In general how happy are you? Are you very happy, fairly happy, not very happy, or not happy at all?	Not every happy or not happy at all.	1	0

TOTAL SCORE

The eight items of this schedule require raters to make a judgment as to whether the proposition in the middle column is satisfied or not. If a proposition is satisfied, then a depressive symptom is present and raters should circle "1" in the right hand column, otherwise "0" should be circled. Each question in the left-hand column must be asked exactly as printed, but follow-up or subsidiary questions may be used to clarify the initial answer until the rater can make a clear judgment as to whether the proposition is satisfied or not. For items that inquire about symptoms over the past month, note that the symptom need not have been present for the entire month nor at the moment of interview, but it should have been a problem for the patient or troubled him or her for some of the past month.

A score of 3 or greater indicates the probable presence of a depressive disorder that may need treatment, and the patient should be assessed in more detail or referred for psychiatric evaluation.

(*Source:* Allen, N, Ames, D, Ashby, D, Bennetts, K, Tuckwell, V, and West, C: A brief sensitive screening instrument for depression in late life. Age and Ageing 23:213–218, 1994.)

If several of these signs and symptoms, especially one of the first two, are present for a couple of weeks, clinical depression may be occurring.[44] The elderly client should be referred to his or her physician. Encourage the client to make an appointment even if he or she does not understand the need for one. As a health care professional, you may want to contact the doctor and/or health care team to let them know of your concern, but be careful not to violate patient confidentiality. A crucial point to keep in mind is that elderly people do not tend to "fake" the signs and symptoms of depression.[46]

Feeling down and depressed is not a natural consequence of the aging process. This mood disturbance must be taken seriously. The suicide rate in the United States is highest among those who are older than 65, with more than 8000 people older than 60 committing suicide each year. Elderly white men are especially prone to suicidal attempts. While suicide is not always a consequence of depression, certainly death is its most serious outcome. Health care professionals need to be aware of the potential for suicide and give serious consideration to *any* indication that the person may be thinking about it. They should listen with great care to the elder's stories and make a referral if there is any cause to think suicide is a possibility.

SUICIDE IN THE ELDERLY

The following are common signals of impending suicide:

- A past history of suicidal attempts, or current/past threats of suicide
- Symptoms of depression or ongoing bodily complaints
- Discharge from a health care facility against medical advice or recommendation
- Spontaneous recovery from a depressed mood, including sudden euphoria
- Depressed mood due to alcohol, barbiturates, or other medications
- Bereavement, severe losses in life, or identifying with a person who is deceased, especially a life-partner
- Psychiatric disorders
- Giving things away or putting one's affairs in order[47]

While it is beyond the scope of this text to discuss the ethical issues raised by suicide undertaken to escape excruciating, irreducible pain and/or terminal illness, it suffices to reiterate that depression is often amenable to treatment. Through medication management, psychotherapy, and/or electroconvulsive shock treatment, there is good potential for restoring the quality of life for elderly people who are depressed. According to Ira Katz,[48] Director of Geriatric Psychiatry at the Hospital of the University of Pennsylvania, 80 percent of the elder persons who are properly diagnosed and treated can recover and return to their usual level of functioning. Depression can happen to anyone; no amount of education, money, or social status can keep it at bay. According to Dr. Katz, as health care professionals our job is "to explain to patients that we think they may have an illness that is treatable, and with treatment they can feel better and function better."

 DEATH AND BEREAVEMENT

Dying and death are natural life events during old age. They are nonetheless events that are at best accepted and at the least feared or dreaded for self and loved ones. Our society has done a good job of neatly tucking away the dying process into institutions, where the final event of death is sometimes forestalled for a very long time. Currently an estimated 80 percent of deaths occur in institutions, whereas a century ago virtually none did.[49] There are many ethical issues related to death and dying that are particularly pertinent for older people. They or their loved ones are more likely to need to make a decision about the level of medical care desired for the eventual times when they would be unable to make a decision for themselves. Living wills and advance directives can outline one's wishes and are encouraged for everyone. They can ease the sense of uncertainty when a loved one must make those "life or death" decisions.

Generally people experience an increased number of losses of significant others as they age. Not only the death of spouses but also the death of siblings and friends occur more frequently as a person reaches toward their own maximal life span. However, just because one lives through these death events more often, this does not imply that the **bereavement** experiences become any easier. The health care professional should keep in mind that grieving persons of all ages may need additional emotional support and that each grieving process is highly individualized.

Several theorists have described the stages of grief. Parkes[50] delineates four stages: numbness, yearning/protest, disorganization, and developing a new identity. Kubler-Ross,[51] on the other hand, describes five stages: denial, anger, bargaining, depression, and finally acceptance. These stages are neither set to specific timelines nor are they completely distinct from one another. However, in our society, grieving is expected to last only a short while, and then those who are grieving are encouraged to "get on with things" or "snap out of it."[52] Unfortunately, the feelings of loss, isolation, and extreme sadness can persist for years—much longer than is socially acceptable.[53] Health care professionals often encounter elders who are in the midst of some stage of bereavement.

Caregivers of dying people are enmeshed in an extremely stressful situation. Health care professionals can ease the burden of caregiving at least a little by promoting wellness practices, by setting limits, and by providing "opportunities for distraction, humor and relaxation."[49] These caregivers are already grieving the impending loss of their loved one, although this may appear to be denial of the upcoming death.

Several recommendations are offered for those working with bereaved individuals or families. The reader is cautioned to keep in mind that each person has his or her own way of handling grief, yet many have found the following suggestions helpful:

- As much as time allows, let the person talk about their loved one and their loss. Asking about the deceased person, even a spouse or child, is generally acceptable and may even be desired. You can assess quickly whether this is a subject the person would rather not broach. Shedding tears is a natural, healthy experience that can aid the healing process.
- Assure the bereaved person that his or her feelings are legitimate. It is not helpful to say "I understand" unless you really have been in a similar situation. It also is not helpful to make comments such as "He was quite old" or "It's all for the best." Even if the person was old, the death of a loved one is never easy.[52] Euphemisms, clichés, and sympathizing remarks are generally regarded as not helpful.
- It is okay not to have the right words or the answers. Just being there and offering your care and support does help.[54]
- Allow the bereaved to make decisions. Alty[55] states that well-meaning individuals often will take over decision-making for grieving persons, but that just because they are grieving does not mean that they cannot function rationally (or that they want to give up decision-making).
- Recommend counseling for those who need additional help. Examples of pathological bereavement include behavior that is harmful to self or others. If the person talks about suicide, tells you that his or her life is now over, or talks about or with the deceased person as if he or she were still alive, a referral is in order.[52] Social workers can be extremely helpful to the grieving individual, as they can assist clients and their significant others "to cope with their feelings, . . . to recognize their choices, . . . to develop and maintain meaningful communication with one another, and to link up with people and services beyond themselves."[56] (Refer to Chapter 11 for a more complete description of the role of social workers working with the elderly.)

Remember that the elderly person may have had to contend with a number of losses in a short period of time. Not only are loved ones dying, but often he or she also may be dealing with the loss of his or her long-term home. In addition, the older person may be demonstrating anticipatory grief of his or her own approaching death.[55] Sensitivity and knowing one's own limits as a health care professional are necessary ingredients for working with bereaved clients effectively.

DEMENTIA

Normal aging does include a slowing down and a gradual wearing out of bodily systems. It does not include dementia, which is considered a pathological aging process. **Dementia** is defined as progressive cognitive impairment that eventually interferes with daily functioning. The prevalence of dementia among 60-year-olds is only 1 to 2 percent, but it becomes increasingly more common with advancing age.[57] Dementia consists of persistent disturbances in cognitive functioning, including memory and intellectual ability. Certain causes of dementia may be treatable, and given the appropriate treatment, cognitive functioning may be restored. While Alzheimer's disease is the most common, accounting for 50 to 75 percent of all senile dementias,[58] other causes of dementia include infections, metabolic and endocrine disturbances, alcohol and/or drug abuse, psychiatric disorders, deficiency states, trauma, Huntington's disease, Pick's disease, and Parkinson's disease.[57]

Dementia encompasses multiple cognitive, psychological, and functional deficits, including memory impairment, which is always present. The following signs and symptoms may be present as well:

- Difficulties with understanding or communicating through language
- Difficulty with problem solving and other high-level cognitive tasks, such as abstract reasoning. A common cognitive test used with people who are suspected to have dementia is the Mini-Mental State Examination, which is a brief cognitive screening tool.
- Impaired visual spatial skills, which can impair the ability to drive safely[59]
- Behavioral disturbances such as depression, anxiety, wandering, and neglect of personal hygiene[60]

A lower educational level has been found to correlate with an increased probability of developing dementia. While the reasons for this are merely conjectural, several have been proposed:

- A lower education level may correlate with certain high-risk behaviors, such as working at higher risk occupations, poorer nutrition, and increased use of alcohol, all of which can affect cognitive functioning.
- A higher educational level may correlate with increased neuronal reserves because of greater brain capacity. This could stave off the noticeable appearance of the onset of dementia. In other words, those who have greater brain capacity could lose proportionately more of that capacity without others taking notice.
- Those with more education may tend to seek out more cognitively stimulating activities, and this productive use of the brain could prevent or postpone neuronal degeneration.[61]

Certainly many well-educated people have also succumbed to dementia; however, while these are only theoretical probabilities at this time, these ideas do tend to lend credence to the "use it or lose it" and other health promotion philosophies. Perhaps by participating in the many informal and formal educational opportunities that are available everywhere, we may be able to slow the progression or even have some control over the onset of this dreaded disease state.

DEMENTIA OF THE ALZHEIMERS' TYPE

The prevalence of **Alzheimer's disease (AD)** in the United States is currently estimated to be at 4 million people, but by 2050, as the proportion of those older than 85 increases, an estimated 14 million people will have AD.[62] The mean age of onset is 81.[60] While the lifetime risk of developing AD is 14.5 to 26.2 percent, those older than 90 have at least a 40 percent chance of getting the disease.[63] Since AD is the most common form of dementia and therefore health care professionals are most likely to encounter people with this type, discussion focuses on this disease specifically.

During the early stages of AD (usually the first few years following onset), physical symptoms are not common. The person is able to walk and displays normal movement patterns and posture. As the disease progresses, all of the deficits of dementia already mentioned may worsen. Those suffering from AD usually regress developmentally until, when near death, they may display some behaviors similar to a newly born infant. Table 4–3 describes some of the progression of features commonly seen in AD. It needs to be pointed out that each person is an individual and may display only a few rather than all of these traits.

AD progresses through three stages: mild, moderate, and severe. Since there is no cure, the current emphasis of medical providers is to prolong the first two stages. The medical community has had some success with this endeavor, including the development of potential medications to enhance memory[64] and other areas of cognitive functioning.[65] Scientists are trying to ward off the third stage, because they believe that initially for those with AD "most of the person is still there." Someone in the initial stages is still physically capable and can still find joy in living.[59] As health care professionals, we need to emphasize these beliefs to caregivers, who greatly need support at this time.

WORKING WITH THOSE WHO HAVE DEMENTIA

There are some general rules to follow when working with persons who have dementia. It is important to always show caring and respect and not to speak about them as if they were not there. This is a time that may try your patience even as a professional, but controlling your emotions is crucial. Remember that the person is not intentionally trying to annoy you. Soothing music may defuse the intensity of the situation. A sense of humor so that you can laugh together is also extremely helpful, although it is important never to let the

TABLE 4–3. *Alzheimer's Disease Symptom Progression*

	Initial	End Stage
General Behavior	Indifferent, may be delusional or depressed	Withdrawn, agitated, mood may change abruptly
Language	Normal or mild word finding difficulties	Severe impairment, words may be meaningless "word-salad"
Memory	Mild short term deficits	Unable to test
Orientation	Fully oriented	Oriented to self only
Personal care/ ADL skills[1]	Inattention to detail, but able to complete	Dependency, may show fear of bathing
Instrumental ADLs[2]	Slight impairment, carelessness, decreased safety awareness, may need supervision	Unable to complete
Mobility	Normal	Abnormal, may not be able to walk or transfer independently
Posture	Normal	Flexed, often preferring a fetal position
Range of Motion/ Movement	Normal	Increased muscle tonus contractures[3] common

1. ADLs include bathing, dressing, self-feeding, grooming etc.
2. IADLs include home management, money management, care of others, etc.
3. A contracture is defined as a decrease of 50% or more of normal passive range of motion. It is a painful condition affecting many in long-term care settings, including more than three-quarters of patients who can no longer walk. Source: Souren, L. E., Frensses, & E. H. Reisberg, B. (June, 1995). Contractures and loss of function in patients with Alzheimer's Disease. Journal of the American Geriatrics Society. *43*(6), 650–655.

Sources: Data from Ham, RJ: Making the diagnosis of Alzheimer's disease. Patient Care 104–120, June 15, 1995; Morris, JC: The Clinical Dementia Rating (CDR): Current version and scoring rules. Neurology 2412–2414, November, 1993; and Cole, SA: Behavorial disturbances in Alzheimer's disease. Patient Care 121–131, June 15, 1995.

person think you are laughing at him or her. Diversion often helps to calm a stressful situation, including the following:

- Involvement in simple activities
- Playing music they enjoyed when they were young
- Looking through old photograph albums
- Giving them an item that they enjoy, for example a doll or stuffed animal (while this may not be considered "age appropriate," it has been helpful to some people with dementia)

Table 4–4 offers some more specific suggestions as well.

TABLE 4–4. Dementia: Problems and Potential Solutions

Functional Problem Area	Potential Solutions
Decreased self-care skills (ADLs)	• Offer supervision. • Simplify clothing/environment. • Gently encourage person to do as much as possible without nagging. • Remove safety hazards. • Occupational therapy referral.
Decreased involvement in daily activities	• Encourage involvement in what person can still do well. • Praise successes and have patience. • Try safe, simple repetitive chores. • Offer items of interest.
Wandering	• Take walks together in safe areas. • Purchase identification bracelet. • Alert neighbors. • Remove obstacles indoors. • If balance is decreased, physical therapy referral.
Impaired communication	• Speak slowly and calmly, do not yell. • Give simple directions, one step at a time. • Use repetition as needed. • Speech therapy referral.
Sleep disturbance	• Establish a bedtime routine. • Make sure person gets enough exercise during the day. • Limit liquid before bedtime. • Toilet immediately before bedtime. • Omit obstacles in bedroom to bathroom route or purchase bedside commode. • A back rub may promote restful sleep.

Problem Behavior	Possible Solutions
Inappropriate behavior	• Always treat person with dignity and respect. • Divert person to another activity. • Watch for signs of overstimulation and try to avoid these situations. • Listen and respond to the feeling behind the words being said, rather than the words themselves. • Ask for help (doctors, support group, adult day care, etc.). • Use humor. • Do not ignore requests for assistance.
Anxiety, agitation	• Structure environment. • Establish daily routine with lots of opportunity for structured activities. • Promote security.

Continued on following page

TABLE 4–4. *Dementia: Problems and Potential Solutions (Continued)*

Functional Problem Area	Potential Solutions
Anger	• Offer a drink or a snack or a favorite item. • Do not confront, tease, or argue with the person. • Listen and divert to new topic if possible. • Limit stimulation. • Remove from disruptive environment. • Take care of your own safety.

Sources: Data from Cole, SA: Behavioral disturbances in Alzheimer's disease. Patient Care 121–131, June 15, 1995; Gwyther, LP: General guidelines for caregivers and tips for communicating with your relative. Patient Care 132–134, June 15, 1995; and Colorado State University: Guidelines for working with people with Alzheimer's disease (class handout). Alzheimer's Disease and Aging Research, Department of Psychology, Fort Collins, CO 80523, 1989.

RELATED DISORDERS

Sometimes what appears to be depression or dementia, is actually another medical disorder in disguise. It is important for the health care worker to be aware of a few of these other problems, not in order to make a diagnosis, but rather to gain a basic understanding of some of these common disorders and to make a referral whenever necessary. Some of the more common ailments associated with symptoms of depression and/or dementia in the elderly are briefly described here.

Malnutrition. Deficiencies of the B-complex vitamins, vitamin C, zinc, magnesium, folic acid, and protein can cause behavioral disturbances, including those implicated in the diagnosis of clinical depression[66] (see also Chapter 5).

Cerebrovascular Accident (CVA) or Stroke. CVA or stroke, especially small infarcts with limited accompanying functional declines, may cause behavior disturbances that may appear to be brought about by depression or AD. In fact, a rather common type of dementia (multi-infarct dementia) is directly caused by a series of small strokes.

Hypothyroidism. This disorder slows metabolic processes, which causes the affected person to respond slowly and to be lethargic.

Failure to Thrive. A related syndrome to the ones previously described is failure to thrive (FTT). An insidious deterioration in functioning that is not related to a specific disease, FTT can be caused by depression, dementia, chronic conditions, or drug reactions. Social isolation, low socioeconomic status, and functional dependency all are predisposing factors of FTT. Case examples are common; perhaps we all know of someone who just seemed to whittle away prior to dying. Common features of FTT include weight loss due to lack of appetite, social withdrawal, lack of concern about appearance, memory loss, impaired ambulation, and incontinence (common in nearly half the cases described).[67] This syndrome is an example of simply giving up on life.

Learned helplessness. Another similar complication that has received a little attention as a problem of aging is learned helplessness. Learned helplessness is a condition that develops when organisms (in this case humans) "learn that their responses are independent of desired outcomes."[68] Consequently they learn to not respond to stimulation from their environments. Seligman[68] related this phenomenon to depression more than 20 years ago. In laboratory experiments, when they could not control electric shocks, dogs eventually gave up and became helpless and apathetic. Similar results can occur in human beings, perhaps especially the aged who receive care from others. A case example illustrates this point.

> Mr. M., an 86-year-old man, came in as a patient for rehabilitation to a long-term care facility because his family had noticed an insidious decline in his functioning ever since he had had a hip fracture about a year before. He was pleasant and cooperative but did demonstrate weakness and dehabilitation, although there did not seem to be any specific cause for his functional deficits. When the occupational therapist evaluated him, she found that although he had decreased endurance, he even surprised himself at being able to complete all the individual tasks during activities of daily living (ADLs). However, he told her that he hadn't completed self-care in several months, stating "Oh, the girls [referring to the home health aides] do that." Through their caring and wanting to help, they had gradually done much more for Mr. M. than he needed, and he had learned to sit back and let them do their job. In so doing, Mr. M. had no useful activities that he had to complete, and he ended up with nothing he was expected to do. They not only dressed and bathed him, they also did all his home management tasks. He became compliant and helpless, and there was little wonder why he also displayed other symptoms of depression on entering rehabilitation. The happy ending is that Mr. M. relearned to take care of himself—again much to his surprise—and he returned home a few months later, independent not only in ADLs but also in light home management tasks.

This case example speaks to the fact that it may be easy to learn helpless behaviors. Many well-meaning caregivers do too much for their patients and therefore may inadvertently "help" them lose the ability to complete vital life tasks.

SUMMARY

Although change is inevitable throughout life, the essential core of the human being is not likely to be altered by the aging process alone. As people age we *tend* to

- Prefer slower paced activities and move more slowly
- Take longer to learn new tasks
- Become more forgetful
- Lose sensory processing skills

However, these changes can be minimal and do not necessarily interfere with daily functioning. In fact, the majority of elders do remain vital contributing members of society throughout most, if not all, of their lives.

Additionally, each age cohort becomes more diverse as their ages increase. Although as a group, the members tend to show the signs of aging already mentioned, within each age group there are those who continue to perform essentially as well as they ever did and those who have succumbed to the ravages of "old age."

While no one is ensured a successful aging process, everyone can take steps to improve the probability of a long and healthy life. The value of human interaction, activity, exercise, and continued involvement in life roles has been written about extensively. In a national study of older adults, Adelmann[69] found that involvement in multiple roles (such as volunteer, worker, spouse, homemaker, family member, hobbyist) was associated with less depression and increased satisfaction with life. In a related study completed in Finland,[70] the researchers found that involvement in physical exercise was also related to increased psychological well-being, while inactivity was associated with a high incidence of depression. Many other studies have corroborated these results; that it, is important to remain active in order to age well or robustly.

As health care professionals, each of us has the responsibility, within our own unique discipline, to foster involvement in purposeful activities and encourage interaction with others. By listening, being supportive and respectful, promoting independence, and making referrals as appropriate, we can help older persons live their best potential quality of life and to remain as productive as they choose to be.

REVIEW QUESTIONS

1. Erikson defines the final era of life as:
   A. Trust vs. mistrust
   B. Wisdom vs. senility
   C. Integrity vs. despair
   D. Doubt vs. faith

2. According to McCrae and Costa, which personality traits tend to remain most stable over the course of adulthood:
   A. Neuroticism and extraversion
   B. Openness to experience and extraversion

    C. Neuroticism and conscientiousness

    D. Conscientiousness and agreeableness

3. Self-efficacy, or the sense that one has control over one's life:

    A. Tends to remain stable over all domains over the course of adulthood

    B. Tends to be lowest in the elderly for the domain of finances

    C. Increases significantly after one retires

    D. Was found to be at a lower level in the elderly as compared with college students

4. Which of the following statements about attention and aging is true:

    A. Sustained attention declines significantly with age

    B. Elderly people have more difficulty dividing attention between complex tasks

    C. Attentional switching does not decline with age

    D. Visual switching of tasks is more difficult for the elderly than auditory attentional switching

5. A&O×2 means a person is alert and oriented to:

    A. Self and others only

    B. Time and self only

    C. Situation and self only

    D. Self and place only

6. Which of the following types of memory tasks is least affected by the aging process:

    A. Implicit (subconscious) memory tasks

    B. Working memory tasks

    C. Short-term memory tasks

    D. Explicit memory tasks

7. Which of the following statements about intelligence is accurate:

    A. Crystallized intelligence is less affected by aging than fluid intelligence.

    B. Fluid intelligence is less affected by aging than crystallized intelligence.

    C. Age-associated memory impairment is less prevalent than age-associated cognitive decline.

    D. Longitudinal studies show a decline in all test areas by age 60.

8. Perceptual skills in the elderly:

    A. Decrease dramatically with age

    B. May be improved for visual closure tasks

    C. Are more accurate and show decreased response time than for younger people

    D. Do not change with the aging process

9. Choose the false statement about sensation and aging:

    A. Men, more than women, lose the ability to hear high frequencies as they age.

    B. The ability to taste sweet and sour is maintained.

    C. Thirst sensation declines with age.

    D. Most older people who have hyposmia are aware of their decreased sense of smell.

10. Older workers tend to:

   A. Be slower and therefore less efficient
   B. Have less of a work ethic driving them
   C. Use past experience effectively to keep up with the work
   D. Withdraw from leadership roles

11. Which of the following tends not to be a factor in depression in the elderly:

   A. Anhedonia
   B. Guilt
   C. Sleep disturbances
   D. Cognitive changes

12. Suicide among the elderly:

   A. Is not common
   B. Is a natural desire due to the aging process
   C. Is highest among older men
   D. Is highest among women

13. Alzheimer's disease:

   A. Always includes memory impairment
   B. Always includes physical symptoms in the first two stages
   C. Always includes language disturbances
   D. Is inevitable for those reaching 100 years old

14. Learned helplessness:

   A. May develop when caregivers do more than necessary for the older person
   B. Is not a phenomenon found in the elderly
   C. Is caused by depression
   D. Is irreversible

15. The stages of bereavement:

   A. Are indistinguishable from one another
   B. Have set time lines
   C. Last longer for the elderly
   D. Are highly individualized

▨ LEARNING ACTIVITIES

1. Think of the role models you know who are at least 60 years old. What personality traits do you appreciate in these older people? How can you ensure that you will have some of these same traits when you are older? Do you think one can develop these traits? Why or why not?

2. It may be interesting to interview a few older people. Ask them how they think their personality and cognition have changed over the course of years. How does this compare with the research data? How do you think you will change as you get older?

3. Discuss the concept of self-efficacy (having a sense of control over one's life). Do you think that for yourself your sense of self-efficacy will increase, decrease, or stay the same as you get older? In one or all domains? Explain your answer.

4. Generally the level of cognition declines as one gets older. How can you ensure that this decline will be minimal? List five things that you can do to improve your cognitive level.

5. Why does driving become more difficult with advancing age? What other life tasks may be more difficult for the elderly and why?

6. Review the seven types of intelligence. Which of these seem most important for your line of work? From your own experience, which of these seem best preserved in the older people you know?

7. Discuss wisdom. What is it, and what makes someone wise? Do you equate being wise with being older? Why or why not?

8. If you could choose which two of your senses to lose (taste, touch, smell, sight, or hearing), which would you choose to lose and why? How would this loss affect your life? (Include safety issues.)

9. Discuss quality of life, which means many things to different people. What aspects of your life give it a high level of quality? Share these with the group. Do you think these will change as you age? Why or why not?

10. Discuss depression in the elderly. What are some of the reasons that older people become depressed? (Include life events and changes that tend to occur.)

11. Handling grief is a personal issue. Discuss with one other person what actions you think would be helpful when you are grieving for a significant other. What actions would cause you to feel worse? Discuss the themes in a larger group. Afterwards discuss how this knowledge will change how you interact with a grieving person as a friend and then as a professional.

▨ REFERENCES

1. Erikson, EH, et al: Vital Involvement in Old Age. WW Norton, New York, 1989, p 36.

2. Erikson, EH: Childhood and Society, ed 2. Norton, New York, 1963.

3. Kogan, N: Personality and aging. In Birren, JE, and Schaie, KW (eds): Handbook of the Psychology of Aging, ed 3. Academic Press, San Diego, CA, 1990, pp 331–335.

4. Papalia, DE, and Olds, SW (eds): Human Development. McGraw-Hill, New York, 1995, p 505.

5. Hayflick, L: How and Why We Age. Ballantine Books, New York, 1994, p 145.

6. Labouvie-Vief, G, et al: Representations of self across the life span. Psychol Aging 10:404–415, 1995.

7. Bandura, A: Self-efficacy: Toward a unifying theory of behavioral change. Psychol Review 84:191–215, 1977.

8. Rhee, C, and Gatz, M: Cross-generational attributions concerning locus of control beliefs. Int J Aging Hum Dev 37:153–161, 1993.

9. McAvay, GJ, et al: A longitudinal study of change in domain-specific self-efficacy among older adults. J Gerontol: Psychol Sci 51B:P243–P253, 1996.

10. Deeg, DJH, et al. Health behavior and aging. In Birren, JE and Schaie, KW. (eds): Handbook of the Psychology of Aging, ed 4. Academic Press, San Diego, CA, 1996, pp 129–149.

11. Zec, RF: The neuropsychology of aging. Exp Gerontol 30:431–442, 1995.

12. McDowd, JM, and Birren, JE: Aging and attentional processes. In Birren, JE and Schaie, KW. (eds): Handbook of the Psychology of Aging, ed 3. Academic Press, San Diego, CA, 1990, pp 222–233.

13. Tun, PA, and Wingfield, A: Does dividing attention become harder with age? Findings for the divided attention questionnaire. Aging and Cognition 2(1):39–66, 1995.

14. Hartley, AA, et al: In McDowd, JM, and Birren, JE (eds): Aging and attentional processes. In Birren, JE and Schaie, KW. (eds): Handbook of the Psychology of Aging, ed 3. Academic Press, San Diego, CA, 1990; pp 224–225.

15. Allen, PA, et al: Adult age differences in attention: filtering or selecting? J Gerontol: Psychol Sci 49:P213–P222, 1994.

16. Kaplan, HI, and Saddock, BJ: Synopsis of Psychiatry: Behavioral Sciences: Clinical Psychiatry. Williams & Wilkins, Baltimore, 1991, p 203.

17. Baddeley, A: Working Memory. Oxford Press, Clarendon, England, 1986.

18. Hultsch, DF, and Dixon, RA: Learning and memory in aging. In Birren, JE and Schaie, KW. (eds): Handbook of the Psychology of Aging, ed 3. Academic Press, San Diego, CA, 1990, pp 258–274.

19. Gorman, WF, and Campbell, CD: Mental acuity of the normal elderly. J Okla State Med Assoc 88:119–123, March, 1995.

20. Lucci, RJ, in Rosenthal, HF: Spring cleaning turns up some leftover news tidbits. Portland Press Herald, Portland, ME, March 26, 1997.

21. Haenninen, T, et al: Prevalence of ageing-associated cognitive decline in an elderly population. Age Ageing 25:201–205, 1996.

22. Gardner, H: Multiple Intelligences the Theory in Practice. Harper Collins, New York, 1993.

23. Schaie, KW: Intellectual development in adulthood. In Birren, JE and Schaie, KW. (eds) Handbook of the Psychology of Aging, ed 3. Academic Press, San Diego, CA, 1990, pp 291–309.

24. Baltes, PB: The aging mind: Potential and limits. Gerontologist 33:580–594, 1993.

25. Baltes, PB, et al: People nominated as wise: A comparative study of wisdom-related knowledge. Psychol Aging 10:155–166, 1995.

26. Albert, M: Neuropsychological and neurophysiological changes in healthy adult humans across the age range. Neurobiol Aging 14:623–625, 1993.

27. Hotz, RL: Probing the workings of hearts and minds. Research. Los Angeles Times, A1, April 3, 1997.

28. Fozard, JL: Vision and hearing in aging. In Handbook of the Psychology of Aging, ed 3. Academic Press, San Diego, CA, 1990, pp 150–170.

29. Lindfield, KC, et al: Identification of fragmented pictures under ascending versus fixed presentation in young and elderly adults: Evidence for the inhibition-deficit hypothesis. Aging and Cognition 1:282–291, 1994.

30. Nordin, S, et al: Unawareness of smell loss in normal aging and Alzheimer's Disease: Discrepancy between self-reported and diagnosed smell sensitivity. J Gerontol: Psychol Sci 50B:P187–P192, 1995.

31. Smolowe, J: Older, longer. Time 148(14): 76–80, Fall, 1996.

32. Booth, DA, et al: Measurement of food perception, food preference and nutrient selection. Ann NY Acad Sci, 561:226–242, 1989.

33. Fozard, JL, et al: Age differences and changes in reaction time: The Baltimore Longitudinal Study of Aging. J Gerontol: Psychol Sci 49:P179–P189, 1994.

34. Spirduso, WW, and MacRae, PG: Motor performance and aging. In Birren, JE and Schaie, KW. (eds): Handbook of the Psychology of Aging, ed 3. Academic Press, San Diego, CA, 1990, pp 183–200.

35. Gunn, EP: Retire today, find a new job tomorrow. Fortune 132(2):102–106, July 24, 1995.

36. Lieberman, S, and McCray, J: The coming of age(ism): Newsrooms should be wary of the generation gap. The Quill 82(3):33–34, April, 1994.

37. Salthouse, TA: Age related differences in basic cognitive processes: Implications for work. Exp Aging Res 20:249–255, 1994.

38. Schalock, RL: Reconsidering the conceptualization and measurement of quality of life. In Quality of Life. American Association on Mental Retardation, Washington, DC 1995, pp 123–138.

39. Kehn, DJ: Predictors of elderly happiness. Activities, Adaptation and Aging 19(3):11–30, 1995.

40. Garfein, AJ, and Herzog, AR: Robust aging among the young-old, old-old, and oldest-old. J Gerontol: Soc Sci 50B:S77–S87, 1995.

41. Ardelt, M: Wisdom and life satisfaction in old age. J Gerontol: Psychol Sci 52B(1):P15–P27, 1997.

42. Johnson, JC: Depression and dementia in the elderly: A primary care perspective. Compr Ther 22:280–285, 1996.

43. Callahan, CM, et al: Depression in late life: The use of clinical characteristics to focus screening efforts. J Gerontol: Med Sci 49:M9–M14, 1994.

44. Diagnostic and Statistical Manual of Mental Disorders, ed 4 (adapted). American Psychiatric Association, Washington, DC, 1994, p 327.

45. McIntyre, LG, et al: Depression and suicide: Assessment and intervention. Home Health Care Management and Practice 9(1):8–17, 1996.

46. Juratovac, E: The Ohio Nurses Association presents "Anxiety and depression in older adults": An independent study. Ohio Nurses Review 4–13, March, 1996.

47. Hemphill, BJ: Depression among suicidal elderly: A life-threatening illness. Occupational Therapy Practice 4(1):61–66, 1992.

48. Adams, RC: Geriatric rehab treat depression to improve function. Advance for Occupational Therapists 19, December 9, 1996.

49. McCue, JD: The naturalness of dying. JAMA 273:1039–1043, 1995.

50. Parkes, CM: Bereavement. Penguin Books, London, 1972.

51. Kubler-Ross, E: On Death and Dying. Macmillan, New York, 1970.

52. Waltman, RE: When a spouse dies. Nursing 92:48–52, July, 1992.

53. Goleman, D: Grief may not follow a predictable pattern. In Dudley, W (ed): Death and Dying: Opposing Viewpoints. Greenhaven Press, San Diego, CA, 1992, pp 139–144.

54. Chessler, BR: Friends can help the grieving cope with death. In Dudley, W (ed): Death and Dying: Opposing Viewpoints. Greenhaven Press, San Diego, CA, 1992, pp 155–160.

55. Alty, A: Adjustment to bereavement and loss in older people. Nursing Times 91(12):35–36, March 22, 1995.

56. Davidson, KW, and Foster, Z: Social work with dying and bereaved clients: Helping the workers. Soc Work Health Care 21(4):3, 1995.

57. Cummings, JL, et al: Dementia. In Cassell, CK, et al: Geriatric Medicine, ed 3. Spring-Verlag, New York, 1997, pp 897–913.

58. Ebly, EM, et al: Prevalence and types of dementia in the very old: Results from the Canadian Study of Health and Aging. Neurology 44:1593–1600, 1994.

59. Ham, RJ: Making the diagnosis of Alzheimer's disease. Patient Care 104–120, June, 15, 1995.

60. Cole, SA: Behavioral disturbances in Alzheimer's disease. Patient Care 121–131, June 15, 1995.

61. Pedersen, NL: Gerontological behavior genetics. In Birren, JE and Schaie, KW. (eds): Handbook of the Psychology of Aging, ed 4. Academic Press, San Diego, CA, 1996.

62. Sunderland, T: Alzheimer's disease statistics. F. Oakley AOTA Institute, March 1, 1994.

63. Drachman, DA: If we live long enough, will we all be demented? Neurology 44:1563–1565, 1994.

64. Riekkinen, M, et al: Tetrahydroaminoacridine improves the recency effect in Alzheimer's disease. Neuroscience 83:471–479, 1998.

65. Rogers, SL, et al: A 24 week, double-blind, placebo-controlled trial of donepezil in patients with Alzheimer's disease. Neurology 50:136–145, 1998.

66. Patenaude, J: Nutrient deficiency-related depression and mental changes in elderly persons. Home Health Care Management and Practice 9(1):29–39, 1996.

67. Palmer, RM: "Failure to thrive" in the elderly: Diagnosis and management. Geriatrics 45(9):47–55, 1990.

68. Seligman, ME: In Fincham, FD and Cain KM: Learned helplessness in humans: A developmental analysis. Developmental Review 6:301–333, 1986.

69. Adelmann, PK: Multiple roles and psychological well being in a national sample of older adults. J Gerontol: Soc Sci 49:S277–S285, 1994.

70. Ruuskanen, JM, and Ruoppila, I: Physical activity and psychological well-being among people aged 65 to 84 years. Age Ageing 24:292–296, 1995.

Thanks in old age—thanks ere I go,
For health, the mid-day sun, the
impalpable air—
for life, mere life.
Walt Whitman
(*Leaves of Grass*, 1892)

Nutrition and the Elderly

Louise D. Whitney

BEHAVIORAL OBJECTIVES

Upon completion of this chapter, the reader will be able to:

1. Demonstrate knowledge of current research of the impact of aging on nutrition status for healthy individuals and individuals with chronic diseases.
2. Describe the importance of early screening and intervention for nutrition risk in the elderly.
3. Describe knowledge of available screening tools.
4. List the physiological impact of aging on nutrition.
5. Understand the special consideration of nutrition in the elderly (energy needs, protein requirements, modifications in the recommended dietary allowances (RDA) for the elderly, dental health, diabetes, constipation, cardiovascular disease, cancer).
6. Understand the multiple influences that affect nutrition status in the elderly (social, psychological, economic, and environmental).
7. Understand the impact of polypharmacy on nutrition status and drug and nutrient interactions in the elderly.
8. Understand the indications for supplemental nutrition in the elderly.

KEY TERMS

Antacids
Antidepressants
Anti-inflammatory
Carbohydrate
  Simple, Complex
Cholesterol
Diabetes
Dietary fiber
Diuretics
Essential nutrients

Exchanges for meal planning
Gastrointestinal
Glucose tolerance
Lactose intolerance
Lipid
Monounsaturated fat
Polyunsaturated fat
Saturated fat
Supplemental nutrition

INTRODUCTION

The importance of good nutrition throughout the life span and its contribution to health and quality of life cannot be overestimated. Good nutrition optimizes health and promotes wellness. A prudent diet strengthens the immune system and helps prevent the onset of many chronic diseases, such as cardiovascular disease, diabetes, and cancer.[1]

Good nutrition is especially important during the elderly years, when the myriad changes caused by aging can compromise health. An evaluation from the Elderly Nutrition Program of the Older Americans Act revealed that 76 to 88 percent of participants were at moderate to high nutritional risk.[1] In addition, it is estimated that 16 percent of the elderly do not have access at all times to a nutritionally adequate diet. However, while growing old is often associated with loss of well-being and mobility, the majority of older adults are able to maintain their health and quality of life. It is imperative that the health care professional show great sensitivity to the wide variation of physiological, socioeconomic, environmental, and psychological changes that accompany aging. Individually or in combination, these factors interact and influence nutritional status in older adults. These factors and their interactions are summarized in Box 5–1.

This chapter discusses the importance of early screening and intervention for nutrition risk in the elderly, an overview of basic human nutrition, the nutrition needs of the elderly, the physiological effects of aging on nutritional status, special considerations in aging and supplemental nutrition, and the impact of drugs on the nutritional status of older adults.

SCREENING AND INTERVENTION

THE NUTRITION SCREENING INITIATIVE

One of the best ways to achieve high-quality nutrition care for the elderly is to promote early screening and intervention. The American Dietetic Association, the American Academy of Family Physicians, and the National Council on Aging have collaborated in an effort called the Nutrition Screening Initiative,[2] to encourage early and routine screening and intervention for nutrition risk in the elderly. The premise of the initiative is that nutrition status is a "vital sign" that is just as important in evaluating a person's health and well-being as the traditional vital signs of blood pressure and pulse.

The result of the Nutrition Screening Initiative is a self-assessment checklist that could be used in a variety of settings to help identify whether the individual is at risk for compromised nutritional well-being. In addition to the self-assessment checklist, the acronym DETERMINE is an educational device that can be used along with the checklist to help identify the warning signs of poor nutritional status in the elderly. The self-assessment checklist and meaning of DETERMINE are presented in Boxes 5–2 and 5–3.

BASIC NUTRITION OVERVIEW

ESSENTIAL NUTRIENTS

There are six classes of nutrients that humans need to eat in order to be healthy: carbohydrates, proteins, fats, vitamins, minerals, and water. We must eat them because our bodies cannot make them. No matter what age, these nutrients are essential for promoting growth, maintenance, and repair of our bodies.

BOX 5–1. SUMMARY OF FACTORS THAT INFLUENCE NUTRITION IN THE ELDERLY

Physiological

Health status
Presence of chronic disease
Changes in appetite
Physical disability
Sensory acuity
Physical activity
Use of alcohol or other drugs
Lifelong diet habits

Socioeconomic

Culture/ethnicity
Income
Education
Lifestyle
Nutrition knowledge and practice
Cooking skills
Susceptibility to food fads
Institutionalization

Psychological

Belief system
Motivation
Self-image
Mental state
Degree of independence
Feeling of usefulness
Presence or absence of spouse
Social contacts
Loneliness

Continued on following page

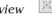

BOX 5–1. SUMMARY OF FACTORS THAT INFLUENCE NUTRITION IN THE ELDERLY (*Continued*)

Environmental

Type and location of housing
Adequacy of cooking facilities
Proximity of family and friends
Availability of transportation
Availability, accessibility, and adequacy of food supply
Health service

Source: Adapted from Boyle, M, and Zyla, G: Personal Nutrition. West Publishing, Minneapolis, MN, 1996, p 400.

Carbohydrates, protein, and fat are the energy nutrients. Vitamins and minerals do not yield energy. Carbohydrates are the preferred source of energy and are the ideal fuel for the body. Proteins too can be used as energy, but they are expensive and offer no physiological advantage over carbohydrates when used for energy. Fats are a dense source of calories but are not used efficiently by the brain and central nervous system. In addition, diets high in fat are associated with increased risk of several chronic diseases.

Measured in calories, 1 gram of carbohydrate yields 4 calories, 1 gram of protein yields 4 calories, and 1 gram of fat yields 9 calories.

Carbohydrates

Carbohydrates are classified as either simple or complex. **Simple carbohydrates** are sugars, and **complex carbohydrates** are starches. Most of our calories, at least 50 percent or more, should come from eating foods that are good sources of complex carbohydrates because they are nutrient rich and have fiber. Complex carbohydrates include grains, legumes (dried beans and peas), fruits and vegetables, cereals, pasta, and rice.

Foods that are high in simple sugars such as cakes, candies, cookies, and sodas are called empty-calorie foods because they are high in calories and low in nutrient value. Fruits and fruit juices also have simple sugars, but they come packaged from Mother Nature with many essential nutrients. No more than 20 percent of total carbohydrate calories should come from simple sugars.

Simple sugars or monosaccharides include

- Glucose, the sugar in our blood
- Fructose, the sugar in fruit and honey
- Galactose, the sugar made from milk sugar

**BOX 5–2. NUTRITION SCREENING INITIATIVE
SELF-ASSESSMENT CHECKLIST**

Answer the following questions as carefully as you can. If you answer
yes, then add up the points and compare with the point evaluation
scale at the end. This checklist will help you determine whether you
are nutritionally at risk.

Question	Yes?
I have an illness or condition that has recently made me change the kind and/or amount of food I eat.	2 pts
I eat fewer than two meals per day.	3
I rarely eat fruits, vegetables, and milk products.	2
I have three or more glasses of beer, liquor, or wine almost every day.	2
I have tooth or mouth problems that make it hard for me to eat.	2
I don't always have enough money to buy the food I need.	4
I eat alone most of the time.	1
I take three or more different prescription or over-the-counter drugs a day.	1
Without wanting to, I have lost or gained 10 pounds in the past 6 months.	2
I am not always physically able to shop, cook, and/or feed myself.	2

Total Score	—

Point Evaluation Scale

0–2 Good! Recheck your score in 6 months.
3–5 You are at a moderate nutritional risk. See what can be done to
improve your eating habits and lifestyle. The Area Agency of Aging,
senior nutrition program, senior citizen center, or health department
may be able to help. Recheck your score in 3 months.
6+ You are at nutritional risk. Bring this checklist the next time you
see your doctor, dietitian, or other qualified health care giver. Ask
for nutrition counseling.

Source: Adapted from the Nutrition Screening Initiative, a project of the American
Academy of Family Physicians, the American Dietetic Association, and the National Council on Aging, Inc.

BOX 5–3. DETERMINE

Use this to help you remember the warning signs of nutrition risk.

D **Disease**—The presence or absence of any disease that causes a change in the eating habits may make it harder to eat right and will increase risk. Four of five adults have chronic diseases that are affected by diet. Confusion and memory loss may make it harder to plan healthy diets and even remember what and when you last ate. Depression and loneliness can cause changes in appetite, digestion, energy level, weight, and well-being.

E **Eating poorly**—Both eating too little and eating too much can cause a decline in health status. Lack of variety, poor quality foods, and poor balance of food types all lead to poor nutritional health. Many elderly skip meals and eat fewer than the recommended five servings daily of fruits and vegetables. Alcohol consumption is a concern, with one in four adults drinking too much.

T **Tooth loss or mouth pain**—Healthy mouth, gums, and teeth are essential to good nutrition. When dental health is compromised, so is nutritional well-being.

E **Economic hardship**—Researchers estimate that 40% of older Americans have incomes of less than $6000 per year. Financial struggles may make it harder to eat right and stay healthy.

R **Reduced social contact**—One third of all older people live alone. For a variety of reasons, aging brings with it fewer meaningful social contacts. This too can affect nutritional well-being.

M **Multiple medicines**—Polypharmacy—the use of multiple drugs—can also compromise nutritional well-being. Almost half of older Americans take multiple medicines daily. Some of the side effects include changes in appetite and taste, constipation, weakness, and nausea.

I **Involuntary weight gain or loss**—Changes in weight (more than just a few pounds) should always be seen as a warning sign that a person's nutrition status may be compromised.

N **Needs assistance in self-care**—One in five elderly needs help with walking, shopping, cooking, and feeding.

E **Elder years past age 80**—Increasing age brings increased risk of health problems. Be sure to see your physician regularly, at least on an annual basis.

Source: Adapted from the Nutrition Screening Initiative, a project of the American Academy of Family Physicians, the American Dietetic Association, and the National Council on Aging, Inc.

Disaccharides include

- Sucrose, the sugar in white or brown sugar
- Lactose, the sugar in milk
- Maltose, the sugar in malt

Polysaccharides or starches include

- Starch, found in plants such as grains, fruits and vegetables, and legumes
- Glycogen, the storage form of complex carbohydrates in animals

Fiber

One type of complex carbohydrate that is important in nutrition is fiber. The major sources of dietary fiber include whole grains, fruits and vegetables, legumes, nuts, and seeds. Unfortunately much of the fiber in our diet in this country is processed away when whole grains are refined and the bran portion is removed.

Fiber, while not an essential nutrient, is necessary to keep our intestinal tract healthy. It binds water, causing softer, bulkier stools that move through the intestinal tract more quickly. Because fiber helps move the waste matter through the intestines quickly, researchers believe diets with adequate fiber help reduce risk of colon cancer.[3] Fiber is also thought to bind carcinogens, or cancer-causing agents, and stools with more water lessen the potency of the cancer-causing agents in the waste material.[4]

Adequate fiber also helps prevent constipation, diverticular disease, and hemorrhoids.[5] In addition, certain types of fiber such as soluble fiber—like that found in legumes, oats, rice, and fruit—may help lower cholesterol levels.[6,7] This benefit of fiber might help lower heart disease risk.

Protein

Proteins are the main substances that the body uses to build and repair tissues such as muscle, blood, internal organs, hair, nails, and bones. Proteins are part of hormones, antibodies, and enzymes. Enzymes are proteins that catalyze the biochemical reactions that take place in the metabolism of the body.

The building blocks of proteins are amino acids. There are 20 amino acids used by the body, but only 9 of them are essential because the body cannot make them. The other 11 can be formed in the body. The presence or absence of the essential amino acids determines the quality of the protein. All animal protein is of high quality, containing all the essential amino acids. Vegetable proteins are all incomplete, meaning that they are missing one or more of the essential amino acids.

How much protein do we need each day? High-quality protein should comprise anywhere from 15 to 20 percent of total calorie intake. But certain physiological situations may dictate that protein intake be higher or lower. (A more complete discussion of protein needs for the elderly follows in the section titled Special Considerations.)

People who are vegetarians must plan their meals carefully so that they include protein of adequate quality and quantity. The primary sources of protein for vegetarians are legumes, grains, nuts, and seeds. But because each of these protein foods lacks one or more of the essential amino acids, they must be combined so that all essential amino acids are eaten. The basic rule is to combine grains with legumes, legumes with nuts or seeds, or grains with nuts or seeds. In addition, any animal protein will complement any plant protein. For example, macaroni (a grain) is complemented with cheese (an animal protein). A good example of a high-quality nonanimal protein source would be red beans and rice. Other examples include, pasta and low-fat cheese sauce, tofu and sesame seeds, or tortilla and black beans.

Fats

The primary function of fats, or **lipids,** in the body is as a rich source of energy. Fat helps insulate and regulate body temperature, it surrounds internal organs and protects them from external injury, and it is the carrier of the fat-soluble vitamins A, D, E, and K. There are two essential fatty acids, linoleic and linolenic acid. They are widely distributed in plant foods, oil, and fish.

In recent years, there has been a heightened interest and awareness of the amount and type of fat in our diets. Research has implicated high-fat diets in a number of chronic, debilitating diseases, such as cardiovascular disease and cancer.[1] In our zeal to reduce the amount of fat we eat, we sometimes forget that fat is a nutrient and that we do need it—in the right quantity. Although recommendations may vary slightly, most health promotion organizations urge a reduction in fat. Fat calories should account for no more than 30 percent of total calories.

About 95 percent of the fat in the foods we eat and the fat in the human body are known as triglycerides. Other types of fats are phospholipids (e.g., lecithin) and sterols (e.g., cholesterol). A triglyceride is made up of three units of fatty acids and one unit of glycerol.

Fatty acids can be further divided into three categories, saturated, polyunsaturated, and monounsaturated. **Saturated fats** are solid at room temperature and are primarily found in animal foods. Beef fat, lard, and butter fat are all examples of saturated fats. **Polyunsaturated fats** are liquid at room temperature and are found in plant products; examples are corn, safflower, and sunflower oils. **Monounsaturated fats,** such as olive, peanut, and canola oils, also tend to be more liquid at room temperature. There are a couple of exceptions. Palm and coconut oils are from plants but they are highly saturated fats.

These distinctions regarding type of fat are important because of the effects these fats have on cholesterol. **Cholesterol** is a waxy substance that is found only in animal products. It is made by the human body and is necessary in making cell membranes, as a building block of some hormones, and is involved in the digestion of fats via bile. Polyunsaturated and monounsaturated fats tend to lower blood cholesterol, and saturated fats tend to elevate blood cholesterol, thereby elevating risk for cardiovascular disease.

Another type of lipid that is important in determining risk for cardiovascular disease is lipoproteins. Lipoproteins are compounds that are involved in carrying fats around the body. Research has shown that as important as it is, total cholesterol is not the only predictive factor in risk for heart disease.[1] Knowing the amounts of the two types of lipoproteins are also important. High-density lipoproteins (HDL) are associated with reduced risk for heart disease, and low-density lipoproteins (LDL) are associated with increased risk. A summary of fats follows.

Polyunsaturated fats

- Are liquid at room temperature
- Are from plants
- Help lower cholesterol levels
- Are corn and safflower oils

Monounsaturated fats

- Are more liquid at room temperature
- Help lower cholesterol levels
- Are olive, peanut, and canola oils

Saturated fats

- Are solid at room temperature
- Are of animal origin
- Elevate cholesterol levels
- Are lard, tallow, butter, and animal fats

When cholesterol levels are high, the health of the arteries and veins is in jeopardy because elevated cholesterol levels cause plaque to build up in the inner lining of the vessel wall. This plaque can harden and restrict the flow of blood. When blood supply is cut off to the heart, part of the heart tissue dies, resulting in a heart attack. When blood supply is cut off to the brain, a stroke occurs.

The general guidelines recommended by the National Cholesterol Education Program is to keep blood cholesterol below 200 mg/dL. LDL cholesterol should be less than 130 mg/dL, and HDL cholesterol should be at or above 45 mg/dL for men and at or above 55 mg/dL for women.

The dietary recommendations to reduce the risk of cardiovascular disease focus on cutting back on fat in general and in particular trying to substitute more monounsaturated and polyunsaturated fat. The following are some suggestions for a heart-healthy diet:

- Choose lean cuts of meat, trim all the fat you can see, and throw away the fat that cooks out of the meat during cooking.
- Use no more than a total of 5 to 8 teaspoons of fats and oils per day for cooking, baking, and salads.
- Use low-fat or nonfat dairy products.
- Try main dishes featuring pasta, rice, beans, and/or vegetables, or create new dishes by mixing small amounts of meats with legumes and/or grains.
- Use no more than 3 to 4 egg yolks a week, including those used in cooking.
- Limit your intake of high-fat meats and organ meats.
- Control the amount of butter, margarine, and cream cheese you add to bread, pasta, and rice.
- Use small amounts of olive oil in cooking, and use oil and vinegar dressings for salads. You could also try reduced-fat or fat-free salad dressings.

Vitamins

Vitamins are substances that are needed by the body to maintain metabolism, growth, and development. There are 13 vitamins, which are divided into two categories. The water-soluble vitamins include vitamins C and B complex. Fat-soluble vitamins include A, D, E, and K. The best way to ensure adequate vitamin intake is through a well-balanced and varied diet. Fruits and vegetables are loaded with vitamins, but vitamins are found in the other food groups too. See Table 5–1 for a summary of the vitamins, their functions, and food sources.

Do the elderly need a multivitamin supplement? In certain circumstances, a multivitamin supplement might be used to ensure adequate intake of nutrients. This is particularly true if the health care practitioner suspects poor or inadequate food intake, if laboratory results reveal a deficiency, or if there is some other reason why an individual may not be getting enough nutrients through the diet. Vitamin supplements should not be used in place of eating good foods, nor should they be carelessly taken. Older patients should always advise their physician if they use a multivitamin (and mineral supplement). Regardless of age, it is always best to eat a balanced and varied diet that is planned with an eye to ensuring adequate intake of essential nutrients instead of relying on supplements.

Of interest to the issue of aging are vitamins that act as antioxidants, beta-carotene (a water-soluble precursor of vitamin A), vitamins C, and E. Antioxidants are thought to help diminish the effects of aging by preventing damage to cells and tissues by free radicals (a by-product of metabolism). They may also be involved as a protective factor in reducing risk for heart dis-

TABLE 5–1. *A Guide to the Vitamins*

Vitamin (Chemical Name)	Best Sources	Chief Roles	Deficiency Symptoms	Toxicity Symptoms
Water-soluble Vitamins				
Thiamin	Meat, pork, liver, fish, poultry, whole-grain and enriched breads, cereals, pasta, nuts, legumes, wheat germ, oats.	Helps enzymes release energy from carbohydrate; supports normal appetite and nervous system function.	Beriberi: edema, heart irregularity, mental confusion, muscle weakness, impaired growth.	Rapid pulse, weakness, headaches, insomnia, irritability.
Riboflavin	Milk, dark green vegetables, yogurt, cottage cheese, liver, meat, whole-grain or enriched breads and cereals.	Helps enzymes release energy from carbohydrate, fat, and protein; promotes healthy skin and normal vision.	Eye problems, skin disorders around nose and mouth.	None reported, but an excess of any of the B vitamins could cause a deficiency of the others.
Niacin	Meat, eggs, poultry, fish, milk, whole-grain and enriched breads and cereals, nuts, legumes, peanuts, nutritional yeast, all protein foods.	Helps enzymes release energy from energy nutrients; promotes health of skin, nerves, and digestive system.	Pellagra: skin rash on parts exposed to sun, loss of appetite, dizziness, weakness, fatigue, mental confusion, indigestion.	Flushing, nausea, headaches, cramps, ulcer irritation, heartburn, abnormal liver function, low blood pressure.
Vitamin B$_6$ (pyridoxine)	Meat, poultry, fish, shellfish, legumes, whole-grain products, green leafy vegetables, bananas.	Protein and fat metabolism; formation of antibodies and red blood cells; helps convert tryptophan to niacin.	Nervous disorders, skin rash, muscle weakness, anemia, convulsions, kidney stones.	Depression, fatigue, irritability, headaches, numbness, damage to nerves, difficulty walking.
Folate	Green leafy vegetables,	Red blood cell formation;	Anemia, heartburn,	Diarrhea, insomnia,

Continued on following page

TABLE 5–1. *A Guide to the Vitamins (Continued)*

Vitamin (Chemical Name)	Best Sources	Chief Roles	Deficiency Symptoms	Toxicity Symptoms
	liver, legumes, seeds.	protein metabolism; new cell division.	diarrhea, smooth tongue, depression, poor growth.	irritability, may mask a vitamin B_{12} deficiency.
Vitamin B_{12} (cobalamin)	Animal products: meat, fish, poultry, shellfish, milk, cheese, eggs; nutritional yeast.	Helps maintain nerve cells; red blood cell formation; synthesis of genetic material.	Anemia, smooth tongue, fatigue, nerve degeneration progressing to paralysis.	None reported.
Pantothenic acid	Widespread in foods.	Coenzyme in energy metabolism.	Rare; sleep disturbances, nausea, fatigue.	Occasional diarrhea.
Biotin	Widespread in foods.	Coenzyme in energy metabolism; fat synthesis; glycogen formation.	Loss of appetite, nausea, depression, muscle pain, weakness, fatigue, rash.	None reported.
Vitamin C (ascorbic acid)	Citrus fruits, cabbage-type vegetables, tomatoes, potatoes, dark green vegetables, peppers, lettuce, cantaloupe, strawberries, mangos, papayas.	Synthesis of collagen (helps heal wounds, maintains bone and teeth, strengthens blood vessels); antioxidant; strengthens resistance to infection; helps body absorb iron.	Scurvy: anemia, atherosclerotic plaques, depression, frequent infections, bleeding gums, loosened teeth, pinpoint hemorrhages, muscle degeneration, rough skin, bone fragility, poor wound healing, hysteria.	Nausea, abdominal cramps, diarrhea, nosebleeds, deficiency symptoms may appear at first on withdrawal of high doses.
Fat-soluble Vitamins				
Vitamin A	*Retinol:* fortified milk and margarine, cream, cheese, butter, eggs, liver.	Vision; growth and repair of body tissues; reproduction; bone and tooth formation;	Night blindness, rough skin, susceptibility to infection, impaired bone growth,	Red blood cell breakage, nosebleeds, abdominal cramps, nausea,

Continued on following page

TABLE 5–1. *A Guide to the Vitamins* (*Continued*)

Vitamin (Chemical Name)	Best Sources	Chief Roles	Deficiency Symptoms	Toxicity Symptoms
	Beta-carotene: Spinach and other dark leafy greens, broccoli, deep orange fruits (apricots, peaches, cantaloupe), and vegetables (squash, carrots, sweet potatoes, pumpkin).	immunity; hormone synthesis; antioxidant (in the form of beta-carotene only).	abnormal tooth and jaw alignment, eye problems leading to blindness, impaired growth.	diarrhea, weight loss, blurred vision, irritability, loss of appetite, bone pain, dry skin, rashes, hair loss, cessation of menstruation, growth retardation; liver disease.
Vitamin D (cholecal-ciferol)	Self-synthesis with sunlight; fortified milk, fortified margarine, eggs, liver, fish.	Calcium and phosphorus metabolism (bone and tooth formation); aids body's absorption of calcium.	Rickets in children; osteomalacia in adults; abnormal growth, joint pain, soft bones.	Raised blood calcium, constipation, weight loss, irritability, weakness, nausea, kidney stones, mental and physical retardation.
Vitamin E	Vegetable oils, green leafy vegetables, wheat germ, whole-grain products, butter, liver, egg yolk, milk fat, nuts, seeds.	Protects red blood cells; antioxidant.	Muscle wasting, weakness, red blood cell breakage, anemia, hemorrhaging.	General discomfort.
Vitamin K	Bacterial synthesis in digestive tract, liver, green leafy and cabbage-type vegetables, milk.	Synthesis of blood-clotting proteins and a blood protein that regulates blood calcium.	Hemorrhaging.	May cause jaundice.

Source: Recommended Dietary Allowances 10th edition National Research Council National Academy Press 1989 and adapted from Boyle, M and Zyla, G: Personal Nutrition. West Publishing Company, Minneapolis, MN, 1996.

ease and cancer.[8] Antioxidants have also recently been linked to changes in visual capacity and macular degeneration.[9,10] Good food sources of these antioxidants include citrus fruits, green peppers, cantaloupe, apricots, carrots, sweet potatoes, and vegetable oils.

Minerals

There are 23 minerals that are essential for human nutrition. They perform numerous functions in the body, including metabolism, maintenance of fluid balance, bone and teeth formation, blood clotting, muscle and nerve function, and formation of red blood cells.

The three most commonly discussed minerals are sodium, because of its association with hypertension; calcium, because of its association with bone health; and iron, because of its association with anemia. See Table 5–2 for a summary of minerals, their functions, and food sources.

The estimated minimum intake of sodium for most adults is 500 mg/day. Sodium intake in the elderly may need to be monitored if hypertension is present. Blood pressure is best controlled with weight reduction (if overweight), moderate exercise, and controlling intake of salt. With elevated blood pressure, the physician will recommend specific guidelines for sodium restriction.

Water

Last, but certainly not least, is water. Approximately 70 percent of total body weight is water. Water is the most important nutrient and is involved in almost every vital body process. Everyone is encouraged to drink at least eight 8-ounce glasses of fluid a day.

PLANNING MEALS WITH GOOD NUTRITION IN MIND

One of the challenges of nutrition is applying the knowledge of what is necessary to eat on a day-by-day and meal-by-meal basis. There are some important nutrition concepts that should be applied when planning meals. Keeping these meal planning principles in mind will help ensure good nutrition:
    These are:

- **Adequacy**—A diet that provides enough of the essential nutrients, fiber and energy.
- **Balance**—A diet that does not overemphasize one food at the expense of another
- **Calorie control**—A diet that has enough calories to maintain a healthy weight
- **Moderation**—A diet that does not contain excess amounts of unwanted items such as sugar, salt, and fat
- **Variety** A diet that has many different nutrient-rich foods

TABLE 5–2. *A Guide to the Minerals*

Mineral	Best Sources	Chief Roles	Deficiency Symptoms	Toxicity Symptoms
Major Minerals				
Calcium	Milk and milk products, small fish (with bones), tofu, certain green vegetables, legumes.	Principal mineral of bones and teeth; involved in muscle contraction and relaxation, nerve function, blood clotting, blood pressure.	Stunted growth in children; bone loss (osteoporosis) in adults.	Intestinal gas, kidney stones, constipation.
Phosphorus	All animal tissues.	Part of every cell; involved in acid-base balance.	Unknown.	Can create relative deficiency of calcium, tetany and convulsions.
Magnesium	Nuts, legumes, whole grains, dark green vegetables, seafoods, chocolate, cocoa.	Involved in bone mineralization, protein synthesis, enzyme action, normal muscular contraction, nerve transmission, lung function.	Weakness, confusion, depressed pancreatic hormone secretion, growth failure, behavioral disturbances, muscle spasms.	Not known.
Sodium	Salt, soy sauce; processed foods: cured, canned, pickled and many boxed foods.	Helps maintain normal fluid and acid-base balance.	Muscle cramps, mental apathy, loss of appetite.	High blood pressure (in salt-sensitive persons).
Chloride	Salt, soy sauce, processed foods.	Part of stomach acid, necessary for proper digestion, fluid balance.	Growth failure in children, muscle cramps, mental apathy, loss of appetite.	Normally harmless (the gas chlorine is a poison but evaporates from water); disturbed acid-base balance; vomiting.
Potassium	All whole foods: meats, milk, fruits, vegetables,	Facilitates many reactions, including protein synthesis,	Muscle weakness, paralysis, confusion; can cause	Causes muscular weakness; triggers

Continued on following page

TABLE 5–2. *A Guide to the Minerals (Continued)*

Mineral	Best Sources	Chief Roles	Deficiency Symptoms	Toxicity Symptoms
	grains, legumes.	fluid balance, nerve transmission, and contraction of muscles.	death; accompanies dehydration.	vomiting; if given into a vein, can stop the heart.
Sulfur	All protein-containing foods.	Component of certain amino acids; part of biotin, thiamin, and insulin; acid-base balance, drug detoxifying pathways.	None known; protein deficiency would occur first.	May depress growth.
Trace Minerals				
Iodine	Iodized salt, seafood, bread.	Part of thyroxine, which regulates metabolism.	Golter, cretinism.	Very high intakes depress thyroid activity.
Iron	Beef, fish, poultry, shellfish, eggs, legumes, dried fruits, fortified cereals.	Hemoglobin formation; part of myoglobin; energy utilization.	Anemia; weakness, pallor, headaches, reduced immunity, inability to concentrate, cold intolerance.	Iron overload: infections, liver injury, possible increased risk of heart attack.
Zinc	Protein-containing foods: meats, fish, poultry, grains, vegetables.	Part of many enzymes; present in insulin; involved in making genetic material and proteins, immunity, vitamin A transport, taste, wound healing, making sperm, normal fetal development.	Growth failure in children, delayed development of sexual organs, loss of taste, poor wound healing.	Fever, nausea, vomiting, diarrhea.
Copper	Meats, drinking water.	Absorption of iron; part of several enzymes.	Anemia, bone changes (rare in human beings).	Unknown except as part of a rare hereditary disease (Wilson's disease).

Continued on following page

TABLE 5–2. A Guide to the Minerals (Continued)

Mineral	Best Sources	Chief Roles	Deficiency Symptoms	Toxicity Symptoms
Fluoride	Drinking water (if naturally fluoride containing or fluoridated), tea, seafood.	Formation of bones and teeth; helps make teeth resistant to decay and bones resistant to mineral loss.	Susceptibility to tooth decay and bone loss.	Fluorosis (discoloration of teeth).
Selenium	Seafood, meats, grains.	Helps protect body compounds from oxidation.	Anemia (rare).	Digestive system disorders.
Chromium	Meats, unrefined foods, fats, vegetable oils.	Associated with insulin and required for the release of energy from glucose.	Diabetes-like condition marked by inability to use glucose normally.	Unknown as a nutrition disorder. Occupational exposures damage skin and kidneys.
Molybdenum	Legumes, cereals, organ meats.	Facilitates, with enzymes, many cell processes.	Unknown.	Enzyme inhibition.
Manganese	Widely distributed in foods.	Facilitates, with enzymes, many cell processes.	In animals: poor growth, nervous system disorders, abnormal reproduction.	Poisoning, nervous system disorders.
Cobalt	Meats, milk, and milk products.	As part of vitamin B_{12}, involved in nerve function and blood formation.	Unknown except in vitamin B_{12} deficiency	Unknown as a nutrition disorder.

Source: Recommended Dietary Allowances 10th edition National Research Council National Academy Press 1989 and adapted from Boyle, M and Zyla, G: Personal Nutrition. West Publishing Company, Minneapolis, MN, 1996.

THE FOOD GUIDE PYRAMID

The Food Guide Pyramid is an excellent tool for planning meals with good nutrition in mind (Fig. 5–1). The pyramid provides general information and was designed so that the placement of the food groups on the pyramid emphasizes their role in the diet. In addition, the pyramid was designed to incorporate the dietary guidelines stressing the preference for foods low in fat, saturated fat, sugar, and sodium.

Food Guide Pyramid

A Guide to Daily Food Choices

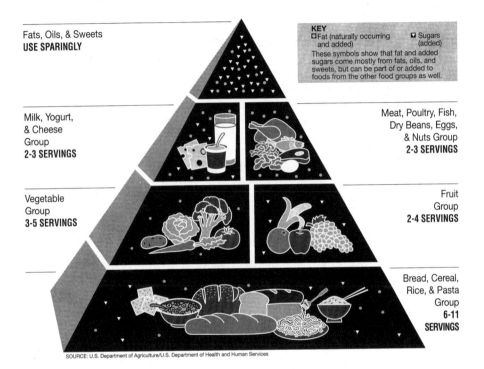

Fats, Oils, & Sweets
USE SPARINGLY

KEY
☐ Fat (naturally occurring   ☐ Sugars
and added)   (added)
These symbols show that fat and added
sugars come mostly from fats, oils, and
sweets, but can be part of or added to
foods from the other food groups as well.

Milk, Yogurt,
& Cheese
Group
2-3 SERVINGS

Meat, Poultry, Fish,
Dry Beans, Eggs,
& Nuts Group
2-3 SERVINGS

Vegetable
Group
3-5 SERVINGS

Fruit
Group
2-4 SERVINGS

Bread, Cereal,
Rice, & Pasta
Group
**6-11
SERVINGS**

SOURCE: U.S. Department of Agriculture/U.S. Department of Health and Human Services

FIG. 5–1. The Food Guide Pyramid. (Courtesy of U.S. Department of Agriculture, Center for Nutrition Policy and Promotion, Washington, DC.)

The foundation of the pyramid includes bread, cereal, rice, and pasta, and these are the foods that should form the foundation of our diets. Choose 6 to 11 servings a day based on caloric needs, and choose whole grains whenever possible.

The next groups are fruits and vegetables. Each day, choose a green and a vitamin C–rich fruit or vegetable such as oranges, green peppers, or papaya. Also choose a deep orange fruit or vegetable such as carrots, sweet potatoes, and apricots. Note that the recommended number of servings from the combined fruit and vegetable group is from five to nine. The recommended minimum from both groups together is five.

The next group is the milk, yogurt, and cheese group. The recommended number of servings is from two or three, and the best choices are low in fat. Next to dairy is the meat, poultry, fish, dry beans, eggs, and nuts group. To reduce fat intake, choose low-fat meats and use legumes in place of meats whenever you can. Healthy individuals not on protein restriction should have two to three servings daily. At the top, are fats, oils, and sweets, which should be used sparingly.

FOOD PREPARATION TIPS FOR THE ELDERLY

There are several suggestions for food preparation specifically for the elderly:

- Eat regular meals. Small, frequent meals may be best. Use nutrient-dense foods as the basis for each meal.
- Put the focus on foods that are low in fat, sugar, cholesterol, and salt. Read labels so you know what you are buying.
- Don't be hesitant to check out convenience foods that are healthy and tasty. Many grocers now carry already prepared fruits and vegetables in single portions. Look for meats that have already been trimmed and cut up and are ready for cooking.
- Keep some quick and easy snacks on hand for times when you don't feel like cooking. There is nothing wrong with making a meal of snacks, as long as they are healthy.
- Make your eating environment cheerful. Perhaps you could read a book, listen to music, or watch television when eating.
- Keep food preparation simple. This will make clean-up easier too.
- Keep moving. Engage in regular exercise, it will help stimulate your appetite.
- Consider shopping, preparing, and eating cooperatively with neighbors and friends. It will put some excitement back into your meals.
- Steam vegetables or fruits (rather than boiling). This will make them easier to chew.
- When you do cook, prepare a double portion and freeze half for later use.

RECOMMENDED DIETARY ALLOWANCES

If the health care provider needs more specific information regarding individual nutrients and the recommended amounts, the recommended dietary allowances (RDA) could be consulted. The RDA are guidelines set by the National Academy of Sciences/National Research Council and are based on the latest scientific evidence regarding health and diet. They are recommendations, not requirements, and are not intended to be used by individuals in planning meals to meet nutrient needs. Rather, they are used to estimate adequacy of an individual's food intake or the adequacy of an eating plan. See Box 5–4 for a summary of the RDA.

BOX 5–4. HOW MANY SERVINGS DO YOU NEED EACH DAY?

	Women & some older adults	Children, teen girls, active women, most men	Teen boys & active men
Calorie level*	about 1,600	about 2,200	about 2,800
Bread group	6	9	11
Vegetable group	3	4	5
Fruit group	2	3	4
Milk group	†2–3	†2–3	†2–3
Meat group	2, for a total of 5 ounces	2, for a total of 6 ounces	3 for a total of 7 ounces

*These are the calorie levels if you choose lowfat, lean foods from the 5 major food groups and use foods from the fats, oils, and sweets group sparingly.

†Women who are pregnant or breastfeeding, teenagers, and young adults to age 24 need 3 servings.

Based on USDA Food Guide Pyramid and the US RDA.

🔲 SPECIAL CONSIDERATIONS

There are some special considerations when planning meals to meet nutrient needs for the elderly.

ENERGY NEEDS

When considering energy needs for the older adult, changes in metabolic rate due to decreasing physical activity and loss of lean tissue translate into decreased calorie needs. There is an estimated reduction in need of nearly 400 calories per day from age 26 to 60.[1] Therefore the RDA for energy is lower for adults beginning at age 51. The estimated average energy allowance for men 51 years and older is 2300 kcal, and for women, 1900 kcal. These figures are only estimated averages and cannot be applied to every individual in every situation. Coming to specific conclusions regarding daily calorie needs requires knowledge of an individual's recent weight history, current goals, activity levels, lifestyle, eating habits, and the presence or absence of diseases that might affect energy needs. In general, older adults need to be mindful that it is important to choose nutrient-dense foods and limit their intake of high-calorie, low-nutrient foods.

If, however, the older adult chooses to participate in regular physical activity, calorie needs may be adjusted upward, allowing for more flexibility in meal planning. Increased calorie intake would also provide more opportunities to ensure adequate nutrient intake.

When weight loss is indicated, under no circumstances should caloric intake fall below 1200 kcal/day unless the individual is under the direct supervision of a physician. Intakes of less than 1200 kcal/day make it very difficult to meet basic nutrient needs. Weight loss should always be undertaken with the direction of a dietitian or physician and should include regular moderate activity, and a balanced diet. Limiting the consumption of high-fat and high-sugar foods and controlling intake of alcohol will stimulate weight loss. Weight loss should not exceed 1 to 2 pounds per week.

If weight loss is a concern, then calories would need to be increased to reestablish a healthy body weight. This could mean increasing intake from between 500 and 1000 kcal per day. It is often much more difficult to gain weight than it is to lose it, so creativity is called for in helping an individual think of ways to increase calorie intake (see Liquid Nutritional Supplements later).

PROTEIN

Research has suggested that it is possible that the current RDA for protein for the elderly is low.[11] While an intake of protein at 0.8 g/kg of body weight is sufficient for younger adults, the elderly are encouraged to increase protein intake slightly to 1 g/kg body weight. This increased need is due in part to reduced protein digestion and absorption with aging. In addition, stressful situations such as infection or chronic disease reduce the efficiency of protein use. Increased protein intake may also help stave off lean tissue loss that accompanies aging. Protein deficiency results in chronic eczema, fatigue, muscle weakness, reduced resistance to disease, slower wound healing, and tissue wasting.

Because protein-rich foods are often more expensive, they are often eaten less often by the elderly. In addition, if overall food intake is low, then protein intake is likely to be low. Along with reduced protein intake also comes lower intakes of several vitamins and minerals.

CARBOHYDRATES

Aging also brings about reduced **glucose tolerance**. There may be more susceptibility to temporary hyperglycemic and hypoglycemic episodes. With a high sugar load, glucose levels return much more slowly in the elderly. High-sugar treats and sweets should be limited so as to avoid these sugar highs and lows.

The older person who has **diabetes** needs regular help in adhering to a diet to manage blood-glucose levels, whether or not she or he is insulin dependent. The individual needs to work with his or her physician and dietitian in order to formulate a diet plan. The dietitian and patient need to work together to develop workable menus that provide good control and take into consideration the food and lifestyle habits of the patient.

One of the best ways to plan a diabetic diet is with diabetic **exchanges for meal planning.** This allows freedom of choice for the patient at the same time that calories and carbohydrate intake are controlled.

The exchange method was developed in 1950 by the American Diabetic Association, the American Dietetic Association, and the U.S. Public Health Service. The method groups foods according to their carbohydrate, protein, fat, and calorie content. The exchange groups include:

- Milk—milk, yogurt
- Vegetables—fresh, frozen, canned vegetables
- Fruit—fresh, frozen, canned, dried fruits, and fruit juices
- Breads—breads, cereals, grains, legumes, crackers
- Meat—lean, medium, and high fat
- Fats—butter, margarine, bacon, cream cheese, olives, oils, dressings
- Beverages, seasoning, condiments, and foods allowed as desired

Within each group are specified foods and their portions. So, for example, if an individual is allowed 2 bread exchanges, 1 fruit exchange, and 1 milk exchange for breakfast, he or she could have a serving of cereal, bread, or muffins, a serving of a fruit or juice, and a serving of milk or yogurt.

Nutrition counseling is required to instruct the patient how to use the exchanges to plan their eating. Most patients also benefit from additional counseling a few months after the initial session. This will help the patients refine their diet plan so that it really works for them. The exchange method can also be adapted to use for patients requiring fat, cholesterol, sodium, or protein restrictions.

A special note is needed here regarding nutrition counseling in general. First, counseling provides the patient with an opportunity to make the diet prescription from the physician fit his or her individual needs. The dietitian will take into consideration all the factors that influence a person's eating habits and will structure an eating plan to provide for optimal nutrition. The American Dietetic Association can provide physicians and patients with the names and telephone numbers of registered dietitians in their area.

Another concern for many elderly individuals is **lactose intolerance,** an inability to break down the carbohydrate (lactose) found in most dairy products. This can cause intestinal disturbances such as gas, bloating, diarrhea, and cramping.

VITAMINS AND MINERALS

Research has led some to suggest that the RDA for several vitamins and minerals may need to be modified to meet the changing needs of the elderly. The following is a summary of the changes in vitamin and mineral needs with aging:[11]

- **Vitamin A**
  Use caution with supplements because there is increased absorption and toxic levels may occur.

- **Vitamin D**
  Increase intake to 400 to 800 IU. Current RDA is 200 IU. There is less exposure to sunlight in the elderly, reduced dermal synthesis of vitamin D, and reduced metabolism of vitamin D in the kidney.
- **Vitamin B$_6$**
  Although no recommended amount has been suggested, there is a reduction in blood levels of vitamin B$_6$ that accompanies aging.
- **Vitamin B$_{12}$**
  Increase to 3 μg. Current RDA is 2 μg. There is debate in this area. Some researchers believe that increasing intake will not change serum levels because there is decreased absorption due to changes in gastric acidity. Therefore, researchers recommend aggressive screening for low serum levels of vitamin B$_{12}$ followed by intramuscular injections to correct the problem.
- **Calcium**
  Increase to 1500 mg. Current RDA is 800 mg. There is decreased absorption of calcium in women especially after menopause. Additional calcium intake will help prevent bone loss in nonvertebral bones such as the hip.

LIQUID NUTRITIONAL SUPPLEMENTS

As has been discussed, there are a myriad of changes that occur with aging that affect nutritional well-being. When weight loss occurs or food intake is compromised, or if multiple vitamin or mineral deficiencies are suspected, liquid nutrition supplements are often an ideal way to correct the situation.

Products such as Ensure by Ross or Sustacal by Mead Johnson are **supplemental nutrition** formulas that can help correct inadequacies in several areas. These products are liquid and can be consumed as is, or added to recipes, soups, or other liquids. They are flavored and are easy to use.

These companies all have consumer hotline numbers with staff available to answer questions about composition. They also have ideas for including the product into the meal plan. See Table 5–3 for a summary of these products.

TABLE 5–3. *Summary of Liquid Supplementals*

Product	Company	Calories per 8 ounces	Protein	Fat
Ensure	Advanced Formula Ross Products	250 calories	9 g	6 g
Sustacal	Mead Johnson	240 calories	14.5 g	9 g
Boost	Mead Johnson	240 calories	10.2 g	4.1 g
ChoiceDM*	Mead Johnson	250 calories	10.6 g	12 g

Prepared with material provided by Ross Products and Mead Johnson.
*For use with diabetics.

PHYSIOLOGICAL IMPACT OF AGING ON NUTRITION

DECREASED APPETITE, FOOD INTAKE, AND WEIGHT LOSS

One of the critical physiological changes that accompany aging is decreased appetite, food intake, and subsequent loss of body weight. Decreases in body weight are common in adults ages 65 to 90, and this should always be seen as a warning that the individual may be at nutritional risk. There are several explanations for a decrease in appetite and food intake that may lead to weight loss.

First, aging brings about changes in the endocrine system that regulate hunger, appetite, and satiety. In addition, loss of lean tissue because of decreased physical activity and the normal aging process reduces metabolic rate, and this too may result in decreased appetite. Changes in taste and smell, which begin around age 60 and become pronounced at age 70, may also account for reduced appetite. Reduced taste and smell acuity can also be caused by certain drugs and medications. Additionally, zinc deficiencies can also lead to loss of taste. Table 5–4 presents a summary of the effects of certain categories of drugs. Table 5–5 lists food sources of zinc.

In addition to physiological changes, for many the elderly years are a time of great change socially. With the death of a spouse and or friends, many elderly find themselves living alone and eating meals alone. Changes in income due to retirement can mean that fewer resources are available for food purchases. Both of these can contribute to reduced food intake.

When weight losses of 5 percent or more in 1 month or 10 percent or more

---

TABLE 5–4. *Drugs That Affect Appetite*

Depress and or delay appetite:

- Phenylpropanolamine (decongestant)
- Amphetamines
- Mazindol (appetite suppressant drug)

Depress appetite and enhance satiety: (meaning shorter meal periods)

- Fenfluramine (appetite suppressant drug)

Stimulate appetite:

- Cyproheptadine (appetite stimulant)
- Lithium (psychiatric)
- Tranquilizers
- Corticosteroids

Source: Physician's Handbook of Nutrition Support. Department of Dietetics, The University of Michigan Hospitals, 1988.

TABLE 5–5. Food Sources of Zinc

RDA:		
Females 51+	12 mg	
Males 51+	15 mg	
Oysters	3 ounces	77 mg
Sirloin steak	3 ounces	5.5 mg
Raisin bran	1 cup	2.97 mg
Yogurt	1 cup	2.20 mg
Swiss cheese	1.5 ounces	1.66 mg
Peanuts	⅓ cup	1.61 mg
Black beans	½ cup	1 mg

Source: Nutritive Value of American Foods in Common Units. Agriculture Handbook No 456. U.S. Department of Agriculture, Washington, DC, 1988.

in 6 months occur, the health care provider needs to aggressively pursue ways to stimulate appetite and increase food intake. Sensitivity to the possible causes of the weight loss will aid in finding ways to make foods appealing and attractive. New food combinations, and new and stronger seasonings may make old favorites more palatable. Modifying food preparation techniques may also help stimulate interest in eating. Great care should be given to being sure that nutrient-dense foods are eaten. To encourage weight gain, healthy snacking and a high-calorie nutritional supplement might be in order. (For additional information see section on Liquid Nutritional Supplements earlier.)

Suggestions to increase appetite for those who need to do so include the following:

- Suggest regular moderate exercise, which will stimulate appetite and hunger
- Encourage testing of new recipes, use of fresh herbs, and communal food preparation gatherings
- Encourage eating with friends and neighbors
- Locate assistance if financial needs are limiting intake of food (a referral to a social worker may be in order)
- Refer to physician to determine whether drugs or zinc deficiency is the cause and suggest increased intake of zinc-rich foods

DENTAL HEALTH

There is a total loss of teeth in 55 percent of adults older than age 85, in 44 percent of those 75 to 84, and 30 percent in those age 65 to 74.[8] Changes in dentition can be a real challenge for many elderly. Mouth pain, loss of teeth, ill-fitting dentures, and difficulty in chewing and swallowing all can make eating less than enjoyable. Obviously, this too can lead to decreased food intake.

When modifications can be made to improve dental health by early intervention, many of the problems listed here can be avoided. Otherwise the health care professional needs creativity to assist elderly people in finding foods that can be eaten with little difficulty but that also meet their nutritional needs. Modifications in consistency can help, as can choosing nutrient-dense foods such a yogurt and custards, bananas, and peanut butter. Often, just encouraging more time for chewing and swallowing will help.

THIRST

With aging comes a change in sense of thirst and diminished activity in the hormonal regulation of fluid balance. Together this results in changes that may make dehydration more likely, and this can lead to confusion and hospitalization.[8] Signs and symptoms of dehydration are listed later.

The elderly may need help remembering to drink enough fluids, especially during illnesses and hot weather. The recommended amount of fluid per day is the same as for younger adults—at least eight cups a day (2000 mL). Water, juices, milk, decaffeinated coffee, and teas all contribute to fluid needs, but it is also good to encourage drinking water frequently to ensure adequate intake of fluids.

DEHYDRATION

Dehydration causes several specific signs and symptoms:

- Dry lips
- Sunken eyes
- Swollen tongue
- Increased body temperature
- Decreased blood pressure
- Constipation
- Decreased urine output
- Nausea

THE GASTROINTESTINAL TRACT

The primary change in the gastrointestinal tract for the elderly is constipation. Many complain of decreased frequency of bowel movements, painful defecation, stools that are hard and difficult to pass, or a feeling of incomplete evacuation. The causes include reduced motility in the gut, reduced intake of fiber-rich foods, insufficient fluid intake, physical inactivity, and medications.

The best way to remedy this is to encourage more **dietary fiber** intake with the goal being 10 to 13 g/1000 kcal of food intake but not to exceed 35 g daily. Fiber, while not an essential nutrient, aids in moving waste material through the large intestine. It acts to soften the stools and make them much easier to pass. Ensuring adequate fiber intake also reduces the incidence of diverticulosis and may also lessen the risk of certain types of colon cancer. Foods that are rich in fiber are whole grains, nuts, seeds, legumes, fruits, and vegetables. Some of the foods that are high in fiber are listed in Table 5–6.

In addition to adequate fiber, regular physical activity will stimulate regularity, as will heeding the call of nature when the urge is felt. Adequate hydration is also important, as discussed earlier. Mineral oil as a laxative should be taken with care, because it binds the fat-soluble vitamins A, D, E, and K and can limit their absorption. Other types of over-the-counter laxatives should be used with caution too, because they can foster dependence and really do little to resolve the problem.

Other changes in the gastrointestinal tract include lactose intolerance due to decreased lactase production. Lactase enzymes can be added to milk products, or specially treated milk can be used to alleviate the problem. These products are available at most grocers and pharmacies. (See also Carbohydrates under Basic Nutrition Overview.)

Acid production in the stomach decreases with age, and this can contribute to reduced absorption of vitamin B_{12}. It is important to note vitamin B_{12} deficiencies can take some time to develop, but early diagnosis can prevent the anemia that may result. Less acid in the stomach also impairs the absorption of iron. In addition, chronic aspirin use may cause blood loss in the stomach, and chronic antacid use possibly binds iron. Ulcer, hemorrhoids, and colon cancer can also increase blood loss and risk of anemia. If iron deficiency anemia is diagnosed, supplements can be taken with vitamin C–rich foods, which will increase absorption.

TABLE 5–6. *Fiber Sources in Foods*

1 medium apple	4.3 g
1 medium banana	3.3 g
½ cup kidney beans	10.2 g
½ cup blackberries	4.9 g
½ cup cooked broccoli	3.3 g
1 ounce brazil nuts	2.5 g
½ cup cooked carrots	2.9 g
1 ounce all bran cereal	8.5 g
1 ounce cheerios	1.1 g
1 ounce wheaties	2 g
1 medium orange	3 g
1 cup popcorn	1.5 g
1 medium baked potato with skin	3.9 g
½ cup strawberries	1.6 g

Source: Anderson, J.: Nutrition and Your Health. Dietary Fiber. Michigan State University Cooperative Extensive Service, 1990.

LIVER, GALLBLADDER, AND PANCREAS

As with other systems, there are age-associated changes in the liver, gallbladder, and pancreas.

The liver functions less efficiently with age. This is complicated if there is a history of alcohol abuse. There may be fatty build-up or outright cirrhosis of the liver that will greatly diminish function and make it harder for the liver to metabolize alcohol. Continued use and abuse of alcohol in later life may be brought on by the many social changes that the elderly experience, such as death of a spouse, loss of friendship, and feelings of loneliness and isolation.

The health care professional needs to be sensitive to these problems and be ready to make referrals to other appropriate health care professionals and community support groups. Nutritionally speaking, alcohol abuse compromises health and leads to malnutrition for several reasons. First, alcohol replaces food in the diet. Alcohol is a source of empty calories, and when limited resources are spent on alcohol instead of healthy foods, health will definitely be compromised. Second, alcohol interferes with the normal absorption of vitamin B_{12}, folic acid, and vitamin C. Alcohol also interferes with the metabolism of vitamins D and B_6. Alcohol also increases the need for B vitamins and magnesium. All of these may result in multiple deficiencies that would require a multivitamin and mineral supplement.

In contrast, diminished liver function may also result in vitamin A toxicity. Elderly people with liver disease should be warned not to take excessive amounts of vitamin A because their livers are less able to manage large doses.

Changes in the function of the gallbladder may lead to the formation of gallstones, which may result in fat malabsorption. A low-fat diet or surgery may be required to correct the situation.

One of the first signs of diminished function of the pancreas is a high blood-glucose level. The pancreas secretes insulin, which controls the amount of glucose in the blood. With diminished pancreatic function, people may require oral hypoglycemic agents, exogenous insulin, and dietary modification to control blood glucose.

CARDIOVASCULAR HEALTH

Cardiovascular health can diminish in the elderly as a result of long-standing atherosclerosis, hypertension, and physical inactivity. The best way to maintain heart health is a lifelong commitment to a heart-healthy diet and regular exercise. Even in the elderly years, encouraging patients to follow a diet low in fat, saturated fat, and cholesterol, control salt intake, and eat adequate amounts of fruits, vegetables, and fiber will help them keep cholesterol levels down and HDL levels within a desirable range. In addition, make sure patients eat foods with sufficient vitamin B_6, B_{12}, and folate to help avoid elevated homocysteine levels, which are a known risk factor for heart disease.[12]

Care needs to be taken, however, whenever extrememly low-fat diets are used in the elderly as a means to control hyperlipidemia (high levels of fats in the blood that can lead to atherosclerosis). A diet too low in fat could cause weight loss and a lack of a variety in the types of food eaten. This could easily compromise nutritional status. Careful evaluation of the patient's current diet usually reveals opportunities for moderate changes that will help correct concerns with hyperlipidemia.

TABLE 5–7. *Drug/Nutrient Interactions*

Drug	Use	Nutrient	Potential Side Effect
Digoxin	Antiarrhythmic	Potassium, calcium, magnesium	Drug toxicity if potassium is deficient
Anticoagulant	Prevention blood clots	Vitamin K	Poor utilization
Antihistamine (Benadryl)	Treatment of allergies Nausea		Weight gain
Beta-blocker	Decrease hypertension		Some can elevate cholesterol
Cathartics	Induce bowel excretion	Calcium, potassium, vitamins A, D, E, K	Poor absorption
Cholestyramine	Reduce blood cholesterol	Vitamins A, D, E, K	Poor absorption
Cimetidine (Tagamet)	Ulcer treatment	Vitamin B_{12}	Poor absorption
Colchicine	Gout treatment	Vitamin B_{12} magnesium, fat Protein, potassium	Decreased absorption
Corticosteroids	Anti-inflammatory	Zinc, calcium	Poor absorption and utilization
Isoniazid (INH)	Tuberculosis	Vitamin B_6	Poor utilization
Phenobarbital	Sedative, epilepsy	Vitamin D, folate, calcium	Reduced metabolism and utilization, possible osteomalacia
Phenytoin (Dilantin)	Epilepsy	Vitamin D, folate, Vitamin B_{12}, K	Reduced metabolism and utilization
Tricyclic antidepressants (Elavil)	Depression		Weight gain
Antibiotics:			
Penicillin	Bacterial infection	Potassium	Hypokalemia
Neomycin		Fat, protein, vitamins A, D, E, K	Decreased absorption
Cephalosporins		Vitamin K	Deficiency

Source: Merck Manual of Geriatrics, ed 2. Rahway, NJ, 1995; Elbe, D: Reference Guide to Drug and Nutrient Interactions, Columbia Dietitian's and Nutritionists' Association, Vancouver, British Columbia, 1993; Wardlaw, G, and Insel, P: Perspectives in Nutrition. Mosby, St. Louis, 1996, p 679.

Hypertension in the elderly is usually treated with medication, sodium restriction, weight loss (if overweight), and moderate exercise (if possible.) Encourage patients to avoid high-sodium foods such as fast foods, snack foods (chips, salted popcorn, nuts), salty meats (cured pork products, salted fish), pickles, and cheese and not to add salt at the table.

DRUG AND NUTRIENT INTERACTIONS

Forty-five percent of the elderly regularly take prescription medications, and many take six or more at one time. The most widely used drugs by the elderly are cardiac medications, followed by arthritis, psychiatric, respiratory, and gastrointestinal drugs.[5] Long-term use of medications can interfere with nutritional well-being. **Diuretics** (furosemide [lasix]) used to promote fluid excretion may increase need for potassium. **Antacids** reduce stomach acidity which decreases absorption of calcium, vitamin B_{12}, and iron. **Antidepressants** such as monoamine oxidase (MAO) inhibitors (Parnate) can lead to hypertension as a result of changes in lysine metabolism. **Anti-inflammatory** analgesics such as aspirin may induce anemia because of blood loss. These are but a few examples. See Table 5–7 for more drug nutrient interactions.

🔡 SUMMARY

In summary, the value of appropriate nutrition screening and intervention cannot be underestimated in providing quality care for the elderly. Good nutrition not only optimizes health and well-being, it helps prevent the onset of many chronic diseases.

It is imperative that the health care provider be sensitive to the many changes that occur with aging and to the ways in which nutrition can affect the quality of life in the elderly. The first step is to understand the basic principles of nutrition and how these can be applied in encouraging healthy eating. Second, health care professionals need to be aware of how the aging process can alter nutrition status. With careful screening, counseling, and referral if necessary, health care professionals can be certain that their patient's nutritional well-being is optimal. Ensuring quality nutrition is invaluable in providing the best health care for the elderly.

🔡 REVIEW QUESTIONS

1. What are the essential nutrients?

  A. Vitamins, fiber, water, protein, carbohydrates
  B. Protein, carbohydrate, fat, water
  C. Protein, carbohydrate, fat, vitamins, minerals, water
  D. Protein, carbohydrate, fat, vitamins, minerals, water, fiber

2. What type of fat is associated with increasing blood cholesterol?

   A. Polyunsaturated

   B. Monounsaturated

   C. Saturated

   D. Glycerol

3. What is the current amount of protein that is recommended for the elderly?

   A. As much as a person can consume

   B. 0.8 g per kilogram of body weight

   C. 1 g per kilogram of body weight

   D. There is no current recommendation regarding protein intake

4. How many servings each day from the fruit and vegetable group are recommended for the elderly?

   A. 4

   B. 8

   C. 5

   D. 2

5. If a person is lactose intolerant, it means:

   A. He or she cannot digest the carbohydrate in milk.

   B. He or she can digest the protein in milk in limited quantities.

   C. He or she cannot digest the fiber in plant materials.

   D. He or she cannot eat any animal protein.

6. Some of the warning signs of nutrition risk in the elderly include:

   A. Obesity, loss of weight, chronic disease

   B. Mental confusion, recent surgery, loss of appetite

   C. High intake of alcohol, limited nutrition knowledge

   D. All of the above

7. What foods are good sources of fiber?

   A. Meat, fish, and poultry

   B. Fruits, vegetables, and whole grains

   C. Whole-fat dairy products

   D. None of the above

8. If you want to diet to lose weight:

   A. Eat as little as possible and keep calories down to about 800–1000 kcal/day.

   B. Eat a balanced diet, get regular moderate exercise, and watch out for fats and sweets.

   C. Use appetite suppressants and liquid diet formulas to ensure rapid weight loss.

   D. Cut back on carbohydrates, because they are fattening.

9. A diabetic is an individual who has:

   A. Abnormal heartbeat and inhalation
   B. Inadequate intake of protein
   C. Insufficient lean body mass
   D. Abnormal glucose levels and insulin response

10. The water-soluble vitamins include:

    A. Vitamin B_{12}, folic acid, and vitamin E
    B. B complex vitamins and vitamin C
    C. Vitamins K, A, and C
    D. Vitamins A, D, E, and K

🔲 LEARNING ACTIVITIES

1. You have just met with an elderly patient who will be included in your case load. The patient is an 82-year-old man whose wife died last year. He has no family members who live in the community. He was referred to you by his physician, who is concerned that the patient has lost 20 pounds in the past year. The patient is 5'10" and his current weight is 158 lb. What additional information do you need in order to assist this patient? What do you believe is the cause of his weight loss? What are your recommendations?

2. You have just met with a new patient at the practice where you work as a medical assistant. Your new patient is a 75-year-old female who is 5'4" and weighs 105 lb. She has a medical history of chronic pain due to arthritis. She reports that she has recently lost interest in cooking for herself and her husband. She adds that she has little appetite and often forgets to eat. What would you suggest?

3. You have just interviewed an 80-year-old male who has high cholesterol. His total cholesterol is 225 mg/dL, his HDL is 40 mg/dL, and the LDL component is 155 mg/dL. Does this indicate risk for heart disease? If so, what would your recommendations be?

4. You are asked by your employer to give a presentation to a senior citizen women's group, who regularly meet at their local church for evening meals that are financed by the church and prepared by volunteers. You agree to join them and note that the meal consists of roast beef, mashed potatoes and gravy, biscuits with butter, coffee, and apple pie. During dinner you ask and find that most of their meals are similar to this pattern. You present your talk on osteoporosis and agree to come back in a month for another talk. What would you want to focus on next time? Why?

🔲 REFERENCES

1. US Department of Health Human Services, Administration on Aging. Older Americans Act, Elderly Nutrition Program, 1972.

2. The Nutrition Screening Initiative, a project of the American Academy of Family Physicians, the American Dietetic Association, and the National Council on Aging, Inc., 1989.

3. Weisburger, JH, and Williams, GM: Causes of Cancer. American Cancer Society Textbook of Clinical Oncology. American Cancer Society, Atlanta, GA, 1995.

4. Giovannucci, E, et al: Relationship of diet to risk of colorectal cancer adenoma in men. J Nat Cancer Inst 84:91–98, 1992.

5. Boyle, M, and Zyla, G: Personal Nutrition. West Publishing, Minneapolis, MN, 1996, pp 89, 399.

6. Glore, SL, et al: Soluble fiber and serum lipids: A literature review. Journal of the American Dietetic Association 94:425–436, 1994.

7. Eastwood, MA: The physiological effects of dietary fiber: An update. Annual Review of Nutrition 12:19–35, 1992.

8. Wardlaw, G, and Insel, P: Perspectives in Nutrition. Mosby, St. Louis. 1996, pp 410–411, 673.

9. Vitae, S, et al: Plasma antioxidants and risk of cortical and nuclear cataract. Epidemiology 4:195–203, 1993.

10. West, S, et al: Are antioxidants or supplements protective for age-related macular degeneration? Arch Ophthalmology 112:222–227, 1994.

11. Ausman, LM, Russell: Nutrition in the elderly. In Shils, ME, et al (eds): Modern Nutrition in Health and Disease. Lea and Febiger, Philadelphia, 1994.

12. Selhub, J, et al: Vitamin status and intake as primary determinants of homocysteinemia in an elderly population. JAMA 270:2693, 1993.

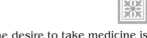
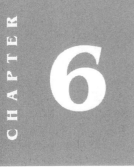

CHAPTER

6

Drug Therapy in the Elderly

Thomas D. Nolin

CHAPTER OUTLINE

BEHAVIORAL OBJECTIVES

Upon completion of this chapter, the reader will be able to:

1. List the four pharmacokinetic parameters, all of which change in the elderly.
2. Describe the primary alterations occurring with each of the parameters listed in #1.
3. List five drugs/drug classes that require dosage adjustment in the elderly.
4. Contrast pharmacokinetic and pharmacodynamic changes.
5. Describe factors contributing to polypharmacy and explain why polypharmacy is not desirable.
6. Define the term adverse drug reaction (ADR) and differentiate it from side effect.
7. Identify three risk factors for the development of ADRs, and list at least three drugs/drug classes that are commonly implicated in their development.
8. Define medication noncompliance, list the types of noncompliance, and discuss the primary causes of it.
9. Discuss an effective means of medication management in the elderly.

KEY TERMS

Adverse drug reaction	Lipophilicity
Compliance	Pharmacodynamics
Hyrophilicity	Pharmacokinetics

INTRODUCTION

Twenty-five years has been added to the average American life span since the turn of the century, resulting in the rapid growth of the elderly cohort, those older than 65 years of age (see Chapter 1).[1] They represent only 12 percent of the population, yet consume more than 30 percent of all medications.[2,3] The majority of elderly individuals have at least one chronic disease and consequently take more medications than younger people, accounting for approximately 25 percent of drug expenditures in developed countries and nearly $3 billion per year in the United States alone.[1,3–5]

The elderly undergo well-documented age related physiologic changes (see Chapter 3) that directly influence drug disposition and response,[1,6–9] a phenomenon that makes them susceptible to often preventable drug-related problems, particularly adverse drug reactions (ADRs).[7,10–14] An increased number of chronic illnesses, which may occur simultaneously, contributes to polypharmacy.[1,7,10,15–17] This also leads to the development of ADRs[10–14] and noncompliance.[1,7,18,19] An understanding of each of these issues is important in ensuring safe and effective pharmacotherapy. Clinicians familiar with them are better prepared to evaluate and individualize drug therapy in the elderly.

PHARMACOKINETIC CHANGES

Pharmacokinetics is the study of how drugs travel through the body over time. It deals with all aspects of drug disposition in the body, including *absorption* from the administration site, *distribution* into various body compartments, hepatic *metabolism* to active and inactive metabolites (by-products of drug metabolism), and *excretion* of parent drug and metabolites from the body.[1] In short, clinical pharmacokinetics strives to reduce drug toxicity without compromising efficacy and/or to increase efficacy while avoiding toxicity.[20] This is accomplished by maintaining blood concentrations of drugs within a proven therapeutic range.[21] Age-related physiological, and hence, pharmacokinetic changes affect the manner in which the body responds to medications (Table 6–1). Careful consideration of these changes, combined with knowledge of which drugs are affected and how those drugs are influenced, allows estimation of the most appropriate dosing regimen.

TABLE 6–1. *Changes Affecting Drug Disposition in the Elderly*

Pharmacokinetic Parameter	Physiological Change
Absorption	↑ Gastric pH ↓ Gastric emptying time ↓ GI motility ↓ GI blood flow
Distribution	↓ Lean muscle mass ↑ Total body fat ↓ Total body water ↓ Serum albumin ↓ Cardiac output
Metabolism	↓ Liver mass ↓ Hepatic blood flow ↓ Enzyme activity
Excretion	↓ Renal blood flow ↓ Glomerular filtration rate ↓ Renal tubular function

Data from references 1, 5–7, and 27.

ABSORPTION

Drugs are administered most frequently via the oral route. Because of this, the effects of functional gastrointestinal (GI) changes on drug absorption need to be examined. Age-related changes in the GI tract include increased gastric pH, delayed gastric emptying times, and decreases in both intestinal motility and blood flow.[1,5,22] In general, however, despite these changes, the *extent* of absorption of most drugs is not significantly affected in the elderly.[5,7] Because of the delay in gastric emptying and decreased motility, the *rate* of absorption may potentially be reduced, but any reduction is usually clinically insignificant.[1,5]

An increase in gastric pH can interfere with the dissolution or breakdown and subsequent pharmacological response of some drugs. For example, ketoconazole, a common antifungal agent, requires a low gastric pH to be broken down and subsequently available for systemic absorption. When used in the setting of an increased gastric pH, the drug exhibits lowered responses because of incomplete dissolution. Other drugs like penicillin are normally less stable in acidic environments but are used in appropriate doses to successfully treat infections. When used in the setting of an increased pH, less drug breakdown may occur, and hence more of the drug is available for absorption with subsequent exaggerated pharmacological responses.[1]

The delay in gastric emptying allows more contact time between drugs and the stomach. This can be problematic with potentially ulcerogenic drugs such as the nonsteroidal anti-inflammatory agents (e.g., ibuprofen, naproxen).[22] Increased drug-drug interactions are also possible, as is the case with antacids and other compounds containing a cation or positively charged element (e.g., calcium carbonate, magnesium hydroxide, aluminum hydroxide, iron or ferrous sulfate), as a result of increased binding (chelation) of the cation to other medications, such as tetracycline and quinolone antibiotics.[22] This can generally be avoided by administering them at least 2 hours apart from one another. Decreased motility and transit time through the GI tract can also diminish the overall absorption of sustained-release products.

Decreased cardiac output and blood flow may slightly affect the rate of absorption of drugs administered orally, as well as those administered topically, intramuscularly, and subcutaneously, as a result of reduced regional blood perfusion.[23]

DISTRIBUTION

Various changes in the composition of the aging body influence the distribution of drugs. The volume of distribution is a term that refers to the extent to which a drug distributes throughout bodily tissues.[24] It does not represent a specific body fluid or volume, per se, but is dependent on several factors, including the extent of water solubility (**hydrophilicity**), fat solubility (**lipophilicity**), and plasma protein binding.[5–7,23,24] Because body composition changes with age, each of these factors is affected, and thus the volume of distribution of many drugs also changes.

The ratio of lean body mass to total body fat changes with age. Lean muscle mass decreases and total body fat increases as we grow older.[17] As a result, lipophilic agents, which distribute extensively into adipose tissue, may exhibit increased volumes of distribution.[17,22,24] This is the case with some common tranquilizing agents such as diazepam (Valium) and chlordiazepoxide (Librium). Consequently, lipid-soluble drugs often accumulate over time, resulting in a prolonged duration of action and longer elimination half-lives due to delayed release from fat tissues. Therefore, it is not surprising that use of these agents has been associated with increased morbidity in the elderly (e.g., falls and delirium).[25,26]

Other drugs are hydrophilic, and their volumes of distribution are proportional to lean body weight.[5,22] Lean body weight primarily reflects muscle mass and total body water.[27] The decrease in both of these as we age reduces the volume of distribution of water-soluble compounds. Failure to reduce doses accordingly results in elevated serum drug levels and potentially can lead to toxicity. Examples of hydrophilic drugs include ethanol, the antibiotics gentamicin and tobramycin, the antiulcer drug cimetidine, and lithium, a common antipsychotic medication.

As one ages, decreases in serum albumin concentrations may occur secondary to chronic disease states, malnutrition, and/or severe debilitation.[17] Since only the free, non-protein-bound fraction of a drug is active, a reduction in serum albumin levels may result in higher free drug concentrations and intensified pharmacodynamic effects.[5,17] Acidic compounds, including oral antidiabetic agents, the antiepileptic agents phenytoin (Dilantin) and phenobarbital, and the anticoagulant warfarin (Coumadin), bind primarily to albumin and should be used cautiously in patients with hypoalbuminemia.[5]

METABOLISM

Metabolism or biotransformation by the liver is a crucial step in the elimination of drugs from the body. During biotransformation, the liver converts drugs through various metabolic pathways to more hydrophilic metabolites, which can then be excreted by the kidneys.[1] Hepatic metabolism of drugs is dependent on the organ's mass, microsomal enzyme activity, and blood flow.[7] Hepatic mass decreases by approximately 1 percent per year after the age of 40, and blood flow to the liver may be reduced by up to 40 percent between the ages of 25 and 75.[1,17] This reduction in blood flow results in less drug presented to the liver and decreased drug metabolism.

In addition to changes in blood flow, age influences the hepatic clearance of drugs by causing alterations in the intrinsic activity of selected microsomal enzymes. Metabolism occurs primarily via two enzyme systems: phase I reactions (oxidation, reduction, and hydrolysis) and phase II conjugation reactions (glucuronidation, acetylation, and sulfation).[1,5,22] Phase I reactions are reduced or unchanged in the elderly, while phase II pathways remain unaffected. Benzodiazepine anxiolytic and hypnotic agents are metabolized via these pathways. For instance, chlordiazepoxide (Librium), diazepam (Valium), clorazepate (Tranxene), and prazepam (Centrax) all undergo phase I metabolism and have prolonged elimination half-lives in the elderly.[1,5,22,25] Conversely, oxazepam (Serax), lorazepam (Ativan), and temazepam (Restoril) undergo phase II conjugation, are not affected by age, and are preferred for use in the elderly.[5,22,25,28]

EXCRETION

Renal function is probably the single most important determinant of drug elimination from the body.[1] It is also the best documented and most predictable.[5] Reductions in kidney mass, renal blood flow, and the subsequent number of functioning nephrons, glomerular filtration rate (GFR), and the rate of tubular secretion account for the decreased renal excretory capacity observed with aging.[5,29] Between the ages of 30 and 70, renal mass decreases by about 20 percent, and renal blood flow and GFR decline approximately 1 percent per year.[29] An otherwise healthy 70-year-old person may have a 40 to 50 percent decrease in renal function, even in the absence of renal disease.[5]

Many drugs are renally excreted and require dosage adjustments in the elderly in order to avoid toxicity. Drug dosage adjustments are typically based on an individual's kidney GFR. GFR is easily estimated from creatinine clearance, which in turn is calculated from a patient's serum creatinine concentration.[30] This must be done with caution in the elderly, however. Serum creatinine is a by-product of muscle that is almost completely excreted by the kidneys, so it is an excellent endogenous marker of renal function. In normal young individuals, a decline in renal function results in a predictable rise in serum creatinine level. However, since muscle mass decreases with aging, creatinine production and presence in the serum also decreases, so that the serum creatinine value may not accurately reflect the true level of renal function in the elderly.[29] It is not uncommon for elderly patients with markedly reduced renal function to have apparently normal serum creatinine concentrations.

Renally excreted drugs requiring dosage adjustments in the elderly include numerous antimicrobials, the cardiovascular drug digoxin (Lanoxin), lithium, and several antiulcer medications like cimetidine (Tagamet), famotidine (Pepcid), and ranitidine (Zantac). Many drugs also require dose adjustment because of the production of active metabolites that are renally eliminated. These include the narcotic agents morphine, meperidine, and propoxyphene, the antiarrhythmics procainamide and disopyramide, and allopurinol, a drug used to prevent gout.

🔲 PHARMACODYNAMIC CHANGES

Most age-related changes in drug response are a result of pharmacokinetic changes that alter the concentration of drug reaching the site of action or receptor site rather than changes at the site of action itself.[31] In the setting of altered pharmacokinetics, target drug concentrations remain the same, and the dose or dosing interval is adjusted to compensate for this age-related alteration in order to achieve the desired concentration.[31]

Despite these dosage adjustments and attainment of the desired drug concentrations, altered drug responses may still occur because of age-related pharmacodynamic changes.[21] Equal concentrations of drug at the site of action produce different effects in the young and the old.[21] **Pharmacodynamics** refers to the action of drugs, or the biological effects resulting from the interaction between drugs and its receptor site.[32] Although poorly studied, age-related pharmacodynamic changes in the elderly can greatly influence drug response, usually leading to increased sensitivity or an exaggerated pharmacological response to a given drug.[8] This is seen with sedatives such as barbiturates and benzodiazepines (e.g., diazepam, chlordiazepoxide, flurazepam), narcotic analgesics (e.g., morphine), anticoagulants (e.g., warfarin), and many antihypertensive agents.[7,8] Diminished pharmacological responses may also be seen with certain cardiovascular drugs including beta-blocking (e.g., propranolol), beta-adrenergic (e.g., isoproterenol), and calcium channel blocking agents (e.g., verapamil).[7] Altered responses may be due to depletion of neurotransmitters and changes at the receptor site, including a decreased number of receptors and a decreased affinity or sensitivity of receptors overall.[8] Changes in the sensitivity of the elderly to drug therapy often requires new target drug concentrations and/or more aggressive or alternative means of monitoring drug response in order to achieve the desired effects.[1] Generally speaking, in an effort to minimize adverse outcomes, it is always best to "start low and go slow" when initiating treatment with new drugs—that is, start new drug therapy with low doses and slowly titrate doses upward until the desired effects are seen.

🔲 POLYPHARMACY

Polypharmacy, in simple terms, refers to the use of multiple medications in one individual.[16,33] Although the use of multiple medications may often be perfectly appropriate, the term *polypharmacy* usually connotes the use of more drugs than are clinically indicated or the excessive and unnecessary use of drugs, which in turn increases patient morbidity.[16,33] Indeed, as the number of medications taken increases, the likelihood of adverse drug reactions and drug-drug interactions also increases.[34] Furthermore, as the complexity of the drug regimen increases, the risk of noncompliance increases.[35] As mentioned previously, age-related pharmacokinetic and pharmacodynamic changes in the elderly make them uniquely susceptible to drug-related problems. For these reasons, the added element of polypharmacy is often detrimental to geriatric patients.

There are many possible reasons for polypharmacy, including an increased number of chronic illnesses or physical ailments, a lack of one primary health provider to coordinate medical care and drug use, subsequent use of multiple physicians (i.e., specialists), use of multiple pharmacies, and self-treatment, primarily with over-the-counter (OTC) drugs.[10,15–17,33] Elderly individuals take an average of 2.8 drugs per day.[17] Those in nursing homes take 3.4, and the hospitalized elderly are prescribed more than 9 medications per day.[17] The geriatric population consumes 30 percent of all prescription and nearly 50 percent of all OTC drugs in this country.[33] Interestingly, physicians have a strong tendency to prescribe medications for many common ailments. American physicians write about 1.8 billion prescriptions per year, an average of 6.2 for each person, young and old, in this country.[36] Societal pressures, upbringing, and training lend to the "pill for every ill" mentality, illustrated by the fact that approximately 60 percent of all doctor's visits result in a prescription for a medication.[10] Similarly, 68 percent of visits by the elderly are associated with initiation or continuation of a prescription drug.[12]

Studies have focused on establishing and quantifying the use of inappropriate medications in the elderly and on discouraging their use.[37–39] One approach to minimize polypharmacy requires shifting attention from specific "inappropriate medications" and refocusing on the "appropriate use of medications" in the elderly.[40] It is important to distinguish between excessive and unnecessary drug use and a well-controlled drug regimen that appropriately and justifiably contains several agents. There is no magic number above which the number of medications becomes polypharmacy. We must resist the temptation to simply count the number of drugs a patient is taking, determine it to be polypharmacy, and pass judgment on providers or the patient.

Other strategies for reducing polypharmacy have been suggested.[15,16,40] A pharmacotherapeutic plan should be devised for every patient for whom drugs are prescribed.[22] Initially, nondrug therapies should be considered. Medications should only be prescribed with clear therapeutic goals in mind. Those with minimal side effects, the simplest dosing schedules, and the lowest cost should be selected whenever possible. Patients need to be educated regarding their drug regimens, and these should be routinely reevaluated with every health care visit. Polypharmacy can be managed if the prescriber assesses each patient's drug regimen every time a patient is seen.[33] It is entirely possible for a drug that was appropriately prescribed initially to subsequently become inappropriate for various reasons, including the development of adverse effects or therapeutic failure.[40] If these situations are identified, geriatric patients will receive maximal benefits from the fewest number of medications.

ADVERSE DRUG REACTIONS

An adverse drug reaction (ADR) is defined as any unexpected, unintended, undesired, or excessive response to a drug when it is used in the approved manner.[41] ADRs are difficult to predict or prevent. They typically:

- Require a modification in drug therapy (e.g., drug discontinuation or dosage change)
- Cause or prolong admission to the hospital
- Require supportive treatment
- Negatively affect prognosis
- May result in disability or death[41]

It is important to differentiate ADRs from normal side effects of drugs, which are extensions of the known pharmacological activity of the drug in question and are therefore expected and predictable (Table 6–2).[42]

ADRs result in approximately 1 million hospitalizations and 140,000 deaths annually.[43] The elderly experience a disproportionately high percentage of these. It is estimated that as many as 3 to 5 percent of all hospital admissions are related to an ADR. In the elderly the percentage may be as high as 16.8 percent. Up to 10 to 20 percent of all hospital inpatients experience an ADR at some time during their admission. Again, in the elderly this is increased to as much as 35 percent.[36,44–46] Unfortunately, as many as 6 to 7 percent of all adverse reactions in the elderly contribute directly or indirectly to death.[27]

ADVERSE DRUG REACTION RISK FACTORS

There are several risk factors for the development of an ADR:[7,12,13,36,48]

- An increased number of chronic illnesses
- Severity of illnesses

TABLE 6–2. *Commonly Observed Adverse Drug Reactions*

Delirium	Tardive dyskinesia, akathisia
Confusion	Pseudoparkinsonism
Lethargy	Visual/hearing disturbances
Fatigue	Orthostatic hypotension
Arrhythmias	Syncopal attacks, falls
Nausea, vomiting	Constipation, diarrhea
Incontinence	Electrolyte abnormalities
Tremor	Urinary retention

Data from references 12, 14, 36, and 48.

- Pharmacokinetic changes
- Pharmacodynamic changes
- Polypharmacy

Although a correlation exists between chronological age and the incidence of ADRs, age, per se, has not been shown to be an independent risk factor for the development of adverse reactions.[7,12,13,36,47] However, ADRs have been directly related to polypharmacy, clearly the most important and preventable risk factor.[14,36,48] The incidence of adverse reactions increases from 10 percent in patients taking one drug, to 50 percent in patients taking five drugs and essentially 100 percent in those receiving eight or more.[14,48] ADRs often lead to medication noncompliance. The financial impact of ADRs on the health care industry has been estimated at $3.4 billion annually.[49]

Inappropriate drug selection, as well as overprescribing, contribute to the development of ADRs. As mentioned previously, studies investigated the use of as many as 20 medications deemed inappropriate in the elderly.[38,39] Incredibly, it was found that nearly 25 percent of people 65 years or older living in the community (representing about 6.64 million people in the United States), received at least one of the contraindicated medications.[39] The problem is exaggerated in geriatric nursing home residents with about 40 percent receiving at least one inappropriate drug.[38] The most commonly prescribed offending agents were the long-acting benzodiazepines diazepam and chlordiazepoxide, the analgesics propoxyphene and indomethacin, the antidepressant amitriptyline, and the antihypertensive agents methyldopa and propranolol.[38,39] Other drugs frequently implicated in adverse reactions are medications that are commonly used in the elderly, including those with narrow therapeutic windows such as digoxin and theophylline. Still others include diuretics, nonsteroidal anti-inflammatory agents, antihypertensives, anxiolytics, antipsychotics, narcotics, and corticosteroids.[38,39]

Adverse reactions are difficult to diagnose in the elderly because symptoms often mimic common complaints and stereotypes of "old age" as well as the characteristics of disease states (see Table 6–2).[7,14,36] All patient complaints and symptoms should be reviewed along with their medication regimen to detect possible adverse drug effects and subsequently discontinue the offending agent. Individualizing patient pharmacotherapy and reducing polypharmacy is the most effective method of treating and preventing ADRs.

NONCOMPLIANCE

Medication **compliance** has been defined as the extent to which a patient's behavior coincides with a prescriber's planned medical regimen.[23] Any deviation from this is, obviously, noncompliance. Reports indicate that more than half of the 1.8 billion prescriptions written each year are taken incorrectly by patients for various reasons, leading to therapeutic failure in 30 to

50 percent of them.[18] Up to 90 percent of the noncompliance is due to patients underusing or taking too little medication.[50] The economic impact of medication noncompliance is in excess of $100 billion per year, because of increased hospital and nursing home admissions, lost productivity, premature deaths, and other necessary treatments.[18]

Several forms of noncompliance exist, including:[18,51,52]

- Failure to have initial prescriptions filled and/or obtain subsequent refills
- Failure to take daily doses exactly as prescribed
- Discontinuing the medication prematurely

Noncompliance may or may not be intentional. It is often viewed as the patient's problem and ignored by practitioners. Noncompliance can be decreased by taking into consideration the reasons for it and identifying individuals less likely to be compliant prior to prescribing medications. Compliance, or lack thereof, is an important medical issue in all patients, and everyone taking medication is at risk. Although age alone is not a good predictor of noncompliance, many characteristics common to geriatric patients contribute to it.[19] Specific factors associated with poor compliance in the elderly include the following:[18,19,49,51]

- Female gender
- Low socioeconomic status
- Solitary living
- Lack of a support person
- Cognitive impairment
- Drug costs
- Multiple disease states
- Physical disabilities
- Complex drug regimens
- Polypharmacy
- Poor communication

Studies of geriatric patients indicate that less than 50 percent take their medications as prescribed, more than 20 percent take one or more drugs that were not prescribed, 20 percent fail to have initial prescriptions filled, and 40 percent stop taking their medications prematurely.[18,27,52]

CAUSES OF NONCOMPLIANCE

Polypharmacy and Complex Drug Regimens

Perhaps the easiest way to improve compliance is to reduce polypharmacy and the complexity of drug regimens. In particular, compliance has been shown to improve dramatically as the prescribed dose frequency decreases.[35] Probably the single most important action prescribers can take is to select medications with the lowest daily dose frequency possible. The pharmaceutical industry recognizes this, illustrated by the fact that nearly all new medications marketed allow administration once or twice daily. Also available are new long-acting or timed-release formulations of drugs that originally had to be taken multiple times per day. Combination products containing more than one drug in one dosage form (i.e., tablets, capsules) are also available. This minimizes the number of different dosage forms taken by a patient. Medications used for the same purpose should be eliminated. When the number of medications or the frequency of administration cannot be reduced, every attempt should be made to minimize the different times throughout the day that medications are to be taken. For example, the use of "with meals" and "at bedtime" usually helps standardize drug administration and serves as memory aids to those taking several medications and should help improve compliance rates. Medication containers or holders of varying types also serve to simplify daily drug administration. The containers are usually divided into days of the week so that an individual's medications can be placed into the corresponding day they are to be taken. They are particularly useful when traveling away from home. Similarly, medication calendars also serve to remind patients when to take their drugs. Lastly, doses of medications should be maximized before adding additional drugs for the same condition, provided adverse reactions are not experienced at the higher, single-drug dosage.[19]

Physical Disabilities

Physical disabilities, however seemingly minor, greatly affect the manner in which patients take their medications. Visual impairment is the most common sensory deficit in elders with more than 90 percent requiring corrective lenses.[49] This leads to problems reading medication labels or instructions and seeing individual dosage forms. Large readable type should be used on labels, and all drugs should be shown to patients with an explanation of what they are.

Hearing impairment occurs in 25 to 40 percent of the elderly, with 90 percent of individuals older than age 90 having impaired hearing.[49] Health care practitioners should anticipate that this will interfere with communication and the patient medication counseling process, and they should speak slowly, in a lower tone, and as clearly as possible (see Chapter 4).[1]

Chronic conditions, particularly those that affect manual dexterity (e.g., arthritis, Parkinson's disease, stroke), create drug administration problems. Safety caps on medication vials and bottles are very difficult for many elderly to remove, especially those with reduced grip strength, arthritic hands and fingers, and tremors.[21,52] This often leads them to either keep the caps off the vials or store the drugs in inappropriate containers. Non-safety caps should be used when possible. Further problems include an inability to break tablets, measure and/or shake liquids, administer eye drops, handle syringes, and properly coordinate the use of inhalers.[52] Patient capabilities should be assessed by all practitioners involved and drug regimens should be tailored accordingly.

Poor Communication

When communication between practitioners and patients breaks down, patients are prone to noncompliance.[51,52] Inaccurate or incomplete information is often relayed to patients, or they get the correct information in a form they cannot readily comprehend or remember.[51] Intimidated patients frequently fail to express concerns and questions, and providers often fail to provide opportunities for them to do so, further compounding the miscommunication and subsequent compliance problem.

Cognitive Impairment

Unfortunately, part of normal aging involves the gradual reduction in cognitive function. Memory functions and the ability to understand and remember text often declines with age (see Chapter 4).[51] Combined with the host of common drugs that also adversely cause cognitive dysfunction of one type or another, the seemingly simple task of understanding and following instructions suddenly becomes much more difficult. Cognitive impairments combined with poor communication practices often leaves the elderly without the necessary tools to comply with complex medication regimens.[51] Various means of improving compliance through better communication have been suggested, including educational programs like "brown bag" sessions, in which patients bring in their prescriptions and are allowed to ask questions of the health care practitioner present.[16,51] Provision of simple, well-written instructions and drug calendars and thorough counseling by pharmacists also have been shown to improve compliance.[16,51]

Drug Costs

Drug costs are a common barrier to compliance, simply because patients, particularly those of low socioeconomic status, cannot afford to have prescriptions filled as frequently as the prescription dictates. Low income is associated with low compliance rates.[19] As mentioned previously, 20 percent of elderly patients fail to have even the initial prescription filled.[18,52] Sadly, it is not uncommon for patients, with several prescriptions in hand, to pick and choose which to have filled based on their associated costs and available funds. The use of generic medications, as well as various medication assistance or indigent patient programs provided for qualified individuals by pharmaceutical companies, is encouraged.[18,19] Pharmacists and social workers are excellent sources for this type of information.

MEDICATION MANAGEMENT

Development of a pharmacotherapeutic plan for the elderly facilitates the routine and efficient management of their medication regimens.[22] Whenever a patient presents with a complaint or symptom, the drug regimen should be reviewed to identify any adverse drug reactions or rule out drug toxicity as a cause.[22] Adverse reactions are often completely reversible when the offending agent is discontinued.[22] Before initiating new drug therapy, nondrug treatment should be used, including lifestyle modification like diet and exercise programs, physical therapy, and psychotherapy. When medically justified, drugs should be prescribed with clear therapeutic goals in mind for each agent, including dosing schedule, monitoring parameters, duration of therapy, and desired outcome or endpoint. Medications should be stopped when desired goals or outcomes are not met. Individual patients should be evaluated for issues that may contribute to noncompliance. Factors to consider when initiating new drug treatment include the drug's efficacy and side effect profile, cost, dosing schedule, and ease of administration. The effect of pharmacokinetic and pharmacodynamic changes and the likelihood of developing ADRs should be considered. The lowest possible effective dose should be started. Patients should be well informed regarding their new medications and provided with opportunities to express concerns or questions. The indications, benefits, potential adverse effects, and directions for use should be clearly explained. Written instructions should also be provided. At subsequent visits, monitoring parameters should be reviewed and endpoints or outcomes desired initially should be assessed to determine whether they have been met.

▨ SUMMARY

Drug therapy offers tremendous benefits to elderly people when used appropriately. However, inherent risks associated with suboptimal drug use in this tenuous population creates challenges for professionals working with them. The effective management of medication regimens in the elderly requires knowledge of the relevant issues. Pharmacokinetic and pharmacodynamic changes necessitate unique dosing and the careful selection of medications in order to minimize polypharmacy, adverse effects, and subsequent noncompliance. We must become attuned to reviewing medication regimens with these issues in mind and develop a high index of suspicion for drug-related problems.[10] In doing so, we will ensure that elderly patients receive maximal benefits from drug therapy while minimizing potential adverse outcomes.

▨ REVIEW QUESTIONS

1. Despite numerous pharmacokinetic changes in the elderly, the extent of drug _____ is not significantly affected in the elderly.
   A. Absorption
   B. Distribution
   C. Hepatic metabolism
   D. Renal excretion

2. Which of the following is the most predictable pharmacokinetic change in the elderly:

   A. Absorption
   B. Distribution
   C. Hepatic metabolism
   D. Renal excretion

3. Pharmacodynamics refers to:

   A. Movement of drugs through the body
   B. The inability of drugs to move through the body
   C. The biological effects of drugs on the body
   D. Constantly changing pharmacokinetic parameters

4. Pharmacodynamic changes in the elderly usually result in _____ pharmacological responses.

   A. Diminished
   B. Unchanged
   C. Exaggerated
   D. None of the above

5. Possible reasons for polypharmacy include which of the following:

   A. Lack of chronic illnesses
   B. Self-medication
   C. Use of a primary care physician
   D. Financial wealth

6. Which of the following are risk factors for the development of adverse drug reactions (ADRs):

   A. Polypharmacy, inappropriate drug selection, several chronic illnesses, aging
   B. Polypharmacy, inappropriate drug selection, low socioeconomic status, pharmacokinetic changes
   C. Inappropriate drug selection, several chronic illnesses, aging, noncompliance
   D. Polypharmacy, inappropriate drug selection, several chronic illnesses, pharmacokinetic changes

7. Commonly observed ADRs that often mimic common complaints or symptoms in the elderly include:

   A. Confusion, hypnosis
   B. Orthostatic hypotension, falls, lethargy
   C. Diarrhea, constipation, bladder obstruction
   D. Leukopenia, thrombocytopenia

8. Medication noncompliance is a significant issue in the elderly. Which of the following statements is FALSE:

   A. Most noncompliance is due to patients' underusing their medication.
   B. Failure to have initial prescriptions filled and discontinuing the medication prematurely are types of noncompliance.

C. Noncompliance is directly related to an individual's personality and is usually intentional.

D. Causes of noncompliance include polypharmacy, drug costs, physical disabilities, and poor communication.

9. Probably the single most important action prescribers can do to improve compliance is:

A. Prescribe medications with the lowest daily dose frequency possible (e.g., once daily)

B. Prescribe generic medications

C. Speak slowly

D. Provide drug containers with non-safety caps

10. Development of a pharmacotherapeutic plan facilitates medication management in the elderly. Essential components of such a plan include:

A. Reviewing the patient's drug regimen every other visit

B. Continuing medications whose therapeutic goals have been met

C. Educating patients regarding their medications

D. Ignoring patient's complaints

LEARNING ACTIVITIES

1. Role playing; two individuals required. One person plays an elderly patient with several chronic diseases, including arthritis and visual impairment, and limited income. Another plays a health care provider counseling the patient how to take the medications. Generally speaking, what are the problems encountered by each individual and how can they be minimized?

2. Design a pharmacotherapeutic plan for the patient in activity #1. What strategies can be used by the health care provider to minimize noncompliance?

3. Assume each of the following scenarios occurring in an elderly patient. Describe what the primary problem is and how it may be avoided or corrected.

A. A patient taking their expensive medication every other day, versus daily as prescribed, so it will "last longer."

B. A patient started on a new H_2 antagonist for a peptic ulcer at normal dosing; a few days later develops confusion.

C. A patient receiving multiple medications, all of which are taken at different times of the day. When asked, he or she has no idea what each medication is, what they are used for, or when to take them.

REFERENCES

1. Pucino, F, et al: Pharmacogeriatrics. Pharmacotherapy 5:314, 1985.
2. Helling, DK, et al: Medication use characteristics in the elderly: The Iowa 65+ rural health study. J Am Geriatr Soc 35:4, 1987.

3. Phillips, SL, and Carr-Lopez, SM: Impact of a pharmacist on medication discontinuation in a hospital-based geriatric clinic. Am J Hosp Pharm 47:1075, 1990.

4. Comorbidity of chronic conditions and disability among older persons—United States, 1984. MMWR 38:788, 1989.

5. Williams, L, and Lowenthal, DT: Drug therapy in the elderly. South Med J 85:127, 1992.

6. Schumacher, GE: Using pharmacokinetics in drug therapy VII: Pharmacokinetic factors influencing drug therapy in the aged. Am J Hosp Pharm 37:559, 1980.

7. Montamat, SC, et al: Management of drug therapy in the elderly. N Engl J Med 321:303, 1989.

8. Lamy, PP: Pharmacodynamic changes with advancing age. Pharmacy Times 82, August, 1990.

9. Ozdemir, V, et al: Pharmacokinetic changes in the elderly: Do they contribute to drug abuse and dependence? Clin Pharmacokinet 31:372, 1996.

10. Beers, MH, and Ouslander, JG: Risk factors in geriatric drug prescribing: A practical guide to avoiding problems. Drugs 37:105, 1989.

11. Schneider, JK, et al: Adverse drug reactions in an elderly outpatient population. Am J Hosp Pharm 49:90, 1992.

12. Chrischilles, EA, et al: Self-reported adverse drug reactions and related resource use: A study of community-dwelling persons 65 years of age and older. Ann Intern Med 117:634, 1992.

13. Walker, J, and Wynne, H: Review: The frequency and severity of adverse drug reactions in elderly people. Age Aging 23:255, 1994.

14. Stein, BE: Avoiding drug reactions: Seven steps to writing safe prescriptions. Geriatrics 49:28, 1994.

15. Stewart, RB: Polypharmacy in the elderly: A fait accompli? Drug Intell Clin Pharm 24:321, 1990.

16. Carlson, JE: Perils of polypharmacy: 10 steps to prudent prescribing. Geriatrics 51:26, 1996.

17. Patel, KB, et al: Drug interactions in the elderly: The role of polypharmacy. P&T 19S, April, 1994.

18. Berg, JS, et al: Patient compliance. Ann Pharmacother 27:S5, 1993.

19. Arcangelo, VP, and O'Conner, TW: Compliance in the elderly: What factors contribute to medication misuse? Pharmacy Times 21, September, 1994.

20. Evans, WE: General principles of applied pharmacokinetics. In Evans, WE, et al (eds): Applied Pharmacokinetics: Principles of Therapeutic Drug Monitoring. Applied Therapeutics, Vancouver, WA, 1992, p 1–1.

21. Nagle, BA, and Erwin, WG: Geriatrics. In Dipiro, JT, et al (eds): Pharmacotherapy: A Pathophysiological Approach. Appleton & Lange, Stamford, CT, 1997, p 87.

22. Sloan, RW: Principles of drug therapy in geriatric patients. Am Fam Physician 45:2709, 1992.

23. Anderson, RJ, and Miller, SW: Geriatric drug therapy. In Herfindal, ET, et al (eds): Clinical Pharmacy and Therapeutics. Williams & Wilkins, Baltimore, 1992, p 1489.

24. Greenblatt, DJ, et al: Pharmacokinetic aspects of drug therapy in the elderly. Ther Drug Monitor 8:249, 1986.

25. Closser, MH: Benzodiazepines and the elderly: A review of potential problems. J Subst Abuse Treat 8:35, 1991.

26. Demaagd, GA: Review of the pharmacologic causes of delirium in the elderly. Consult Pharm 10:461, 1995.

27. Adamcik, BA, and Rhodes, RS: The pharmacist's role in rational drug therapy of the aged. Drugs & Aging 3:481, 1993.

28. Maletta, G, et al: Guidelines for prescribing psychoactive drugs in the elderly: Part 1. Geriatrics 46:40, 1991.

29. Bennett, W: Geriatric pharmacokinetics and the kidney. Am J Kidney Dis 26:283, 1990.

30. Cockroft, DW, and Gault, MH: Prediction of creatinine clearance from serum creatinine. Nephron 16:31, 1976.

31. Garnett, WR, and Barr, WH: Geriatric pharmacokinetics. The Upjohn Company, Kalamazoo, MI, 1982, p 1.

32. Lalonde, RL: Pharmacodynamics. In Evans, WE, et al (eds): Applied Pharmacokinetics: Principles of Therapeutic Drug Monitoring. Applied Therapeutics, Vancouver, WA, 1992, p 4–1.

33. Kovach, LJ: Polypharmacy in the elderly. P&T 1709, November, 1992.

34. Col, N, et al: The role of medication noncompliance and adverse drug reactions in hospitalizations of the elderly. Arch Intern Med 150:841, 1990.

35. Eisen, SA, et al: The effect of prescribed daily dose frequency on patient medication compliance. Arch Intern Med 150:1881, 1990.

36. Bosker, G, and Albrich, JM: Emergency detection of adverse drug reactions in the elderly. Resident & Staff Physician 35:25, 1989.

37. Beers, MH, et al: Explicit criteria for determining inappropriate medication use in nursing home residents. Arch Intern Med 151:1825, 1991.

38. Beers, MH, et al: Inappropriate medication prescribing in skilled-nursing facilities. Ann Intern Med 117:684, 1992.

39. Wilcox, SM, et al: Inappropriate drug prescribing for the community-dwelling elderly. JAMA 272:292, 1994.

40. Plushner, S, and Helling, DK: Identifying inappropriate prescribing in the elderly: Time to refocus. Ann Pharmacother 30:81, 1996.

41. ASHP guidelines on adverse drug reaction monitoring and reporting. Am J Health-Syst Pharm 52:417, 1995.

42. Turner, WM, and Milstein, JB: Drug-induced diseases. In Dipiro, JT, et al (eds): Pharmacotherapy: A Pathophysiological Approach. Elsevier, New York, 1989, p 60.

43. Etzel, JV, et al: Impact of the development of a multidisciplinary adverse drug reaction committee. Hosp Pharm 30:1083, 1995.

44. Ladshmanan, MC, et al: Hospital admissions caused by iatrogenic disease. Arch Intern Med 146:1931, 1986.

45. Einarson, TR: Drug-related hospital admissions. Ann Pharmacother 27:832, 1993.

46. Cantu, TG, and Tyler, LS: Development of a hospital-based adverse drug reaction reporting program. Hospital Formulary 23:658, 1988.

47. Gurwitz, JH, and Avorn, J: The ambiguous relation between aging and adverse drug reactions. Ann Intern Med 114:956, 1991.

48. Korrapati, MR, et al: Adverse drug reactions in the elderly. P&T 1762, November, 1992.

49. Jinks, MJ, and Fuerst, RH: Geriatric drug use and rehabilitation. In Young, LY, and Koda-Kimble, MA (eds): Applied Therapeutics: The Clinical Use of Drugs. Applied Therapeutics, Vancouver, WA, 1995, p 101–1.

50. Cooper, JK, et al: Intentional prescription nonadherence (noncompliance) by the elderly. J Am Geriatr Soc 30:329, 1982.

51. Morrow, D, et al: Adherence and medication instructions: Review and recommendations. J Am Geriatr Soc 36:1147, 1988.

52. Salzman, C: Medication compliance in the elderly. J Clin Psychiatry 56(suppl 1):18, 1995.

The two great needs for vital aging
are control over one's own life and
those bonds of intimacy.
Betty Friedan
(*The Fountain of Age*)

Sexuality and Aging

Nancy MacRae

BEHAVIORAL OBJECTIVES

Upon completion of this chapter, the reader will be able to:

1. Recognize the importance of intimacy in feelings of sexuality.
2. Define sexuality.
3. Describe gender differences in sexual functioning caused by aging.
4. Recognize complications from common diseases that can interfere with expression of sexuality.
5. List techniques to ameliorate complications in the expression of sexuality.
6. Recognize the role prescription drugs can play in sexual expression.
7. Identify two approaches to deal with sexuality issues.

KEY TERMS

Estrogen Replacement Therapy (ERT)
Gay
Intimacy
Lesbian

Menopause
PLISSIT model
Sexuality

INTRODUCTION

The demographics of the United States underscore the graying of the American population with 70 million elderly (those 65 years or older) predicted in 2030; this is projected to be 20 percent of the population.[1] Issues of aging must to be faced. Providing accurate information about the effects of time and development on the body, mind, and spirit is crucial to keep people informed about what to expect and perhaps, more importantly, what can be done to prolong health and to become a successful ager. Health care practitioners need to be vigilant about remembering the fact that only a small portion of the elderly are institutionalized. The vast majority of elders are leading active lives. Each cohort has benefited from more education and better health care practices. It will be fascinating to see what more knowledgeable and demanding elders will require of themselves and their health care practitioners in terms of health in the future decades.

With a high quality of life potentially continuing longer in each elder's life, it can be expected that there will be activity in each significant area of one's life. One wellness perspective[2] artificially divides life into occupational, intellectual, spiritual, social, physical, and emotional (includes sexuality and relationships) dimensions. An individually determined balance among these areas dynamically changes as one matures. Physical activities may decrease in importance as spiritual and social ones increase, for example. Changes likely will occur in the sexual area, if only because of decreased opportunities.

However, an awareness of each of these areas and how one can participate in each throughout life can enrich one's life. This chapter provides information about sexuality and aging, knowledge about specific acute and chronic conditions elders experience, and how these can be combined with two recommended approaches to help health care practitioners deal with sexuality issues of their elderly clients. Addressing these issues may well help such clients regain intimacy and a sense of autonomy or control in their lives, both crucial for a meaningful existence.

SEXUALITY

Sexual innuendo pervades our society. We see sexual images and stereotypes portrayed in our daily lives in advertisements, in print, in song, and in movies and on television. Jokes with sexual connotations are also a frequent occurrence in our day-to-day activities. Yet as prevalent as sex is within our society, little time or attention is devoted to sexuality.

Sexuality is much more than a eight-letter word. It is a core characteristic of who we are; it is a state of mind; it is a holistic concept. We can be sexual without engaging in sex. Learning about sexuality is a lifelong process, a lifelong adventure. What we learn about sexuality, whether explicit or not, frames how we perceive ourselves and can greatly influence how we act. Taking stock of what constitutes sexuality can help us realize how very basic it is to our sense of self.

Sexuality includes the ability to be intimate with another person in a mutually satisfying manner. Obvious components of sexuality are our feelings and beliefs about what it is to be male or female, how we relate to people of our own or the opposite gender, how we establish relationships, especially close and intimate ones, and how we express our feelings. The familial, cultural, and religious environments in which we develop influence the growth of sexuality. If we were loved and nurtured and our sense of competence was fostered and strengthened by those we love, it is likely that we will have healthy self-images and a fair amount of success in both initiating and sustaining personal relationships. If abuse of any sort was present in our background it is conversely likely that we will not develop a positive sense of self-worth and may have difficulty with trusting relationships.

How our first exposure to overtly sexual feelings was handled by others also colors our perception of ourselves as sexual beings. Embarrassment, ridicule, or censure as reactions to sexual expressions can leave lasting scars. Acceptance, encouragement, and enjoyment of such feelings obviously lead to a different conclusion. Fostering the ability to say "no" and accept the responsibility that accompanies the expression of sexuality can only strengthen one's feeling of self-efficacy.

AGING AND SEXUALITY

Deeply embedded in our youth-oriented society is the assumption that sex and sexuality are provinces only for the young. Aging men are depicted as "dirty old men" if they show any interest in sex, while aging women are characterized as sexless old hags. Yet the feelings of sexuality do not disappear as the years pass. Hopefully, these feelings change and grow as we change and grow.

Betty Friedan, in her book *The Fountain of Age,*[3] challenges us to look at how social values victimize both sexes: women by the feminine mystique; men by a lifetime of machismo. Images of youthful erection that always leads to intercourse and an excessive emphasis on performance are a heavy burden for both men *and* women to bear, as these youthful sexual measures impose barriers to intimacy for those who are aging. Pleasuring, cuddling, and touching have been found to be more important among elders,[4] who tend to view the total sexual experience through a qualitative rather than a quantitive lens. Successful sexuality experiences are more than meeting or exceeding a standard of performance. First, the two people involved in a sexual relationship define the parameters. Second, there is an infinite variety of possibilities that may prove satisfying to one or both partners.

INTIMACY

What becomes clear in the recent literature on sexuality and the elderly is the importance of **intimacy.**[5] Sexual intimacy requires self-acceptance and risk taking. It is purposely losing control of oneself and acquiescing with what is happening. When the result of sexual intimacy is a satisfying one, feelings of self-esteem and safety are reinforced.

Intimacy needs to be included as a component of meaningful sexuality. Women, as kin keepers, have traditionally nurtured a capacity for connection and engagement with others in all forms of intimacy. Men may have many friends, but deep and honest disclosure, so vital to intimacy, may not be a part of these friendships. Jung in describing the years after 40 called them the "afternoon" of life and suggests each gender comes to know their polarities, the sexually opposite side of their nature—for the male, his feminine qualities; for the female, her male traits. Coming to grips with these unused and unfamiliar characteristics can involve stress and anxiety, but ultimately the emergence of them can lead to a freedom of expression previously unknown.[5] This "crossover" may be a key to vital aging. "Disengagement from the roles and goals of youth and from activities and ties that no longer have any personal meaning may, in fact, be necessary to make the shift to a new kind of engagement in age."[3] It can enhance sexual activity, with the woman showing more initiative but also expecting more closeness and disclosure from her partner. Couples that persevere through these growth trials can find a new depth and richness to their relationships. They will then be ready to reinvest in different ways of communicating with each other. They want to genuinely touch, know, and love each other. Such renewed ties of intimacy can lead to a sense of control of life and an acceptance, rather than a fear, of aging.

PHYSIOLOGICAL CHANGES FOR WOMEN

There are undeniable changes that occur to both men and women in the physiological aspects of their sexual functioning as they age. The effects of gravity begin to be seen in both men and women as bodies begin to sag and waistlines begin to widen. The changes that each gender encounters do not need to preclude sexual activity, as reduced sexual hormones only affect response time and may affect the intensity of the physical response. Knowing about and understanding the effect of these changes, combined with appropriate adaptations, can actually enhance rather than deter sexual satisfaction.

Menopause, a natural consequence of getting older, is the cessation of menstruation. It is part of the climacteric, a period of time lasting from 6 to 15 years leading up to and following the experience of the last period. It is usually accepted as the beginning of a woman's second half of life and is a physiological marker for changes in her sexual functioning. The average age of the last period of a woman is approximately 52, with a range from 45 to 55.[7]

Much has been written in feminist texts[3,7,8] about the "medicalization" of menopause with large portions of the medical field viewing it as a "deficiency" disease. How menopause is approached and dealt with by women is significantly influenced by a combination of their cultural, religious, and family experiences, as well as their acceptance or denial of the aging process. Ironically, during the first half of the century in this country, medical intervention was seldom used for menopause, since it was viewed as a natural event. Now that 50 million women are nearing menopausal age, an incredible market for manufactured hormones exists.[3] **Estrogen replacement therapy (ERT)** is recommended by physicians to treat this "deficiency disease" with its accompanying hot flashes, sweating, and vaginal dryness and to reduce the likelihood of developing osteoporosis or heart disease. Debates regarding the necessity for ERT abound because of an increased likelihood of developing uterine or breast cancer with this treatment, with the final decision needing to be made by the individual woman based on her particular health status and unique family medical history. More natural approaches (use of homeopathic and herbal remedies, diet, exercise, and the like) are also now preferred to help women experience the menopausal years.[7,9]

Decreasing amounts of estrogen account for many of the signs exhibited at menopause. They include:

- Vaginal changes
    - Thinning of walls
    - Decreased lubrication
    - Foreshortening of vagina
    - Delayed and reduced expansion of the vagina
- Vasomotor changes leading to hot flashes or flushes
    - Blood flows to skin causing a 4°F to 8°F skin temperature increase
    - Sweating
    - Increased heartbeat
    - Chills
    - Tingling of skin
- Less rapid and extreme vascular responses to sexual arousal
    - Waning of flush
    - Reduced increase in breast volume during arousal[9]
- Orgasm—fewer contractions
- Bladder and urethral changes
    - Increased need to urinate, particularly immediately after intercourse
    - Irritability—a variant of "honeymoon cystitis"[9]

- Diminished fatty tissue of mons
    - Labia majora—make them susceptible to mechanical trauma from repetitive bumping or rubbing during intercourse
- Clitoral area more susceptible to irritation by forceful manipulation[7,8,10,25]

An obvious omission from this list of changes is a decrease in libido. Sexual desire and activity do not need to decrease during this period as " sex drive is *NOT* related to estrogen levels."[7] Libido can actually increase postmenopausally because of the elimination of pregnancy fears, decreased child care responsibilities, an increase in energy and a zest for life, and improved self-knowledge.

PHYSIOLOGICAL CHANGES FOR MEN

Sexual functioning also changes for men as they age. These changes are less dramatic than those experienced by women perimenopausally. A gradual decrease in circulating testosterone after 60 years of age accounts for these changes; they do not signal a decrease in potency. Changes include:

- Arousal
    - Delayed and less firm erection with longer intervals to ejaculation
    - Less clear sense of impending orgasm
- Orgasm
    - Abbreviated ejaculation
    - Decreased expulsive urethral contractions

Decreased force of seminal fluid expulsion
Reduced amount of semen ejaculation; ejaculation may not occur
with every intercourse
- Postorgasm
Rapid loss of erection
Longer time needed between erections
- Extragenital
Decreased swelling and erection of nipples
Absence of flush
Reduced elevation of testicles[7,9]

Knowing about these changes can diminish a man's fears of performance and can in fact contribute to increased sexual pleasure. Realizing the need for more prolonged and direct stimulation can lead to lengthened and more engaging lovemaking sessions, sessions that may offer even a more profound sense of pleasure than when the partners were younger. The technique of "stuffing," when a partially erect penis is stuffed into the vagina and the woman tightens her vaginal muscles rhythmically to stimulate both partners, can be an effective alternative.

GENDER DIFFERENCES

New meanings regarding sexuality may emerge as one ages. Despite the fact that men and women develop distinctive sexual styles and that gender differences persist throughout life, some older women have been affected by the current cultural expectations for sexual behavior. These cultural changes may include different sexual scripts,[11] whereby the women can assume the lead, asking for dates or paying her share of expenses on dates. Occupational accomplishments can lead to secure managerial jobs, increased self-esteem, role transitions (loss or change of partner), and an increase in sexual agency, including the ability to choose and have control over one's sexual life.[12]

Masturbation occurrences increased significantly over time for unmarried women, according to a nonrandomized sample of 102 respondents aged 60 to 85 in a 1985 Adams and Turner study.[12] Besides preserving sexual functioning when a partner is not available, masturbation may enhance feelings of autonomy. However, masturbation was not a favored sexual activity of the majority of those, both men and women, who engaged in it. It was viewed as a substitute sexual activity. In this same study, 85 percent of the women and 89 percent of the men preferred interpersonal rather than solo sexual activity if given a choice. Adams and Turner conclude their article on a hopeful note. A substantial minority of women in their study experienced an increase in the frequency of orgasm, subjective pleasure, and overall satisfaction. These changes in sexuality occurred in late middle life and beyond.[1]

Interviews with elders reveal a lasting difference in how men and women view sexual activity. Duke Longitudinal Studies[13,27] have found that sexual activity is more stable over time than previously thought. They found three quarters of men in their 70s engaged in intercourse at least once a month, while over a third of men in their early 60s and nearly 30 percent of men in their late 60s engaged in weekly intercourse. The majority of women were not sexually active, primarily because of a paucity of partners or their male partner's decreased desire. However, from the same Duke University Studies, it was found that nearly one half of married 66 to 71-year-old women were sexually active. Nearly 30 percent of those closer to 80 were sexually active.

In interviews with 10 high functioning, healthy and active, married and divorced, or single women older than 60, Crose and Drake[14] found a decrease in incidence but a constant or increased level of sexual satisfaction from when they were younger. These women also felt they displayed more positive sexual attitudes over time. Sexual encounters had become less pressured, pregnancy was no longer a fear, and seeking pleasure for themselves was an acceptable goal. Masturbation was increasingly used by these women to relieve sexual tension. They indicated a stimulating relationship was a prerequisite to sex. Women maintain and renew ties of intimacy (with both men and women), and this may help them to maintain a sense of control in their later lives.[3]

Prevailing public attitudes that women, after disability, are less interested in sex and their physiological response is less affected led Nosek and colleagues[15] to survey the top concerns of women (1150 women aged 18–65) with physical disabilities. They found that these women were concerned about the following issues:

- The satisfaction of their partners
- Feeling sexually unattractive
- Others viewing them as sexually unattractive
- The physical issues of urinary or bowel accidents

They wanted to receive information about:

- Coping emotionally with the changes in sexual functioning
- Helping a partner cope emotionally with limitations on sexual activity
- Methods and techniques to achieve sexual satisfaction

Despite these findings, women were less likely to have received information about sexuality after injury. This report underscores the importance of psychosocial factors in sexual functioning.

Recognition of the importance of continuing sexuality in the lives of older adults can help to enhance self-esteem and to increase the options for intimacy. Combined with more realistic expectations about age-related changes, it can assist in the development of adaptive coping strategies.

🔲 OLDER LESBIANS AND GAYS

Older **lesbian** and **gay** people are a diverse group—a group whose popular image is often a negative one. Their issues with sexuality are both similar to those that heterosexuals confront and different. Ageism added onto homophobia increases the challenges faced by aging lesbians and homosexuals as they deal with their changing and developing sexuality. Negative stereotypes of lonely, depressed, oversexed, unattractive, and unemotional old lesbians and gays are myths.

Friend,[16] in an article on older lesbian and gay people, reports that a substantial portion of older gay men were found to be "psychologically well-adjusted, self-accepting, and adapting well to the aging process," while a majority of older lesbian women studied were found to be happy and well-adjusted.

Friend, using a social construction theory, proposed that the concept of heterosexuality shaped or constructed the homosexual identity as one of sickness during the turn of the century. Elder lesbian and gay individuals have had to manage heterosexism for the greater part of their lives. They have had to reconstruct the meaning of a homosexual identity in an attempt to control their own sexuality. The attempts to do this have often involved conflicts with family and friends and active attempts to initiate social change. Efforts to find a niche in society have often led to high levels of adjustment where they have developed skills that facilitate their adjustment to the aging process. Such experience develops a "crisis competence" flexibility in gender role, and a redefinition of family,[16] that both provide a unique perspective on other crises in one's life. Knowledge that they may not be able to count on family in old age has encouraged them to more carefully plan for older age.

Lesbian women can and do experience sexual difficulties. Instead of one woman undergoing menopausal changes, there may be two, and at the same time. One may experience a decreased interest in sex.[11] Same gender relationships can, because of a certain closeness that comes from being the same gender, become extremely close and confining, necessitating the establishment of a healthy balance between togetherness and aloneness. Expectations, because of being the same gender, that the other will intuitively know what is wanted and needed may be unrealistic and, as with heterosexual relationships, require good communication between partners to be met.

🔲 ADDRESSING SEXUAL ISSUES

With sexuality such a primal core of our lives, it is a necessary part of a functional evaluation. It is identified as an activity of daily living and falls within the domain of practice of many health care practitioners.[17] When the issue of sexuality is viewed as another aspect of the day-to-day activities in which a client will be involved and when its psychosocial importance is understood, it needs to be included in assessment procedures. Mentioning it as yet another aspect of daily life to be considered provides an opportunity for the client to talk about his or her functioning in this area and to pursue any desired intervention.

It is crucial for the practitioner to have a clear comprehension of his or her comfort level in dealing with issues of sexuality. An obvious first prerequisite is an acceptance of one's own sexuality which requires a level of maturity and a period of introspection. A helpful tool is Annon's four-level **PLISSIT model,**[18] which not only identifies the level of intervention needed by a client but also can assist the practitioner in understanding the level at which he or she can comfortably provide intervention.

Annon's model is a conceptual scheme for differentiating and treating sexual problems and concerns. His schema can help discern those who are likely to respond to sex education and brief sex therapy from those who need intensive psychotherapy. Each descending level requires more expertise from the clinician so the approach can be geared to his or her own level of competence. Knowledge of resources available within their treatment site or community is necessary so referrals can be handled smoothly.

The four levels of treatment within the PLISSIT model are:

Permission — Where the client is given permission to discuss any concerns and is reassured as a sexual being; affords an opportunity for the practitioner to provide a nonjudgmental and relaxed environment in which to share his or her knowledge.

Limited **I**nformation — Where specific factual information directly relevant to the particular sexual problem of concern is provided on a one-on-one basis; myths and misconceptions, particularly about disabilities, can be dispelled.

Specific **S**uggestions — Where strategies or alternatives are provided to change or influence the specific problem behavior; partner needs to be involved at this level; positioning and adaptive equipment are examples.

Intensive **T**herapy — Where long-term treatment for chronic sexual problems is provided.

Health care practitioners need to proceed only to the level to which they feel comfortable and for which they feel prepared. Many will feel able to deal effectively with the first three levels. Inherent in this is preparation for the requisite referral information and knowledge about myths and various disabilities. What is crucial, however, is being able to calmly relay information in an accepting and nonjudgmental manner and to smoothly refer to others, such as occupational therapists and psychologists, for their expertise when necessary.

For practitioners to be able to help clients deal with their sexual concerns they need to be:

- Sensitive
- Understanding of the effect of losses on the mind, spirit, and body
- Knowledgeable of the processes of the diagnosis, as well as possess a knowledge of available resources
- Respectful of differences in sexual expression
- Familiar with a wide number of possible strategies for intervention

They also need to be aware of the following assumptions:

- That the client will bring up sexuality issues
- That chronological age may indicate an increased or decreased libido
- The client's sexual preference
- That the client is monogamous
- That the client shares your views on morality

In other words, you may need to make the first move and to be aware of indirect attempts on the part of the client (jokes, as an example) to bring up the topic.

With aging comes an increase in both chronic and acute physical problems and disabilities. Typical elders have a number of chronic conditions that can affect them not only physically but also emotionally and sexually. Some of the most prevalent chronic conditions of those 65 years or older are arthritis, hypertension, heart disease, deformity or orthopedic impairment, and diabetes.[19]

Another approach is to look at the areas of sexual concern for those who are physically challenged, whether from a recent injury or chronic problems. These fall into four general categories: self-esteem; body image; relationships; and family.[20] Questions about continued worthiness as a man or woman can arise soon after the disability or appear gradually as a chronic condition worsens with age. Issues about whether one's body can be trusted or respected again are likely to coincide with questions regarding self-esteem. Anxiety about the ability to maintain or initiate new relationships, from social to intimate, also surfaces. Options for sexual relations and for continuing to effectively fulfill family roles may need to be addressed.

A practitioner prepared with a foundation of healthy acceptance of his or her sexuality and a desire to holistically treat those who are aging can effectively use his/her clinical knowledge and skills to help in the recovery of a client and/or in the client's ability to learn to live with one or more disabilities. Approaching sexuality from a positive viewpoint, based on what does work rather than on what the person cannot do, and from a base of open communication and intimacy can make a crucial difference.[21]

SAMPLE DIAGNOSTIC CATEGORIES

Knowledge about specific diagnostic categories likely to be associated with being elderly, as well as the coexistence of multiple chronic illnesses, is necessary to effectively and sensitively deal with sexuality issues. Building on psychosocial issues that have been mentioned earlier, using Annon's PLIS-SIT model, and taking into account the areas of sexual concern for those who are physically challenged can help a health care practitioner assist a client. The combination of these two approaches will be used to demonstrate how sexual issues can be dealt with in the following three diagnostic categories, chosen for their prevalence in the elderly.

Arthritis

Limitations by arthritis and rheumatism affect more than 30 percent of people aged 65 and older. Sore joints, range of motion limitations, loss of mobility, and pain with movement can impede sexual performance, yet regular sexual activity can lead to adrenal gland production of cortisone and can decrease stress and lead to less pain, discomfort, and depression.[21] The following are suggestions to deal with the problems this diagnosis may cause:

- Resting prior to sexual activity to prevent fatigue
- Placing a pillow under limbs that are painful
- Using aspirin prophylactically for pain before sexual activity
- Using a hot shower or other heat source before sexual activity
- Experimenting with alternative positions, ones that do not put prolonged pressure on involved joints
- Using alternatives to intercourse such as mutual masturbation or oral sex
- Emptying bladder before sexual activity to increase comfort
- Exercising regularly to increase or maintain joint mobility
- Communicating with partner about fears
- Using a warm waterbed[22]

Heart Disease

Heart disease can lead to anxiety about and avoidance of sexual activity. However, the energy costs of the average sexual act approximates walking rapidly or climbing one or two flights of stairs. A client 4 to 5 weeks after a coronary attack is usually ready to resume these activities. It is not uncommon for men to have sexual difficulties for up to 6 to 12 months after recovery. Fear of sudden death during sex, low endurance, and medication-induced erectile problems feed a man's anxiety. In fact, death during coitus accounts for less than 1 percent of sudden coronary deaths, and, of these, 70 percent occur during extramarital relations.[23] Women are less likely to develop subsequent sexual problems. Suggestions include:

- Taking a less active role in sexual act
- Learning and using relaxation techniques
- Masturbating as an alternative
- Taking time with foreplay to allow the heart to warm up slowly
- Avoiding sexual activity when anxious or fatigued or when weather is extremely hot, cold, or humid
- Using positions that conserve energy and are non-weight-bearing (sitting, side-lying, for example)[22]

Cerebrovascular Accidents and Stroke

Cerebrovascular accidents (CVAs) lead to sensation loss, perceptual problems, loss of strength and mobility, visual problems, and/or communication problems. Suggestions for older people with this diagnosis include using altouch, smell and vision rather than speech.

- Experimenting with comfortable positions
- Having partner stay within the visual field
- Using a waterbed
- Using a vibrator to compensate for weakness or incoordination
- Stimulating areas that remain responsive to touch[22]

An alternative way to list helpful possibilities is one that does not rely on diagnostic categories but rather on symptomatology. The chart in Table 7–1 is self-explanatory.

THE INFLUENCE OF MEDICATIONS

Knowledge of how medications can affect sexual functioning is also important for effective intervention with sexuality concerns. Honest reporting of concerns to the physician is necessary. Alternative medications, ones that may eliminate or reduce any sexual problems, may be available. A list of commonly used drugs and their possible side effects is included for your reference (Table 7–2).

SEXUALITY ISSUES FOR THE INSTITUTIONALIZED

When elders become dependent and institutionalized, the need for intimacy and sexual expression does not disappear. Their needs for intimacy may in fact increase as they make efforts to cope within a constrained environment. Acknowledging these needs and taking steps to accommodate them are important signs of respect and are normally done on a case-by-case basis. Some institutions have set aside one room where couples may spend time alone to

TABLE 7–1. Presenting Problems and Potential Solutions

Presenting Problem	Possible Diagnoses	Precautions	Potential Solutions
Decreased endurance	Arthritis Cardiac disease Post CVA Parkinson's disease	Avoid extreme temperatures, heat, cold, humidity. Avoid anxiety and fatigue. Avoid sexual activity until 1 hour after a large meal. Avoid alcohol.	Rest prior to sexual activity. Schedule sexual activity forbest energy time during day. Utilize sexual positions and techniques that require less energy: • Affected partner lying on back (no energy expended to support weight on arms) • Both partners in spoon side-lying position with back of one to front of another (no overworking of muscles to support weight) • Ample direct genital foreplay Use masturbation as alternative.
Pain, stiff joints, or decrease range of motion	Arthritis	Pain: Respect pain. Support painful area. Do not continue painful motion. Avoid staying in one position too long. Be well rested.	Place pillow under affected limbs. Precede sexual activity with warm bath, hot shower, or other heat source. Take aspirin prophylactically for pain prior to sexual activity. Exercise regularly to increase or maintain joint mobility. Use warm waterbed. Use relaxation techniques. Experiment with alternative positions, ones that do not put prolonged pressure on involved joints: • Rear entry supported by woman • Nonaffected partner on top

Continued on following page

TABLE 7–1. *Presenting Problems and Potential Solutions*

Presenting Problem	Possible Diagnoses	Precautions	Potential Solutions
Sensory changes	Post cerebral vascular accident (CVA) (sight, touch, proprioception)	Be aware of involved body parts and extent and type	Stimulate adjacent areas that may have become more sensitive.
	Cataracts, glaucoma, diabetic retinopathy, macular degeneration	of involvement. Avoid prolonged pressure on any body part with decreased sensation.	Experiment to find new pleasurable focal points. Experiment with different types of stimulation: • Vibration • Temperature • Lotions/oils
	Hearing impairments	Slowly change positions to prevent injury.	Rely on other sensory channels: • Verbal • Visual, erotic imagery Have partner stay within visual field
Loss of motor control Muscle weakness Paralysis	Post CVA Multiple sclerosis Parkinson's disease		Use firm surface (for better balance and transfers). Use pillows and rolled pillows for added support. Use bed rails, trapeze, etc. for safety and assistance with position changes. Search for positions that provide stability, as well as comfort and pleasure.
Abnormal muscle tone	Cerebral palsy (CP) Post CVA		Use positions that decrease tone: • Supine with flexed knees • Lying on affected side • Quadruped Use firm surface and pillows and rolled towels to assist in maintaining position. Use relaxation techniques as part of foreplay: • Rocking • Slow massage Use warm comfortable room with soft music and low lighting.

Continued on following page

TABLE 7–1. *Presenting Problems and Potential Solutions*

Presenting Problem	Possible Diagnoses	Precautions	Potential Solutions
			Use prescribed muscle relaxants for high tone prior to sexual activity.
Contractures	Arthritis Post CVA	Avoid stress to contractures.	Use comfortable positions. Work within pain-free range of movement.
Tremors	Parkinson's disease Medication-related side effect		Use positions that incorporate weight bearing on affected limbs. Either decrease or increase movement, depending on which produces fewer tremors.
Bladder/bowel dysfunction	Post CVA Spinal cord injury	Have towels nearby in advance.	Discuss fears and concerns with partner before sexual activity. Determine safest time during urinary schedule for sexual activity. Use protective covering on mattress. Man can wear condom for small amounts of urinary incontinence during sexual activity. Empty bladder before sexual activity. If on catheterization program, catherize and empty bladder before sexual activity. Secure indwelling catheter prior to sexual activity (woman, to abdomen; man, to penis) Use extension on tubing for bedside drainage bag for more maneuverability.

Data from references 8, 11, 22–24.

TABLE 7–2. *Drug-Induced Sexual Dysfunction*

Drug	Potential Effects
Alcohol (ethanol)	Libido enhanced at low doses; dose-related progressive decline due to central nervous system depressant effects; can result in failure of erection in men and reduced vaginal vasodilation and delayed orgasm in women; can also cause disinhibition, impaired judgment, and decreased ability to enjoy sexual encounter
Amphetamines	Libido enhanced at low doses; possible erectile dysfunction in men with higher doses may cause hyperexcitability, tremulousness, and anxiety
Anticonvulsants	Reduced libido; can cause drowsiness, irritability, dizziness, confusion, ataxia, and slurred speech, as well as nausea, constipation, and/or diarrhea, which may interfere with sexual activity
Antidepressants	
Tricyclics; monoamine oxidase inhibitors	Decreased libido, erectile dysfunction, impotence, delayed and/or painful ejaculation, and anorgasmia in men; decreased libido, delayed orgasm, and anorgasmia in women
Selective serotonin rouptake inhibitors	Delayed orgasm, anorgasmia (primarily with fluoxetrine)
Trazodone	Priapism, increased libido in women
Antihypertensives	
Diuretics	Decreased libido, erectile dysfunction, impotence, gynecomastia
Beta-blockers	Erectile dysfunction, decreased libido, impotence
Alpha-blockers	Erectile dysfunction, priapism
Calcium-channel blockers and methyldopa, clonidine, hydralazine	Erectile dysfunction
Barbiturates and Benzodiazepines	Libido enhanced at low doses; progressive decline with higher doses due to central nervous system depressant effects
Cocaine	Erectile dysfunction, ejaculatory dysfunction, anorgasmia

Data from material by Thomas D. Nolin, RPh, MS; and Aldridge, SA: Drug-induced sexual dysfunction. Clin Pharm 1:141–147, 1982; Lee, M, and Sharifi, R: More on drug-induced sexual dysfunction. Clin Pharm 1:397, 1982; Smith RJ, and Talbert, RL: Sexual dysfunction with antihypertensive and antipsychotic agents. Clin Pharm 5:373–384, 1986; Thompson JF: Geriatric urological disorders. In Young, LY, and Koda-Kimble, MA (eds): Applied Therapeutics: The Clinical Use of Drugs. Applied Therapeutics, Vancouver, WA, 1995, p 103–1; Troutman, WG: Drug-induced sexual dysfunction. In Anderson, PO, and Knoben, JE (eds): Handbook of Clinical Drug Data. Appleton & Lange, Stamford, CT, 1997, p 686.

pursue whatever course of intimacy they choose; other organizations help schedule time alone in shared rooms when the roommate is regularly out of the room.[26] Staff are educated to be accepting of expressions of intimacy and sexuality (masturbation, hand holding, kissing, touching, petting)[27] and to know when to guide the involved people into more private areas.

Special needs may also be apparent in the community partners of those institutionalized. Providing time and space for intimacy when desired is important, as is offering counseling and understanding from the medical staff.[28]

A primary issue of concern is that of competence. Determining whether an elder is capable of making a choice and not being taken advantage of is crucial. Guidelines have been proposed for use in long-term care settings by Lichtenberg. They are based on a Mini-Mental State Examination score of at least 14 and a subjective interview that addresses awareness of others, capacity to decline uninvited sexual contact, and realization that a relationship may be time-limited.[29]

RESPONSIBLE SEXUAL BEHAVIOR

Age is not an excuse for failure to follow safe sex practices. Sexually transmitted diseases and HIV cases do exist in the elderly population. Statistics from the Centers for Disease Control and Prevention show that approximately 10 percent of the diagnosed cases of acquired immunodeficiency syndrome (AIDS) are among Americans 50 years or older. This incidence is rising faster among this group than in younger age groups with a male/female ratio of approximately 9:1.[30]

This elder group differs from those who are younger with AIDS. They show the largest proportion of cases in any adult age group attributed to heterosexual transmission[31]; other cases are ascribed to blood transfusions occurring before 1985[32]; and approximately 16 percent in a study[31] of older adults became infected from IV drug use. However, homosexual or bisexual behavior remains the predominant risk factor for HIV infection up to the age of 70.[32] An additional startling difference is that the proportion of AIDS cases diagnosed in the same month of death rises with age,[32] indicating both a more rapid disease progression and lack of awareness by medical personnel. Nonspecific symptoms are frequently overlooked, because of the high level of chronic illnesses in the older population. AIDS dementia complex may be the initial manifestation of HIV infection and needs to be part of any differential diagnosis of elders with diffuse cognitive dysfunction.[33] This type of dementia progresses more rapidly than that of Alzheimer's disease.

Educational efforts regarding safe sexual practices have been almost exclusively directed to younger cohorts, at least partially explained by the societal stereotype that elders are no longer sexual. Consequently, safe sex practices are not subscribed to by this age group. At-risk persons older than 50 were only one sixth as likely to use condoms as compared with at-risk persons in the 20- to 29-year group.[30] Atrophic vaginal tissue changes in older women make them particularly susceptible to lesions that may readily admit HIV.[32]

Recommendations include an increased awareness on the part of health care practitioners, particularly physicians, of the need to routinely make sexual histories a part of their medical examinations.[32,33] This involves demystifying the stereotype that elders are sexually inactive. Health care practitioners also need to be aware of the different ways this disease may be manifested in elders, the appropriate modes of treatment, and a sensitivity to how this information is acknowledged by the client and shared with significant others.[31] Support, in all forms, must be nurtured in this group, as in any age group.

SUMMARY

Acknowledging the importance sexuality plays in all of our lives and displaying a sensitivity to the personal nature of this component of our lives can help health care practitioners assist the elderly to effectively deal with sexuality issues. Providing empathy and appropriate information, devising adaptations, and encouraging experimentation to find resolutions can be an invaluable service to clients. Tact, discretion, and sometimes judicious use of humor are also effective tools on which a health care practitioner can rely. Routinely discussing sexuality as another one of the activities of daily living gives the client permission to talk about and deal with any issues in this area. Collaborative problem solving can help to empower the client to gain control over this most intimate of areas. The resulting feelings of wholeness and connectedness to another are gifts we can give ourselves.

REVIEW QUESTIONS

1. Sexuality is not only an eight letter word. It can best be defined by which of the following phrases?

   A. Sexual intercourse
   B. Is basic to our sense of self
   C. Intimacy is a prerequisite
   D. A dynamic concept defined in a mutually satisfying way by both partners

2. Choose the statement that is NOT true. Aging:

   A. Causes physiological changes in both genders
   B. precludes sexual activity
   C. for women has become medicalized (in its treatment of menopause)
   D. causes a decrease in testosterone in men, but it does not signal a decrease in potency

3. Choose the TRUE statement that best completes the following sentence. Sexuality changes in later life for women can include:

   A. An increase in orgasm frequency, subjective pleasure, and overall satisfaction
   B. Masturbation as a favored sexual activity
   C. Increased lubrication of the vaginal walls
   D. Few vasomotor changes

4. Choose the FALSE statement that best completes the following sentence. Sexuality changes in later life for men can include:

   A. A rapid loss of erection
   B. A reduced amount of ejaculate
   C. An increase in potency
   D. Less dramatic changes than those experienced by premenopausal women

5. Which of the following issues do older lesbian and gay people face that heterosexuals do not encounter?

   A. Homophobia
   B. Ageism
   C. Aging bodies
   D. Negative stereotypes

6. Which of the following is NOT helpful to a practitioner about to deal with issues of sexuality?

   A. A sense of humor
   B. An understanding of own comfort level with issues of sexuality
   C. A knowledge of sexuality resources
   D. Waiting for the client to bring up concerns about sexuality

7. Choose the following phrase that best addresses the areas of sexual concern for those who are physically challenged.

   A. Self-esteem, body weight, appearance and relationships
   B. Family, relationships, body image, and self-esteem
   C. Appearance, family, ability to perform, and friendships

8. The most common diagnostic categories of the elderly that may affect sexuality issues are:

   A. Arthritis, heart disease, and cerebrovascular accident
   B. Spinal cord injury, multiple sclerosis, and burns
   C. Diabetes, glaucoma, and tinnitis
   D. Vertigo, arthritis, emphysema, and macular degeneration

9. Utilizing sexual positions and techniques that require less energy is a method that is helpful for all people with the following diagnoses EXCEPT:

   A. Parkinson's Disease
   B. Post cerbrovascular accident

C. Glaucoma
D. Cardiac disease
E. Arthritis

10. Fill in the blank with the best choice. Exercising regularly, using a warm waterbed, using relaxation techniques, and experimenting with alternative positions are examples of potential solutions for the presenting problem of _____.
   A. Sensory changes
   B. Paralysis
   C. Abnormal muscle tone
   D. Pain

LEARNING ACTIVITIES

Now that some of the basics of sexuality and aging have been presented, it is time to apply the knowledge to the following questions and scenarios.

1. Describe your first discoveries of sexual feelings.

2a. How have your family, culture, and religion affected your own sexuality?

b. How have your family, culture, and religion affected your views on the sexuality of others?

3a. What effects has peer pressure had on your sexuality?

b. How can cohort effects influence one's sexuality?

4. Using the PLISSIT model and considering the four areas of sexual concern, develop a plan that addresses the specific diagnosis, age, and concerns of the following client:
   A. A woman, aged 72, with a total hip replacement and arthritis who is interested in continuing sex with her partner.
   B. A 65-year-old man with congestive heart failure who is very concerned about continuing his sexual relationship with his 55-year-old wife.
   C. A 70-year-old man post right cerebrovascular accident who is experiencing both sensory changes (decreased sensation on the left side; decreased left visual field) and decreased endurance. Despite these, he wishes to maintain an intimate relationship with his wife of more than 50 years.

REFERENCES

1. American Association of Retired Persons: A Profile of Older Americans. American Association of Retired Persons, Washington, DC, 1995.
2. Hettler, B: Test Well Wellness Inventory. National Wellness Institute, Stevens Point, WI, 1979.

3. Friedan, B: The Fountain of Age. Simon and Shuster, New York, 1993.

4. Starr, BD, and Weiner, MB: The Starr-Weiner Report on Sex and Sexuality in the Mature Years. Stein and Day, New York, 1981.

5. Butler, RN, et al: Love and sex after 60: How physical changes affect intimate expression. A roundtable discussion: Part 1. Geriatrics 49(9):21–27, 1994.

6. Bruce, MA, and Borg, B: Frames of Reference in Psychosocial Occupational Therapy. Slack, Thorofare, NJ, 1987, pp 47, 196.

7. Northrup, C: Women's Bodies, Women's Wisdom. Bantam Books, New York, 1994.

8. Siegal, DL, et al: Menopause: Entering our third age. In Doress, PB, and Siegal, DL (eds): Ourselves Growing Older. Touchstone Book, New York, 1987, p 116.

9. Weed, SS: Menopausal years: The Wise Woman Way. Ash Tree Publishing, Woodstock, NY, 1992.

10. Masters, WH: Sex and aging—expectations and reality. Hosp Prac 15 August, p 175, 1986.

11. Leiblum, SR: Sexuality and the midlife woman. Psychology of Women Quarterly 14:495, 1990.

12. Adams, CG, and Turner, BE: Reported change in sexuality from young adulthood to old age. The Journal of Sex Research 21(2):126, 1985.

13. Pfeiffer, E, et al: Sexual behavior in middle life. Am J Psychiatry 128(10):82, 1972.

14. Crose, R, and Dranke, LK: Older women's sexuality. Clinical Gerontologist 12(4):51, 1993.

15. Nosek, MA, et al: Sexual functioning among women with physical disabilities. Arch Phys Med Rehabil 77:107, February, 1996.

16. Friend, RA: Older lesbian and gay people: A theory of successful aging. Journal of Homosexuality 20(3–4):99, 1991.

17. Friedman, JD: Sexual expression: The forgotten component of ADL. OT Practice 20, January, 1997.

18. Annon, JS: The PLISSIT model: A proposed conceptual scheme for the behavioral treatment of sexual problems. Journal of Sex Education and Therapy 1, Spring/Summer, 1976.

19. Adams, PF, and Benson, V: Current estimates from the National Health Interview Survey. National Center for Health Statistics. Vital Health Statistics 10(184), 1991.

20. Fox, S: Dismissing taboos: OT's integrate sexuality into "whole reason" treatment approach. Advance for Occupational Therapists 13–17, June 18, 1990.

21. Joe, BE: Coming to terms with sexuality. OT Week 13, September 19, 1996.

22. Laflin, M: Sexuality and the elderly. Aging: The Health Care Challenge, ed 3. Lewis, CB, F.A. Davis, Philadelphia, 1996, p 364.

23. Lewis, CB: Aging: The Health Care Challenge. F.A. Davis, Philadelphia, 1985, p 293.

24. Montgomery, EA, and Hogan, LS: A New Beginning: Sexuality and Rehabilitation. Spaulding Rehabilitation Hospital, Boston, 1992.

25. Kiernat, M: Occupational Therapy and the Older Adult: A Clinical Manual. Aspen, Gaithersburg, MD, 1991, p 39.

26. Galindo, D, and Kaiser, FE: Sexual health after 60. Patient Care 25–41, April 15, 1995.

27. Steinke, EE: Sexuality in aging: Implications for nursing facility staff. The Journal of Continuing Education in Nursing 28(2):59–63, March/April, 1997.

28. McCartney, JR, et al: Sexuality and the institutionalized elderly. Journal of American Geriatric Society. 35:331–333, 1987.

29. Lichtenberg, PA: A Guide to Psychological Practice in Geriatric Long-Term Care. Haworth Press, New York, 1994.

30. Feldman, MD, et al: The growing risk of AIDS in older patients. Patient Care 61–63, October 30, 1994.

31. Stall, R, and Catania, J: AIDS risk behaviors among late middle-aged and elderly Americans: The National AIDS Behavioral Surveys. Arch Intern Med 154:57–63, 1994.

32. Whipple, B, and Scura, KW: The overlooked epidemic: HIV in older adults. Amercian Journal of Nursing 96(2):23–28, 1996.

33. Wallace, JI, et al: HIV infection in older patients: When to suspect the unexpected. Geriatrics 48(6)61–70, 1993.

🔲 **BIBLIOGRAPHY**

Cole, E, and Rothblum, E: Commentary on "Sexuality and the midlife woman." Psychology of Women Quarterly 14:509, 1990.

Cross, RJ: What doctors and others need to know: Six facts on human sexuality and aging. SEICUS Report, June/July, p 7, 1993.

Doress, PB, and Siegal, DL (eds): Ourselves Growing Older. A Touchstone Book by Simon and Shuster, New York, 1987.

Goldstein, H, and Runyon, C: An occupational therapy educational model to increase sensitivity about geriatric sexuality. Physical and Occupational Therapy in Geriatrics 11(2):57, 1993.

Mooradian, AD, and Grieff, V: Sexuality in older women. Arch Intern Med 150:1033, 1990.

Pedretti, LW: Occupational Therapy: Practice Skills for Physical Dysfunction, ed 4. St Louis, MO, Mosby, 1996, p 275.

The Boston Women's Health Collective: The New Our Bodies, Ourselves. A Touchstone Book by Simon & Shuster, New York, 1992.

Pfeiffer, E, et al: The natural history of sexual behavior in a biologically advantaged group of aged individuals. J Geronto 24:193, 1969.

Schiavi, RC, et al: Sexual satisfaction in healthy aging men. Journal of Sex and Marital Therapy 20(1):3, Spring 1994.

Smedley, G: Addressing sexuality in the elderly. Rehabilitation Nursing 16(1):9, 1991.

The Continuum of Care

Regula H. Robnett

BEHAVIORAL OBJECTIVES

Upon completion of this chapter, the reader will be able to:

1. Describe housing options for people who are able to live independently, including advantages and disadvantages.
2. Define the three different types of continuing care retirement community (CCRC).
3. List other group housing options and relate these to prospective residents' needs.
4. Define assisted living.
5. Describe how home health care and rehabilitation fit into the health care continuum.
6. Discuss past and present opinions on long-term care.
7. List the risk factors associated with needing long-term care.
8. List several components of the Omnibus Budget Reconciliation Act (OBRA).
9. Discuss how health care professionals can ensure a supportive environment for the elderly.
10. Define reminiscence and describe how the health care professional can effectively use this tool.

KEY TERMS

Activities of dail living (ADLs)
Adaptation
Adult day care
American Association of Retired
   Persons (AARP)
Assisted living center
Board and care facility
Congregate housing
Continuing care retirement
   community (CCRC)
Empowerment
Home health care
Independent living units

Instrumental activities of daily
   living (IADLs)
Life care communities
Long-term care
Managed care
Omnibus Budget Reconciliation Act
   (OBRA)
Physiatrist
Rehabilitation
Reminiscence
Residential care
Reverse mortgage
Single-room occupancy (SRO)

INTRODUCTION—HOUSING AND ENVIRONMENT

Housing is intimately related to health care. Healthy, physically able elders can live independently in their own homes, while those with physical and/or cognitive disabilities may need a more supportive environment. This chapter explores the continuum of care for older people, looking at different housing options, along with their limitations and advantages, and relating these options to the health care requirements of the elderly. This chapter also covers the basic tenets of environmental adaptation. At times, adapting the environment is all that is needed for continued safety and independence in the home.

🕸 INDEPENDENT LIVING

Many senior citizens decide to maintain living arrangements in their lifetime homes, even though staying in these homes may present environmental barriers and cause financial hardships. These homes are often the ones in which they raised their children; they frequently offer more room than is needed and involve more than one story of living space. The reasons for staying in these homes can be quite compelling. A few possibilities are listed here:

- Older people may feel that by giving up their home, they are giving up their freedom and independence.
- They may feel emotionally attached to a home that holds years of cherished memories.
- They may like the neighborhood and not want to leave friends.
- They may want to maintain a large house for when family and friends visit.
- Many people, of all ages, either do not like or are even fearful of change.

As health care professionals, we must respect competent older peoples' wish to remain in their own homes, even if we do not believe that this is the best possible plan for them. This can be difficult for families and friends to accept. Morgan and colleagues[1] claim that the majority of elderly householders do wish to remain in their own homes for as long as possible, preferably their whole lives. Well-meaning family members may insist that the elderly person leave the family home, but this kind of interference may be more detrimental than helpful.

Garrett[2] speaks to this difficulty when he describes an elderly woman, Violet, who was forced to leave her home with steep stairs, several cats over whom she regularly tripped, an outdoor toilet, and a gas stove. Her children insisted that she move to a modern apartment that was determined to be much safer. However, because of Violet's hearing impairment and her lack of familiarity with the new surroundings and the way things worked in the apartment, she became isolated and depressed. Garrett contends that, while safety is crucial, the home environment should be of the person's choosing if at all possible. He states that home improvements to increase safety may be a preferred alternative to moving out of the home.

Unfortunately the lack of adequate income among elders precludes some older people, especially women, from staying in their homes even if they want to and are physically capable of doing so. The results of the American Housing Survey conducted by the Department of Housing and Urban Development, which were reported in 1995, indicated that 20 percent of elderly households had incomes below the poverty level.[3] Elderly people often had to pay more than 25 percent of their household income for housing, and consequently about a third of the nation's elderly reported not having enough money left over for essentials like food, clothing, and health care.[3] In 1992, 71 percent of the 4 million elderly poor in this country were women. Their median yearly income was just over $8000, compared with men of the same age who had a median income well over $14,000.[4]

The **reverse mortgage** program, which is just beginning to gain popularity in the United States, is one option that has made it possible for many older people (especially women at or below poverty level) to afford to stay in their own long-term homes. In 1991, the median amount of home equity for those aged 65 to 69 was $50,000, and approximately 3 million women (more than half of them considered low-income) had home equities of $40,000 or more.[1] Through this program, borrowers use their home as collateral, and the bank sets up either an annuity or a line of credit to be used as needed until the home is sold. This allows those with inadequate monthly income, but substantial home equity, to continue to reside in their own homes. When the older person decides to or needs to sell or he or she dies, the bank then recovers its investment.

While reasons for staying in the family home are compelling, the decision to move may be the necessary or preferred option. Older people may decide to move for reasons such as limited finances, wanting fewer home management responsibilities, physical decline, and/or seeking a warmer or more moderate climate. The federal government provides incentives that may make it particularly attractive for an older person to sell the family home. Profits from home sales can be tax exempt following certain guidelines. The government also subsidizes low-cost apartments for lower income people.[5] Often these units are well designed for people who are elderly and/or who have disabilities.

The housing options for the elderly are numerous, but vary in their accessibility both physically and financially. The simplest move may be to a smaller house or apartment. Older people often begin to realize the need to move to more accessible housing, which may have fewer or no stairs and less space. To make accommodations, some begin giving away or selling longtime possessions.

Sometimes these retirement homes, which are generally ranch style houses or condominiums, are located in clusters. A convenient plan is for each individual home to be situated on commonly owned land, which is taken care of by a groundskeeper hired by the housing association. The housing development may also offer a clubhouse for group activities and a pool. The amenities come for a price; besides a mortgage payment, there is also a monthly fee to the association for upkeep of the common grounds.

Apart from the spouse or life partner, a home may be the single most important factor in the life of an elderly person.[2] Therefore, it is crucial that the home environment foster a sense of security and comfort. This is especially important for the remaining spouse after the death of a long-time partner. Unfortunately, this is exactly when it may be difficult for the one left, usually a widow, to afford to "live in the manner to which she has become accustomed."

This may be the time that the elder decides to move in with other family members such as children or grandchildren. Nearly one of five elderly who are not living in a group home reside in multigenerational households. This arrangement may have a cultural bias: studies have found that older people of southern, central, and eastern European descent are more likely to reside with family (other than spouse) than those of northwestern European descent. Ethnicity and the importance of family relationships tend to be stronger among the first group.[6] This finding can have implications for social policy and is of significance to the health care professional. Not infrequently in the United States, homes are being purchased or built with the intention of having a separate "in-law apartment." While this seems to be a good solution for many families, not all elders wish to be in such proximity to their children (or vice versa), and in fact, research findings generally show that most elderly people prefer not to live with their children.[7] If at all possible, the arrangement should be the optimal choice of everyone, especially the elder involved.

Some elderly people (usually widowed or unmarried) choose to live in **single-room occupancy (SRO)** buildings, because these are inexpensive and may be located in familiar neighborhoods. An estimated 400,000 elderly in the United States lived in SROs in 1987. These single rooms are usually found in cities and rarely offer a private bathroom or kitchen facilities. They are considered by some to be a substandard housing type. However, these single rooms do offer a low-cost independent living alternative, especially for those who have little money and weak family ties. Based on survey results, Crystal and Beck[8] conclude that SROs are a needed housing alternative and that an appropriate level of support should be available for elders living in these rooms as their needs change as a result of aging.

🔲 LIFE CARE COMMUNITIES

Health care for life can be obtained at **continuing care retirement communities (CCRCs),** which have existed for more than 100 years, but have just recently gained popularity in the United States. Some view the CCRC idea as a promising living option for elderly people. To join, the person pays an entrance fee and a monthly fee, and in return gets a home and certain services (specific to that CCRC). These homes are arranged in a small community and may be free-standing houses, condominiums, or apartments and can include residential treatment facilities to provide ongoing long-term care. The services may be optional for the resident and may range from no outside services at all to comprehensive health care services as needed. Services that are sometimes available include housecleaning, meals, recreational programs, transportation, grounds upkeep, laundry service, individual medication management, respite care, rehabilitation, nursing services, health promotion and illness prevention programs, recreational programs, and social services. Table 8–1 describes the three categories of CCRCs as explained by Brower.[9]

There are several advantages to living in a CCRC, if it is the choice of the older person to move there.

- CCRCs are becoming more affordable. They were historically viewed as being essentially for affluent elders only, but now with the different types of CCRCs and a menu of services that can be pared down, they are more accessible to those with moderate incomes, especially those who have a substantial sum of money in life savings or home sales equity.

TABLE 8–1. *Features of Continuing Care Retirement Communities (CCRCs)*

Type of CCRC	Fees	Services
Type A Extensive CCRCs	The entrance fee is higher than the other two types (up to or exceeding $300,000). However, the monthly fee does not increase substantially if more health care services are needed.	Provide unlimited long-term care for residents as they need it.
Type B Modified contract CCRCs	Usually have more moderate fees than extensive CCRCs.	Provide a specified level of long-term care in the original contract, but if the amount needed exceeds the specified level, the older person then is responsible for the additional payment.
Type C Fee-for-service CCRCs	Tend to have lower entrance fees (usually at least $5000) and lower monthly fees than types A and B.	The resident pays for all services as needed.

- Those who need health care services can remain in close proximity to friends and family members who are well and are able to live independently.
- CCRCs offer barrier-free environments and a variety of opportunities for social and physical interaction that can improve overall health and quality of life.[9]

Although the CCRC can be the ideal living situation for some elderly people, the concept also has its disadvantages:

- The cost is still out of reach for many elderly people, even with the pared down fee-for-service option.
- The financial risk of joining a CCRC is real. It is based on the idea of risk pooling, which is like an insurance plan. Everyone pays in, but only a few are expected to need to use a large sum of money for extended long-term care. If significantly more residents than expected need extensive health care services, the financial viability of the organization can be threatened. (Fortunately, the bankruptcy rate is quite low. In 1992, only 1.4 percent of CCRCs had reported bankruptcy.[10]) On a similar note, if sales of the CCRC units do not progress as quickly as planned, it can also spell financial hardship for the residents and the organization.
- There is a lack of uniform standardization of regulations for CCRCs, and financial statements about the CCRC can be difficult to obtain or understand.
- CCRCs do not accept all applicants. Sloan and colleagues[10] report that approximately 60 percent do not accept applicants who are incontinent, and 90 percent do not accept applicants who are unable to perform one or more activities of daily living (ADL) tasks.
- Finally, in at least some CCRCs there is little mingling with younger generations.[9] The CCRC may be a tight-knit community, but made up only of senior citizens. One resident had exactly that complaint about her life care community, which she called a "small microcosm of geriatric society, or God's waiting room."[11] On the other hand, in response to this woman's comments about the presence of disability and death at a CCRC, Somers, who is also a woman living in a CCRC, writes: " . . . such tragedies are not limited to those who live in CCRCs but an inevitable part of human experience." The only alternatives to the loss of loved ones—neither very attractive—are to avoid love or to die first.[12]

OTHER GROUP HOUSING OPTIONS

CONGREGATE HOUSING

A concept similar to the life care communities described in the previous section is that of **congregate housing** facilities. This term encompasses a multitude of differing options, including **independent living units,** adult congregate living facilities, rental retirement housing, and senior retirement centers. These units, which are sometimes subsidized by state and federal government programs, are difficult to describe comprehensively since they can vary so much from one another. Generally they do not offer personal assistance or health services, although the resident may be eligible for home care services through an outside agency. The units are usually sponsored by a not-for-profit organization, but the private for-profit sector is becoming more involved. On the average, a congregate housing complex contains 145 units. Aside from added security or safety features, these units may resemble any other apartment complexes. However, they do often offer group dining and socializing centers. Incoming tenants, whose average age is 80, must be capable of living independently.[5]

Unfortunately, a significant portion (estimated at 35% to 40%) of elderly people (those who cannot afford the market price but are not eligible for subsidized housing) are left out of the congregate housing market. It seems, as Golant[5] describes, as if there are indeed "many possibilities" available for senior housing, but "few choices" for those with inadequate income—a substantial portion of the elderly population in this country.

RESIDENTIAL CARE

Residential care facilities also have multiple labels, including adult residential facilities, adult group homes, domiciliary homes, personal care homes, family care, adult foster care, rest homes, board and care homes, and perhaps currently the most popular name, **assisted living centers.** All have the common theme of bridging the gap between independent living and 24-hour-a-per day nursing care.[5]

Assisted living companies are proliferating across the nation, and the business of providing assisted living was listed as one of the four promising industries for 1997 by *Fortune* magazine. Growth is expected in this area for the next 10 to 20 years.[13] The concept is simple: assisted living centers provide senior citizens the opportunity to "age in place."

The Assisted Living Association of America[14] defines assisted living as:

> A special combination of housing and personalized health care (services) designed to respond to the individual needs of those who need help with **activities of daily living (ADLs).** Care is provided in such a way that promotes maximum independence and dignity for each resident.

Residents rent small apartments and receive needed assistance with ADLs and **instrumental activities of daily living (ADLs)** (home management) as part of their monthly rental fee. Some companies provide nursing home level of care (including skilled nursing) in their facilities, while others provide only minimal care. This alternative model of housing seeks to allow independent decision making and risk taking, while promoting the ultimate safety of all residents. The apartments are "homelike" and environmentally accessible. Residents are encouraged to bring personal furnishings.

One study by Armer[15] found that the degree of personalization of the environment was related to the degree of adjustment to the new surroundings. She recommended that caregivers support the relocated older person in adapting his or her own room. When this personalization fails to take place, caregivers should view this as a signal that the person may have some unmet mental health needs. In such a case, further assessment or a referral may be necessary.

Community or shared space is also a feature of assisted living centers. Dining rooms, laundry areas, libraries, and activity/physical fitness areas are conveniently located to promote social interactions.[16] While an initial move is necessary to establish oneself at an assisted living facility, many elderly people find relocating is well worth the consequent security it brings. While residents are encouraged to maintain an optimal level of functioning, they also can trust that if health issues do surface, they will receive the needed care in their new home for as long as possible.

Board and care facilities are also considered to be in this residential care spectrum, but they differ from many assisted living centers in that they tend to be located in older, large single family homes. These homes for elders are typically run by a middle-aged woman or a couple, who provide meals, transportation, other services, and "protective oversight" as needed. A board and care home has generally one to eight beds, which may be located in either private or shared bedrooms. Although licensed board and care facilities account for two thirds of all residential care facilities, they house only one third of the residential care occupants because of their small occupancy numbers. The atmosphere is often family oriented and homelike.[5]

For many, residential care facilities offer a viable alternative to nursing home care. Proponents for assisted living claim that 30 percent of nursing home residents could be more appropriately placed in residential care facilities, if these placements were available.[17] However, there are a few problem areas with assisted living centers that surface under scrutiny:

- The lack of adequate licensing, inspection, and enforcement of these facilities may put residents in danger of abuse or neglect. Governmental agencies blame this deficiency on limited financial resources.
- There is a lack of public funding for assisted living beds, again causing this vital resource to be financially out of reach for many elderly people who need exactly this type of arrangement.
- There is no training or education required for residential care operators. Therefore some caregivers may be ill equipped to care for older people who have physical problems, mental illness or dementia.[5]
- The cost per month can vary from $20 to more than $200 per day, with an average cost of $72 per day (1995).[18] Also the facilities may charge an ini-

tial deposit or entry fee and may not admit someone who does not have substantial assets (to pay for future fees).[19]

These problems are being addressed by the Assisted Living Quality Coalition, an alliance of several interested parties including the American Association of Retired Persons (AARP) and the Assisted Living Facilities Association. The coalition released an initiative that includes recommendations for monitoring standards, while at the same time preserving the flexibility to cater to individual needs and continuing to offer cost-effective services.[20]

HOME HEALTH CARE SERVICES

Home health care is the fastest growing industry in the United States.[21] While home care has existed for well over 100 years to provide primarily nursing services, this health care arena has recently experienced a huge growth spurt. For example, the cost of home care services was $63 million in 1970 but has risen to an estimated $36 billion in 1996, with a growth factor of approximately 13 percent per year. Much of this expansion is due to the rise of **managed care,** which focuses on moving people out of the more costly health care settings, such as hospitals, as quickly as possible.[22] Consumers are also increasing demand for services in their own homes. In a 1991 survey of more than 1000 people, approximately 71 percent of the respondents of all ages reported a preference for being cared for at home for both a serious accident or illness as well as for terminal hospice care.[23]

Home health care has gone far beyond the provision of nursing services alone. Home health care agencies, now numbering more than 9000 that are Medicare certified,[21] offer therapies (including occupational, physical, respiratory, and speech therapy), home health care aides, social work intervention, and sometimes psychological and nutritional counseling, in addition to the long-standing nursing care services. Although the home care client usually does not need the level of care that could be provided in a hospital or nursing home, there are now rehabilitation health care service providers who will arrange for an acute level of rehabilitation in the person's home. This might mean several hours of skilled care in the client's home daily. One such company claims not only reduced costs but also increased patient control and sense of well-being, decreased stress for patients and their families, and "more positive rehabilitation outcomes."[24]

In 1995, approximately 10 million people required home care services.[19] As the population ages, this number is expected to rise. Because of the expansion of the 85-and-over cohort as well as the capability of technological advances to save lives we previously would have lost, we can expect growth in the home care field for at least the next 20 or 30 years.[23]

The escalation of managed care has also had an impact both on home health care and health care for elderly people in general. Traditionally health care services have been provided on a fee-for-service basis; when a patient visited the health care provider, that provider received payment specifically for that visit. Now managed care companies (the payers of the health care services) may decide how much and perhaps even which health care services are needed. These services are usually limited (or capitated). The physician may receive a sum of money every month for each patient on the plan, rather than a set fee per visit. Proponents of managed care claim that such a system promotes health care provider accountability and cost containment because the therapists, nurses, or doctors are expected to achieve the best possible outcome for their services in the shortest possible amount of time. While the service providers do a better job of prioritizing their health care goals, the patients need to take on more responsibility for their own health. [25] Prevention or health promotion is also a major component of many managed care plans, again with an underlying philosophy of cost savings and enhancement of life quality.

REHABILITATION

Rehabilitation is the process of restoring someone to their highest possible level of functioning after an injury or illness. Rehabilitation specialists, including **physiatrists** (who are medical doctors), nurses, and therapists, work with patients or clients in the settings already described as well as in the hospital. Rehabilitation services are provided at different levels of intensity. In an acute rehabilitation hospital, where a patient can stay for a few weeks (rarely a few months anymore), the patients generally receive 3 or more hours of therapy per day, at least 5 days per week. Through medical management and therapy, they are expected to make significant gains in a reasonable and expected period of time. Therapists, rehabilitation nurses, and physiatrists are experts in judging whether or not this has occurred.

For example, after a stroke or cerebrovascular accident (CVA), elderly patients often can make good progress in regaining the strength, balance, and motor control to do the tasks they want or need to do. If they make excellent and quick gains, they may return home directly from the rehabilitation hospital. However, if their gains are slower or not as significant, they may need alternative placement (e.g., board and care facility, long-term care facility) prior to or instead of going home. Also if their level of endurance cannot withstand an acute level of rehabilitation, they may receive fewer hours of skilled therapy services in a subacute rehabilitation center, which is likely to be housed in a skilled nursing facility.

Through rehabilitation, which includes positioning, education, and training in ADLs, instrumental ADLs (e.g., home management), mobility, communication, and other functional tasks as needed, many elderly people have been able to return to their former level of independence. This is accomplished through the restoration of function and/or through the use of compensatory measures to make up for lost skills.

LONG-TERM CARE

Long-term care is needed by those people who have disabilities that interfere with their self-care skills. Because of their physical or cognitive impairments, others must assist them in completing their daily tasks. Many elderly people who have long-term care needs receive assistance from their family members. However, caregiving is an extremely difficult position to hold over an extended period of time, especially when the caregiver does not have the support system to get some respite during the 24-hour-a-day job.

Home care services can help, especially in assisting the patient to attain the highest possible level of independence. Also **adult day care** programs provide a break for caregivers during the day by offering health and social services and supervision for the elderly person who is not safe when left alone. There may come a point when professional full-time services are needed, when the caregiver is "burned out" or physically no longer able to care for his or her loved one alone.

Long-term care facilities, more commonly known as nursing homes, provide round-the-clock care through the use of paid caregivers, primarily nurses and nurse's aides. Currently approximately 1.6 million people in the United States reside in nursing homes. The average age of residents is 83.[26] The average nursing home has 65 beds and is a for-profit facility, although 21 percent are not-for-profit and 6 percent are owned by the government. Approximately 5 percent of the population aged 65 and older are residents in long-term care facilities at any one given time,[27] but approximately one of three people (25% to 50% of the population) will become nursing home residents at some point in their lives.[28]

In the past, people generally entered a nursing home to live out their final days. Indeed, even today people often speak of long-term care as if it only offered a life (or death) sentence. In spite of this reputation, the concept of long-term care is changing, and we have reason to hope the services provided are improving as well. Rehabilitation services are available in most nursing homes through contracted or on-site providers. Elderly people are often admitted to the facility for an anticipated few weeks or months. The goal of a short stay is to improve their functioning enough so that they are able to transfer to a less restrictive environment, usually after receiving skilled nursing services and physical, respiratory, occupational, and/or speech therapy.

Certain risk factors are associated with the need for long-term care services:

- Limitations in ability to complete ADLs.
- Having few informal support services, such as close family and friends, especially when one lives alone and needs regular assistance.
- Limitations in instrumental ADLs, such as home management
- Older age, especially older than 85
- Cognitive impairments, especially those caused by dementia
- Low income[29]

Long-term care is the most regulated industry in the United States, yet nursing homes still have a "reputation for substandard care."[27] Many are working to increase the quality of care for elders in our country. The federal government provided a new set of guidelines for long-term care facilities with the passage of the **Omnibus Budget Reconciliation Act (OBRA)** in 1987. OBRA requirements are quite detailed and strict. A few of the regulation highlights are summarized here:

- All nursing homes must have quality assurance programs.
- Facilities must provide enough staff for residents to attain (and maintain) the highest functional level possible.
- Registered nurses must be available 8 hours a day 7 days per week. Nurse's aides must be certified.
- All new residents must have a clear and individualized plan of care. Assessment forms must be filled out within 4 days of admittance.
- Restraints are to be used minimally and only under doctors' orders.
- There is a residents' bill of rights, which includes their right to refuse any medication or treatment.

If OBRA regulations are not followed, nursing homes can be fined (based on state and federal surveys, approximately $10,000 per day in 1995),[30] or lose their Medicare/Medicaid certification.[27]

Although OBRA requires that nursing homes provide a safe and homelike setting, according to *Consumer Reports*[26] many problems still exist. Forty-five percent of facilities have received a deficiency rating for failing to respect the residents' dignity (e.g., disregarding privacy or allowing people to sit in public places not decently clothed). Twenty-five percent have received a deficiency rating for allowing bed sores to develop. (Bed sores, or decubitus ulcers, occur when a person is not repositioned often enough. They heal only with great difficulty and at great medical expense. Technically, they should never occur.) An equal percentage were cited for failing to provide range of motion and walking activities that prevent muscle atrophy. Unfortunately part of the problem is extremely high employee turnover. In many homes, between 70 and 100 percent of the nursing staff leave every year.[26] Certified nurse's aides (CNAs) have extremely difficult jobs and receive low pay.[25] Little wonder then that many do the work only because it is merely a job, not because it is their chosen vocation.

Some nursing homes are excellent and provide a friendly, homelike atmosphere where residents enjoy numerous, warm interactions among themselves and with the staff (Fig. 8–1). Dedication to quality care and appreciation of the residents certainly exist, but not yet universally. If people have complaints about a specific home or treatment, they do have recourse. Concerns can be addressed to state or local agencies on aging. All states have ombudsmen to "protect the health, safety, welfare, and rights of the elderly in nursing homes."[26]

THE HOUSING AND HEALTH CONNECTION

While certainly not a sole determinant, housing has a significant impact on the health of individuals, especially if we take into account what transpires in one's personal living spaces. Housing is not health care, but "good housing is one of our best health care measures." (M. Halkett)[31] The World Health Organization (WHO) in its charter defines health promotion, which includes the creation of supportive environments, determined at least in part by senior citizens themselves.[32]

What can health care professionals do to ensure a healthy, supportive en-

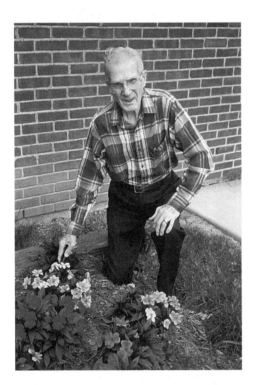

FIG. 8–1. To enhance the quality of life for their residents, Schoellkopf Health Care Center has started a gardening club. Alex, a resident, stays active by working in the garden.

vironment? Several different areas have been highlighted by research and are explained in more depth later. These are to provide:

- Independence
- Empowerment
- Social and emotional support
- Purposeful activity
- Accessibility

INDEPENDENCE

In a study researching the link between health and housing, MacDonald and associates[31] found that the desire for independence was extremely strong among the elderly who participated in their study. However, independence was interpreted in a number of different ways. While some viewed it as living comfortably without needing regular assistance from anyone else, others viewed independence as living in one's own apartment or home rather than a nursing home and the ability to make one's own decisions. Independence was on a relative scale, not an all or nothing construct, at least to this group of senior citizens. Certain participants viewed independence as not being a burden to their family, while others viewed being independent as being able to manage with just the help of their families, not outside resources.

As health care practitioners, our job is to promote the level of independence sought by older people. We must first seek to understand the meaning of independence to the person, and respect his or her particular viewpoint, even if it differs from our own. Then those of us who assist people in gaining their independence (e.g., therapists, nurses) must use all our creative and scientific resources to promote the kind of life the elder is seeking.

EMPOWERMENT

Empowerment is closely related to independence, or perhaps more aptly stated, freedom. It relates not only to older people's ability but also to the privilege of making choices that affect their own lives. Decisions made by the competent older person should garner our respect, as stated earlier, even if these choices do not fit in with our own comprehension of what is right for the person (Box 8–1).

Participants in the study by MacDonald and colleagues[31] clearly stated that they sought control over, and thereby wanted to make choices about, their own lives, particularly in three areas:

1. The type of environment in which they live (housing in general)
2. Where they would go if they needed additional care (continuity of care)
3. Control over their day-to-day lives (reflecting their personal view of independence)

Health care professionals need to keep the idea of empowerment at the forefront when working with and for older people, allowing and encourag-

---

BOX 8–1. MY CHILDREN ARE COMING TODAY

My children are coming today.

They mean well, but they worry.

They think I should have a railing in the hall.

A telephone in the kitchen.

They want someone to come in when I take a bath.

They don't really like my living alone.

Help me be grateful for their concern.

And help them to understand that I have to do what I can.

They're right when they say there are risks.

I might fall. I might leave the stove on.

But there is no challenge, no possibility of triumph, no real aliveness without risk.

When they were young and climbed trees and rode bicycles and went away to camp,

I was terrified. But I let them go.

Because to hold them would have hurt them.

Now our roles are reversed. Help them see.

Keep me from being grim or stubborn about it, but don't let them smother me.

Anonymous

Source: Reprinted with permission from Aging Arkansas. Arkansas Aging Foundation, Little Rock, AR, September, 1995, p 8.

---

ing choices whenever possible. We may need to remind those who have forgotten that choices exist; that it is their right and privilege to guide the course of their daily lives. Along with making choices does come a certain amount of responsibility. At the very least, each person should be given the choice of whether or not to accept this level of responsibility. Indeed many of our problems of aging may be directly related to what theorists call the "environmentally induced loss of control."[33]

Allowing the freedom of choice is allowing people to "gain mastery over their lives."[33] On a community or national level, the results can be dramatic. People come together through support groups, coalitions, organizations, and associations to reach common goals by working collectively. These goals can be as diverse as improving housing conditions and access to health care or lowering the crime rate. Old age is not a stage when one must simply become a victim of fate, but rather a time when well elders can offer years of valuable past experience and current free time to significantly improve the quality of their own and others' lives.

An example, one of many nationwide, of a successful community organizing project is the Tenderloin Senior Organizing Project (TSOP) in California. These low-income senior citizens living in SRO hotels have worked together for more than a dozen years. They have identified and successfully solved many collective problems. For instance, because of their living situations in SROs (without kitchen facilities), malnutrition was a common problem. The TSOP started a "mini-market" food cooperative and a group breakfast program, which then made their hotel eligible for food bank services. In addition, other TSOP members published a "no-cook cookbook" of nutritious recipes that did not require kitchen facilities. Not only did these efforts solve some life-threatening problems, but consequently the participants felt an increased sense of control and purpose in their lives.[33]

SOCIAL AND EMOTIONAL SUPPORT

All these realms (independence, empowerment, social support, and purposeful activities) are hardly distinct from one another. By focusing on one, other areas may also improve. Numerous studies have linked the concept of social support and interaction to better health. The "social support" theory purports that those who are lacking adequate social support systems are more susceptible to disease because of a decrease in functioning of the body's immune system. During tense times, the love and support of other people can decrease stress and may also help to increase a person's sense of control.[33]

Marriage is correlated to a higher level of life satisfaction in elderly people, but one spouse, more often the woman, is nearly always left alone after the death of the other. Widows and widowers usually need to find a replacement social support system after the death of their spouse. In two separate studies Hong and colleagues[34] found that life satisfaction was positively correlated to the frequency of participation in group activities and high level of interaction with friends. Perhaps it is evident that close human interaction is crucial in attaining and maintaining wellness for most people of all ages. People do not thrive in isolation. Yet as people get older, as their senses become impaired and they are less mobile, isolation becomes a common problem. Elders may not want to be a burden on close friends or family or they may be embarrassed that they can no longer hear conversations as well or walk as quickly or as far. For whatever reason, social withdrawal occurs. This, in turn, may lead to further decline both socially and physically.

Health care professionals should attempt to intervene and stop this downward spiral. Not only can we lend a listening ear, but also we can encourage human interaction, either directly by setting up and becoming involved in programs or by making appropriate referrals to those who can (e.g., activity directors, social workers, nurses, recreational therapists). At least one study has found that older people value emotional support and that they feel it is important to feel "cared about" rather than just "cared for."[35]

Structured as well as informal **reminiscence** sessions can give the person the opportunity to speak about their personal history and experiences. Elderly people often enjoy talking about their past and processing their feelings through this sort of life review. The **American Association of Retired Persons (AARP)**[36] gives useful hints for helping someone reminisce effectively:

- Active listening to show someone that you care about what he or she is saying
- Asking open ended questions, such as
    What advice did your parents give you as a child?
    What is the meaning of your family name?
    What was the best time of your family or career life?
- Giving positive and clarifying responses, through appropriate verbal and bodily expressions
- Keeping the conversation focused and redirecting the person when she or he gets caught in repeating memories
- Using tools for reminiscing, such as memorabilia or photographs to engage the person's interest

On a related note, an intergenerational, social interaction program was started by Poole and Gooding.[37] Their program simply brings together isolated senior citizens and 10- to 12-year-olds in nearby schools for social activities and for "programs to do what grandparents and grandchildren used to do naturally." While the youth gain valued friendships and guidance about making decisions, the elderly people benefit from the social involvement, the chance to use their skills and share their wisdom. Both groups improve their awareness of issues facing the other generation. The community also benefits through the utilization of dormant resources.

Perhaps our ancestors would be saddened or oddly amused by the fact that our present-day society needs formal programs to bring elders and youngsters together. Yet with the small, extremely mobile nuclear families of today, much of the multigenerational intermingling, which took place naturally in the large extended families of the past, has been lost. People often seek social and emotional support outside of the immediate family. For all of us, there are many benefits to increasing our level of intergenerational awareness and friendship, even if the introductions are initially contrived.

PURPOSEFUL ACTIVITY

Involvement in enjoyable and productive activity is paramount to successful aging (Fig. 8–2). Lack of participation leads not only to physical but also cognitive and emotional decline. Even if this fails to lead directly to premature physical death (which it may), it certainly leads to a premature death of the spirit. Continued participation of older people definitely involves a shifting of gears. For example, after retirement one cannot stay involved in the same job, or the choice of purposeful activity may need to be altered to accommodate a changing and slowing body.

Nevertheless, as health care practitioners, we can promote an optimal level of participation through our own particular health care provider roles. A significant lack of interest in day-to-day activities or life in general may indicate clinical depression (see Chapter 4). Encourage the older person to seek assistance from a physician if this seems to be the case. At other times the person may need assistance in finding suitable activities or hobbies. A referral to a recreational or occupational therapist may be appropriate if the person can no longer participate in or enjoy past occupations (including hobbies, home management, and work activities).

If one seeks your opinion, remember to remain openminded and creative, although never coercive. Whitgift House, a residential home for the elderly near London, deserves mention for their staff's innovative ideas to foster active engagement of their residents. Whenever someone new moves into their home, they are asked about their unfulfilled ambitions, hopes, and interests. Then the staff members work together with the resident to make these ambitions a reality. Residents from Whitgift House have gone hang-gliding and hot air ballooning. They have been involved in croquet matches, art classes, and flu-injection parties. At a similarly creative residential home also in the vicinity, the residents run a craft center and use their profits to pay for more craft supplies. Also local hostesses have tea parties for small groups of residents to promote community integration. One of the primary goals of the Whitgift House is to have fun and to offer on-going opportunities for residents to lead more fulfilling lives.[38]

An important consideration in fostering the involvement of elders in any activity is to remember to include them in the choice and planning of the activity as well. While encouragement and enthusiasm for participation may be appreciated, one should never be forced to attend an event.

ACCESSIBILITY

Participation is difficult or impossible if activities take place in an environment that is not easily accessible. A supportive environment fosters comfort, safety, and ease of movement. Although many of the basic changes described here may be based on common sense, the concept of universal design (a building design that fits all persons, not just the physically able) is not yet commonplace. Although the ideas presented herein are not difficult to grasp, the process of adapting a home to fit the requirements of a particular indi-

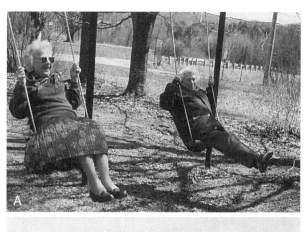

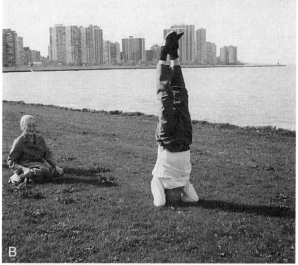

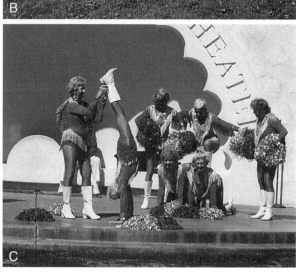

vidual with special needs usually requires technical skills and clinical reasoning. For a full home safety evaluation, a physician should refer the client to an occupational and/or physical therapist.

Environmental design that fits the needs of older people basically falls into two categories:

- Building new, accommodating structures
- Adapting existing structures

Universal Design

The typical newly built home is not designed with aging in mind, even though each of us is headed in that direction. In one survey of building contractors, only 3 percent of the companies had designed and built adaptable housing.[39] With multiple living levels, narrow doorways, and inaccessible spaces (especially for those who use wheelchairs), existing homes are generally not very suitable for "aging in place."

Perhaps the best way to introduce a design that is accommodating for elderly people (as well as everyone else) is to describe an "aging-in-place" residential facility that currently exists in Louisiana.[40] Woldenberg Village provides a "barrier free environment" for the people living in the 60, one- and two-bedroom apartments within its boundaries. Each apartment provides the following features:

- Bright lighting (because people older than age 60 require twice the amount of illumination needed by a 20-year-old).[41]
- Single story construction that includes no stairs and ramps built to Americans with Disabilities (ADA) specifications. (While single story construction may not be feasible everywhere because of space constraints, an accessible, efficient elevator may work just as well for those who have impaired mobility.)
- Total privacy within each apartment (to preserve dignity), but lots of public space (to promote social interaction).
- Raised planters and numerous benches located along the walkways.
- Anti-slip floor finishes.

This village exists in stark contrast to much of the housing currently available for older people, which is described as "a depressing wasteland of Leisure Worlds and Shady Acres subdivisions . . . where older Americans are put out to pasture." Also called institutional, rigid, predictable, and "designed as if the

---

FIG. 8–2. (*A*) Elsie (in her nineties) and Marge (in her seventies) share a swinging session on Marge's swing set. (*B*) Mr. In-Sik Im, an octogenarian, still teaches yoga and relaxation. (*C*) The Sun City Poms are an internationally renowned pom and dance troupe from Arizona. The average age of the performers is 74. (Photograph courtesy of the Sun City Poms.)

market were one monolithic gray block,"[42] currently senior housing does not convey an inviting image.

Perhaps new construction and design plans should consider some relatively minor changes, such as wider doorways, eliminating thresholds, wheelchair accessible bathrooms, and windows that are easy to open and close. In so doing, as long as we preserve the individuality of a personal home, there would be increased opportunity for elders to enjoy aging in place, even with physical disabilities.

Adaptation and Compensation

As stated earlier, most people wish to remain in their own homes for as long as possible. This presents a problem when the home can no longer offer a safe and comfortable living space. A full home evaluation is usually warranted to determine whether changes can be made. At times, the proposed accommodations will involve extensive remodeling such as building a bathroom on the first floor or tearing down walls to increase accessibility. Entry steps may need to be replaced by a ramp to allow for wheelchair access. Ramps are not safe unless they are built to ADA specifications, which are available at local independent living centers. (The grade should not exceed one inch of height per foot.) Doorways may need to be widened to accommodate a wheelchair, and kitchens may need to be remodeled to allow continued use. Chair lifts may need to be added to existing stairways (Fig. 8–3).

Many changes are less drastic and therefore more acceptable and affordable to the home owners. These changes may include:

- Raised toilet seats and grab bars installed in the bathroom (Fig. 8–4A)
- Tacking down or eliminating scatter rugs
- Improving lighting levels
- Using shower seats or bath transfer benches (Fig. 8–4B)
- Eliminating clutter and excess furniture
- Checking smoke alarms and resetting the water heater to a lower temperature (not exceeding 120°F)
- Removing door thresholds
- Moving items commonly used into easily reached spaces

Not all elderly people need to make all these changes in order to be safe, although these accommodations should not cause harm to anyone. Many other minor adjustments in the home or small equipment purchases may also be necessary. A physical or occupational therapist can help the resident in making decisions regarding home safety (Fig. 8–5).

In addition to altering the environment to accommodate the changing needs of the aging adult, the person may also be taught compensatory strate-

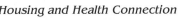

FIG. 8–3. Brockie of Coastal Manor graciously demonstrates the use of a stair lift. This device can be used to make the upstairs of a home accessible to those who have difficulty with stairs.

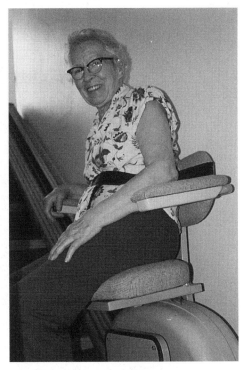

gies to remain as safe as possible in the home. As protection from possible injury, the therapist may help the elderly person learn to:

- Transfer into and out of the tub or shower safely
- Use a walker or cane to accommodate for decreased balance
- Use safer techniques when using kitchen appliances
- Use new, more effective techniques for completing their daily activities
- Use joint protection and energy conservation techniques
- Compensate for the physical changes of aging (such as decreased eyesight, decreased memory, and decreased hearing)

This is just a small sample of accommodations and compensatory strategies that can be used on an individual basis as needed. Through these techniques and others, many people are able to remain in their homes safely.

▨ SUMMARY

The housing and health connection is important for maintaining the quality of life of senior citizens. While safety is the utmost concern, perhaps the next

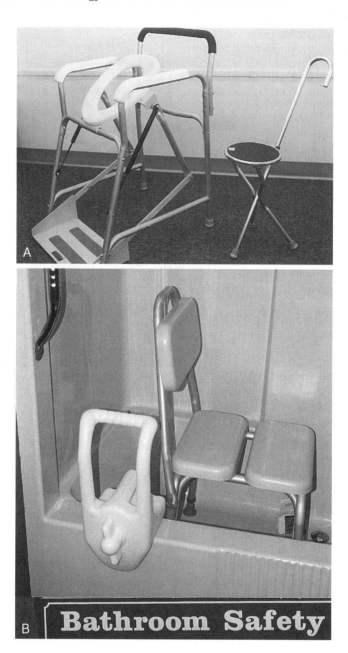

FIG. 8–4. Equipment is available to help people with their activities of daily living. (*A*) A lifting toilet seat and cane seat. (*B*) Shower seat and grab bar. (Equipment courtesy of Black Bear Medical.)

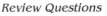

FIG. 8–5. Marge, who is legally blind, has made simple adaptations to her microwave oven so that she can continue to use it. She is in her seventies and lives alone.

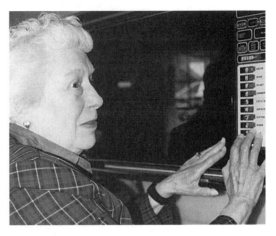

most important consideration is providing elders a home of their own choosing. Such a home, described by Garrett,[2] "fulfills many needs: it is a place of shelter and security, inspires a sense of belonging and mastery, and allows the person to be him or herself, reinforcing (by the presence of significant personal items) their life and identity."

Elderly people should be given every opportunity to live in such a home, whether it is a house, apartment, SRO, CCRC, or just a single room. The home should be as pleasing to the individual, as affordable, and as accessible as possible. Along with safe and enjoyable surroundings, older people also need adequate social support systems (provided by their families or beyond) and plenty of opportunities to participate in personally meaningful activities, for these are the tools to promote successful aging. The environmental influence on physical health can hardly be underestimated.

✳ REVIEW QUESTIONS

1. Most elderly people would prefer to live _____ if widowed.
    A. Alone
    B. With their children
    C. In their own home
    D. In an SRO

2. Approximately what percentage of elderly people (who do not live in institutions) live in multigenerational homes?
    A. 10%
    B. 20%

C. 35%
D. 60%

3. All the following characteristics describe SROs EXCEPT:
   A. Private bathrooms
   B. One room
   C. Limited kitchen facilities
   D. Low cost

4. Which of the following describes all types of CCRCs?
   A. Unlimited long-term care as long as needed
   B. Entrance fees
   C. Condominiums
   D. Rehabilitation services

5. Each of the following is considered an advantage of CCRCs EXCEPT:
   A. Affordability
   B. Barrier-free environments
   C. Remaining in close proximity to friends or family even when needing additional services
   D. They offer a variety of social interactions

6. _____ bridges the gap between independent living and long-term care.
   A. Single room occupancies
   B. Skilled nursing facilities
   C. Subsidized housing
   D. Residential care facilities

7. Home health care is expanding for all the following reasons EXCEPT
   A. Most people prefer to recuperate at home
   B. Most health care workers prefer home health care
   C. Managed care
   D. The aging population

8. Rehabilitation
   A. Can only take place in the hospital
   B. Involves at least 4 hours of therapy per day
   C. Doctors are called physiatrists
   D. Therapists are called physiatrists

9. The Omnibus Budget Reconciliation Act (OBRA) does NOT include:
   A. Regulations regarding restraint use with residents
   B. Staffing requirements for nursing homes
   C. A residents' bill of rights
   D. A daily plan for nursing home residents

10. What may be the most important aspect of environmental life quality for the elderly?

    A. Allowing/encouraging choices
    B. Encouraging independence
    C. Having lots of friends
    D. Maintaining former lifestyle

LEARNING ACTIVITIES

1. Without referring back to the chapter, individually list the five most important things for you when considering your own environment when you are older. Compare your answers with the group. What can you learn from the answers of others?

2. Brainstorm above different ways that older people can improve their quality of life. Be creative. Remember in brainstorming there are no wrong answers. Can you, as health care professionals, assist in the improvement process? How?

3. Spend some time designing a retirement community. You can list features or draw them out. Be specific. Share the designs among the group.

4. Dicuss the poem (Box 8–1) by answering some of the following questions. Do you agree with the writer? Why or why not? Do you agree with the writer's children? Why or why not? What are some of the other risks, besides those mentioned, to living alone? When would you personally decide that it was time to move? What do you think makes a person incapable of making these decisions? How does this compare with the offficial definition of competence? Was the writer displaying competence or incompentence? In what ways?

REFERENCES

1. Morgan, BA, et al: Reverse mortgages and the economic status of elderly women. The Gerontologist 36:400–405, 1996.

2. Garrett, G: But does it feel like home? Accommodation needs on later life. Professional Nurse 7:254–257, January, 1992.

3. Gilderbloom, JI, and Mullins, RL: Elderly housing needs: An examination of the American Housing Survey. International Journal of Aging and Human Development 40:57–72, 1995.

4. Rothstein, FR: Facts about older women: Income and poverty. AARP Fact Sheet, 1994.

5. Golant, SM: Housing America's Elderly: Many Possibilities/Few Choices. Sage Publications, Newbury Park, CA, 1992, pp 7, 229–246.

6. Clarke, CJ, and Niedert, LJ: Living arrangements of the elderly: An examination of differences according to ancestry and generation. The Gerontologist 32:796–804, 1992.

7. Kehn, DJ: Predictors of elderly happiness. Activities, Adaptation & Aging 19:11–29, 1995.

8. Crystal, S, and Beck P: A room of one's own: The SRO and the single elderly. The Gerontologist 32:684–692, 1992.

9. Brower, HT: Policy implications for life care environments. Journal of Gerontological Nursing 20:17–22, 1994.

10. Sloan, FA, et al: Continuing care retirement communities: Prospects for reducing long-term care. Journal of Health Care Politics, Policy and Law 20:75–98, 1995.

11. Greganti, MA: Life Care at Golden Acres. Ann Intern Med 17:867–868, 1992.

12. Somers, AR: Positive views of retirement communities. Ann Intern Med 118:751–752, 1993.

13. Assisted living is "hot" industry for 1997. Industry Update. OT Week 14, January 9, 1997.

14. Fisk, CF: Fact Sheet: Assisted Living. Assisted Living Association of America, Fairfax, VA, 1992.

15. Armer, JM: Research brief: Degree of personalization as a cue in the assessment of adjustment to congregate housing by rural elders. Geriatric Nursing 17:79–80, 1996.

16. Just, G, et al: Assisted living: Challenges for nursing practice. Geriatric Nursing 16: 165–168, 1995.

17. Cerne, F: Consumer choice could give big boost to assisted living. Hospital and Health Networks 72, June 5, 1994.

18. Citro, J: Assisted living in the United States. AARP. Fact Sheet 62, 1998.

19. Can loved ones avoid a nursing home? The promise and pitfalls of assisted living. Consumer Reports 60:656–662, October, 1995.

20. Kerr, T: Coalition seeking better regulation of assisted living facilities. Advance for Occupational Therapists 12–13, December 12, 1996.

21. Halamandaris, VJ: Managing managed care: Controlling our destiny. Caring 4–39, January 4, 1996.

22. Joe, BE: Home care growth and change. OT Week 14–15, November 7, 1996.

23. Gibbons, M: Home care industry: Healthy and looking forward to future. Advance for Occupational Therapists 12–13, December 14, 1992.

24. Pathways Healthcare Services (Brochure). Pathways, Westwood, MA, Undated but distributed in 1996.

25. Marmer, L: How managed care is changing home health. Advance for Occupational Therapists 19, July 16, 1996.

26. Nursing homes: When a loved one needs care. Consumer Reports 60:518–528, August, 1995.

27. Trella, R: From hospital to nursing home: Bridging the gaps in care. Geriatric Nursing 15:313–317, 1994.

28. Lui, K: A data perspective on long-term care. The Gerontologist 34:476–480, 1994.

29. Robert, S, and Norgard, T: Long-term care policy based on ADL eligibility criteria: Impact on community dwelling elders not meeting the criteria. Journal of Gerontological Social Work 25: 71–91, 1996.

30. Licciardello, G: Meeting the needs of the elderly in long term care settings. Maine Occupational Therapy Association Conference Workshop, March, 1997.

31. Mac Donald, M, et al: Research considerations: The link between housing and health in the elderly. Journal of Gerontological Nursing 20:5–10, 1994.

32. World Health Organization, Health and Welfare Canada, and Canadian Public Health Association, Ottawa Chapter for Health Promotion: Presentation at the International Conference on Health Promotion, Ottawa, November, 1986.

33. Minkler, M: Community organizing among the elderly poor in the United States: A case study. International Journal of Health Services 22:303–316, 1992.

34. Hong, LK, and Duff, RW: Widows in retirement communities: The social context of subjective well-being. The Gerontologist 34:347, 1994.

35. Cox, J: It's a lifeline. Elderly Care 8:13–15, 1996.

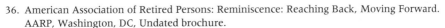

36. American Association of Retired Persons: Reminiscence: Reaching Back, Moving Forward. AARP, Washington, DC, Undated brochure.

37. Pool, GG, and Gooding, BA: Developing and implementing a community intergenerational program. Journal of Community Health Nursing 10:77–85, 1993.

38. Lyall, J: Beyond Bingo. Nursing Times 89:16–17, 1993.

39. Frain, JP, and Carr, PH: Is the typical modern house designed for future adaptation for disabled older people? Age and Ageing 25:398–401, 1994.

40. Thompson, I: Woldenberg Village: An illustration of supportive design for older adults. Experimental Aging Research 20:239–244, 1994.

41. Cannava, E: "Gerodesign": Safe and comfortable living spaces for older adults. Geriatrics 49:45–49, 1994.

42. Gunts, E: Housing the elderly. Architecture 81–87, October, 1994.

One key to health cost containment is
health promotion; another involves
difficult choices, and many elders take
on these challenges gladly.
RHR

Financing Health Care for the Elderly

Edward F. Saxby, Jr.
Regula H. Robnett and Walter C. Chop

BEHAVIORAL OBJECTIVES

Upon completion of this chapter, the reader will be able to:

1. State several reasons why it is imperative for elders to have proper legal authority.
2. Describe financial power of attorney and durable power of attorney.
3. Define advance directives, medical powers of attorney, and living wills.
4. Differentiate the Medicare program from the Medicaid program.
5. Describe elder benefits under Veterans Administration Benefits.
6. Define long-term care insurance.
7. Identify private sources of elder funding.
8. Discuss the benefits of long-term care insurance.
9. Discuss possible cost containment measures for health care financing for the elderly.

KEY TERMS

401(k) plan
Advance directives
Community spouse resource
  allowance (CSRA)
Cost containment
Durable power of attorney
Fiduciary
Financial power of attorney
Geriatric care managers
Health care proxy
Home health care

Individual retirement accounts
  (IRAs)
Keogh plan
Living will
Long-term care
Long-term care insurance
Medicaid
Medical power of attorney
Medicare
Prospective payment system (PPS)
TSA plan
Veterans' benefits

INTRODUCTION

Health care costs in the United States continue to escalate. This is true for several reasons. While burgeoning technology allows us to keep people alive who once would have died, the price of using these advances is high and rising. The sheer number of elders is increasing. Since most people use medical services more toward the end of their lives, this affects overall expenditures in health care (see Table 9–1). In addition, as a society we have tended to believe that life should continue almost at any cost. We may even be obsessed with prolonging life.[1]

TABLE 9–1. *Average Annual Cost per Consumer for Health Care 1995*

Age	Cost in Dollars
≤25	$465
35–44	$1609
65–74	$2617
>75	$2683
Average (all ages)	$1732

Source: Statistical Abstract of the United States, 1997, ed 17. U.S. Department of Commerce, Washington, DC, 1997, p 119.

Elderly people use a large portion of our health care dollars. Much of this money is spent on **long-term care** (see Table 9–2). Long-term care is singled out in this chapter largely because its cost can be overwhelming and the intricacies of making medical decisions involving extended care are complicated and often misunderstood. The chapter also provides an overview of the Medicare and Medicaid programs, because these are the health care services that are most widely used by the older generation.

🔳 FINANCING OPTIONS FOR LONG-TERM CARE

How to pay the costs of long-term care for seniors, whether in their own homes or in institutions (such as boarding homes or nursing homes), is one of the most difficult issues being addressed in our country today, and this issue is likely to become more contentious in the near future. The costs of extended long-term care are staggering (see Table 9–2). The cost of nursing home care for one resident is between $3000 and $5000 a month, while extended around-the-clock home health care costs between $3500 and $6000 a month.[2]

Most elders have lived frugally over the course of their lives. They experienced the Great Depression, lived through rationing during times of war, worked hard to buy their homes, provided their children with a better education than they themselves received, and assisted close family members whenever they could, for example by providing down payments for children's homes or contributions to their grandchildren's education. They paid off their homes and saved to establish estates of between $100,000 and $300,000 liquid assets. The cost of long-term care for these individuals can often dwindle their life savings in a matter of months.

Seniors tend to have great apprehension and fear around these financial issues. They often have difficulty finding current and accurate information regarding options to pay for these types of expenses. The demographics of our aging population clearly show that the situation is likely to deteriorate

TABLE 9–2. Nursing Home Expenditures 1980–1995 in Billions of Dollars

Year	Cost
1980	17.6
1985	30.7
1990	50.9
1995	77.9

Source: Statistical Abstract of the United States, 1997, ed 17. U.S. Department of Commerce, Washington, DC, 1997, p 112.

during the next two or three decades. While there are currently about 37 million Americans aged 65 and older, that figure is expected to more than double (to more than 75 million Americans) within the next 20 to 25 years. Improvements in medical technology have enabled us to extend the average life expectancy in the United States by nearly 20 years over the past half century. People are healthier longer. We have witnessed the joy of many active elders. However, elders also may live in an unhealthier state longer than in the past. Individuals, who in the 1970s would not have survived a debilitating illness such as cancer or a catastrophic health event such as a heart attack, are now able to live for greatly extended periods of time with sometimes many concurrent chronic conditions.

Currently, the public sector, through the federal Medicare and Veterans Administration programs, the federal and state Medicaid partnership, and various state programs, pays for approximately 60 percent of long-term care expenses. The private sector, through insurance vendors and through individual and family savings, pays for approximately 40 percent of those costs.[2] It is unrealistic to expect that ratio to be able to continue in the future, because of the sheer volume of growth of the elder population. Funding of long-term care expenses is an issue that must be addressed.

It is incumbent upon caregivers and care providers alike to begin becoming familiar with the payment system for long-term care. Rumors, folklore, and half truths can be incredibly damaging to seniors and their families. Misinformation can be financially devastating. Care providers also need to be aware of their payment sources. Securing viable payment options for required services is currently an issue for all caregivers, including individuals as well as organizations and institutions. Health care dollars are becoming more squeezed as everyone scrambles to find adequate funds for a growing need in a shrinking pot.

The public sector programs (i.e., Medicare and Medicaid) have typically paid for services, such as medical and long-term care, on a fee-for-service basis. This means that every time a service was rendered, the provider received a set amount of money, usually based on the time spent with the patient. Instigated at least partially by the Balanced Budget Act of 1997, these programs are beginning to consider or are already using a **prospective payment system (PPS),** in which patients may be placed into case mix groups and payment is subsequently received for the level of care expected rather than for specific services. This new payment system incorporates more of the managed care concept and is viewed as one measure to help curtail burgeoning, long-term medical costs. The specific systems of payment vary among states and can involve quite complicated methods of cost calculation.

PROPER LEGAL AUTHORITY

A discussion on paying for long-term care begins with proper legal authority. First one should ask: does the individual require care, and if so do his or her family members have adequate access to funds in order to pay for the individual's care? Do they also have the proper legal authority necessary to make medical decisions on behalf of that individual? If they cannot access a payment source, and if they do not have the ability to assent to treatment on behalf of an individual, a difficult process can evolve into a nightmare.

If an elderly person is deemed incompetent, it is necessary for someone close to that person to make decisions on the individual's behalf under the proper legal authority. Obviously, if a person is competent and can process information effectively, he or she usually will agree to use personal assets to pay for the care needed. However, for individuals who have been frugal and independent for most of their lives and who have enjoyed the benefits of the public sector Medicare program, the reality of having to pay for medical care with their own funds can be shocking and traumatic. Necessary care may be rejected as too expensive. Caregivers and care providers need to be sensitive, well-informed, and firm in helping elders understand what their new financial obligations are.

If an individual is no longer competent or is struggling at the edge of competency, both access to funds and the ability to consent to treatment become looming issues. If preplanning has not occurred, it may be necessary to seek protection for an incompetent individual through the probate court system.

Probate courts are state courts. In most states, they are set up as separate special courts that deal with such issues as wills, trusts, probates, guardianships, and conservatorships. Individual states and jurisdictions may have different names for probate courts or the various petitions that are brought before them. Generally, the care of a person's self under the protection of a probate court is known as a guardianship. Protection of a person's money and other assets is known as a conservatorship.

Each state has different rules regarding the "priority of appointment" that directs the order that may appoint others to represent and protect the incapacitated person's interests. Often a surviving spouse or child of the individual assumes the primary role as guardian or conservator. However, if there is no surviving spouse, or if that individual is also incapacitated, obvious problems arise.

Most state statutes allow the children of the person in question to petition the state for protection of the individual. In families in which everyone is close, in proximity and/or in their outlook in developing a plan of care for their parents, sharing the responsibility as coguardians or coconservators is quite feasible. Unfortunately often this is not the case. Approximately 20 percent of Americans change residences each year. Families are often scattered throughout the country or even the world. Communications are sometimes strained. Consensus can be elusive. Long-standing or quietly smoldering sibling rivalries or disagreements often manifest themselves at the time when parents are no longer able to care for themselves, but are looking to their children for protection and care.

Without consensus among family members—regarding the precise details of plan of care, a plan of asset management, or at least acceding to having one of the family members act as the appointed representative of the court—clarity in determining what care is given to the individual and how it is to be paid for immediately evaporates. Disagreements in this situation create what could be termed a "minority veto." The one individual who is not happy with the plan of care for a parent is able to hold up the process. Ultimately, an older person at some point will be protected by the probate court, although this may occur only at great financial and emotional expense. The costs associated with bringing an action in probate court are usually borne by the protected person's estate. The probate court proceeding is a matter of public record.

It is preferable for an individual or a couple to memorialize their medical and financial instructions while they are competent to do so. Individuals have the right to be able to determine "who will speak for them" if and when they are not able to do so themselves.

The primary document regarding financial decision making is known as a **financial power of attorney** for **durable power of attorney.** This document allows an individual to appoint another person to legally represent them or speak for them in the event that they are physically and/or mentally unable to do so for themselves. This document is designed to "survive the disability for the incapacitated person." The document, once properly signed, witnessed, and executed, directs that the attorney-in-fact or agent named in the document has legal authority to speak for that individual by creating what is called a fiduciary relationship.

A **fiduciary** is legally bound to put the interests of the person for whom he or she is acting ahead of his or her own in making decisions for that person. In this relationship of trust, the fiduciary is bound to ascertain and protect the best interests of the person granting the legal authority under the power of attorney. Generally a power of attorney has to be notarized (i.e., signed in the presence of a notary public), to insure that the individual granting the power is signing the document freely and voluntarily. A financial power of attorney is a revocable document. This means that the individual appointing an attorney-in-fact may change his or her mind and revoke or cancel the document at any time as long as he or she is deemed competent to do so. A well-drafted financial power of attorney will allow the attorney-in-fact to have access to an individual's bank accounts, brokerage accounts, safe-deposit box, and/or real property. It will allow the attorney-in-fact to deal with various third parties in handling the individual's financial affairs.

Individuals also can provide for health care and medical decisions to be made on their behalf through a variety of documents. The primary documents for permitting health care decision-making are called **advance directives** or medical powers of attorney. Many states also use terms such as health care proxy and living wills. A health care provider is well advised to check his or her state's particular requirements for advance directives, medical powers of attorney, and living wills. These matters are considered issues of state law and have a wide variety of subtle differences. Both statutory law and case law concerning these issues are continuing to evolve rather quickly.

A **medical power of attorney** or **health care proxy** is used to appoint an individual to make medical decisions for a person who is no longer able to make them for himself or herself. Usually one of the primary components of such a document includes instructions as to whether or not an individual wishes to be kept alive solely by artificial or extraordinary means in the event that he or she is at the end stage of a terminal illness or is in a permanent vegetative state. This is generally known as a living will provision. The focus for care providers (or their institutions) may be to decide whether or not it is possible or desirable to request a do not resuscitate (DNR) order for the individual following consultation with that person's attending physician. Proper legal authority is required for such an order to be entered.

The authority of a medical power of attorney is broader than the relatively rare circumstances in which it becomes necessary to issue a do not resuscitate (no code) order. Myriad intermediate issues can arise, such as whether or not an individual should receive a specific procedure, therapy, or medication. The medical power of attorney also provides authority to place an individual into different institutional settings (e.g., a hospital, rehabilitation center, boarding home, assisted living center, or nursing home). If an individual is no longer able to process information regarding his or her own medical care or safety, then it is necessary for the person having the power of attorney to use his or her substituted judgment to ensure that the individual remains safe. Also advisable is to name at least one successor individual in the event that the first attorney-in-fact is unable or unwilling to continue to act in the capacity of medical power of attorney.

A document more well known and often confused with the medical power of attorney is a **living will**. Living will provisions are sometimes incorporated into medical power of attorney, advance directives, or health care proxy documents. However, just as often, a living will can exist without the complementary medical power of attorney.

The distinction is an important one for caregivers and for the medical establishment. A living will is a statement of intent. It expresses an individual's desire that he or she not be kept alive solely by artificial or extraordinary means. These documents have become widespread during the 1990s. Every state has some form of statute addressing the issue. A person's express written intent is a useful guide for a caregiver or an attending physician if an individual becomes incompetent or unable to interact with the environment at the end stage of a terminal illness or when he or she is in a permanent vegetative state. However, a living will is not necessarily dispositive; it is only a statement of intent. The living will does not give authority to any individual to carry out or enforce its terms, but it is intended to be the primary instrument directing the person's attending physician. Yet if there is any disagreement between or among family members, and the individual's wishes are no longer clear, a living will alone likely will be insufficient either to direct the termination of life support or for the issuance of a do not resuscitate order. Also a living will does not extend any authority to a family member to participate in issues in which the termination of life are not specifically indicated or to gain access to confidential medical records.

Access to both accurate medical information and financial resources is necessary for any fiduciary to effectuate and fund an adequate plan of care. This is true if the person is acting either in a court sanctioned capacity as guardian and/or conservator or in the capacity of a privately directed medical and financial power of attorney.

PUBLIC SECTOR FINANCING FOR LONG TERM CARE

The majority of long-term care expenses for senior citizens are currently funded through the public sector (Table 9–3).

The federal government's share of these expenses currently dwarfs all state programs. The three primary federal programs funding some level of long-term care are the Medicaid program, the Medicare program, and costs covered by the Veterans Administration. State governments contribute a proportional share of the long term care benefits paid under the Medicaid program. State contributions generally range from 30 percent to 50 percent of the covered costs. In addition, many states have their own programs that

TABLE 9–3. *Percentage of Nursing Home Residents by Primary Payer Source*

Payer	1991	1995
Medicare	5%	8%
Medicaid	68%	68%
Private/Other	27%	24%

Source: Nursing Home Care in the United States. Health Care Financing Administration Office of Research and Demonstration, Baltimore, MD, 1997, p 12.

supplement the federal long-term care initiatives. The state programs primarily center on extending **home health care** benefits to individuals whose Medicare benefits have either expired or who do not qualify for long-term care benefits under the Medicaid program. Because of the continued growth in the senior population, Americans probably should not expect any broad-based increase in long-term care benefits. The United States has not yet attained the political consensus willing to pay higher taxes to ensure any expansion of benefits. Trends at the federal level have revealed a consistent pattern in which federal guarantees and entitlement are becoming more limited or restricted. The health care initiative proposed by President Clinton in his first term, which included a plan to expand home health care benefits, failed.

Eligibility for long-term care Medicaid benefits for middle-class senior citizens has become more restrictive in recent enactment of the federal budget cycles. The 104th Congress proposed but did not adopt a plan that would have ended the federal guarantee of Medicaid benefits and passed those program funds to individual states under block grant financing. Attention has been focused on abuses within the Medicare system, in particular fraudulent or inflated claims made on behalf of home health care providers. We can expect additional federal regulatory scrutiny of this area of health care.

🔳 MEDICARE

The **Medicare** program, enacted in 1966, is a federal health insurance program usually for persons 65 years of age and older. Persons entitled to Social Security or railroad retirement benefits are eligible for Medicare benefits on attaining the age of 65. (The Medicare program also covers certain individuals with disabilities, although that discussion is outside the realm of this chapter.) Medicare provides two different plans for eligible recipients. Nearly all elders have hospital coverage (Part A) and can choose to supplement with Part B, primarily for physicians' visits and outpatient care. The number of enrollees and the amount of money spent on the Medicare program have continued to rise since 1980 (Table 9–4).

Many older persons are under the mistaken impression that Medicare will pay for all of their long-term care needs whether they wish to remain at home or they require institutionalization in a nursing home. The reality is that the Medicare program has very limited long-term care benefits. If an individual requires skilled nursing facility services after a catastrophic health event such as a stroke, heart attack, or broken hip, Part A of the Medicare program will pay for up to 100 days or extended care services in a skilled nursing facility.[3]

There is a mandatory 3-day period of inpatient hospitalization required in order to trigger the 100-day skilled nursing facility benefit. Medicare pays the full cost of the first 20 days of skilled nursing facility care; it covers the majority of costs from day 21 through 100, but the covered individual is required to pay a copayment. In 1997, the coinsurance amount was $95 per day.[3]

Medicare benefits for skilled services are paid only as long as an individual is still making progress toward measurable goals. The services must meet the following requirements:

1. Be ordered by a physician
2. Require the skills of technical or professional personnel such as registered nurses, licensed practical nurses, physical therapists, occupational therapists, speech and language pathologists, or audiologists
3. Be furnished directly by or under the supervision of such personnel
4. Be needed by the patient on a daily or close to daily basis
5. Be provided by the professional, out of necessity on an inpatient basis

Please note that once a patient reaches a plateau, i.e., reaches his or her maximum rehabilitation potential, that individual's status changes from needing skilled (nursing facility) care to custodial care. Medicare does not continue to pay long-term care benefits for custodial care.[4] This can cause

TABLE 9–4. *Medicare Enrollees and Expenditures 1980–1995*

Year	Number of Enrollees in Millions	Expenditures in Billions of Dollars
1980	28.5	36.8
1985	31.1	72.3
1990	34.2	111.0
1995	37.5	181.5

Source: Statistical Abstract of the United States, 1997, ed 17. U.S. Department of Commerce, Washington, DC, 1997, p 115.

great confusion for many elders. A common misperception among elders is that their "Medigap" insurance will continue to pay benefits once Medicare benefits cease. This is simply not true. Medigap policies are designed to pay the deductibles and coinsurance requirements of the Medicare system. However, once Medicare coverage stops, then Medicare wraparound coverage stops as well. Medicare supplemental insurance is just that. The insurance supplements the basic Medicare benefit. It does not generally extend that coverage. Certain private health insurance plans (long-term care insurance plans) do provide extended coverage for long-term care benefits in addition to or instead of Medicare. Currently the Medicare plan is becoming increasingly stringent in reviewing individuals to continue receiving Medicare coverage for skilled nursing facility services beyond the initial 20-day period.

Individuals who are discharged from facilities to their homes, who are homebound and continue to require skilled nursing care and/or physical, speech, or occupational therapy, are entitled to services of a home health agency under a physician's treatment plan. The cost of these services can be covered by Medicare without the requirements of prior hospitalization. Home health services may be furnished to a beneficiary under the following conditions:

1. The beneficiary is confined to home or an institution that is not a nursing facility, hospital, or skilled nursing facility (e.g., a boarding home or residential care facility).
2. The beneficiary is under the care of a doctor who establishes a plan of care.
3. The beneficiary is in need of intermediate skilled nursing care, physical, speech and/or occupational therapy.
4. The services are provided by a Medicare certified home health agency.[3]

Services covered under this plan are intended to provide for an individual who has skilled care needs. If a person reaches a point when services received by physical, occupational, and/or speech therapists no longer help in improving his or her condition, or if the need for skilled nursing care is alleviated by improvements in the medical condition (e.g., the healing of an open wound), then Medicare benefits are likely to be discontinued. For many individuals, the need for continuing custodial care remains. Those expenses are not paid for under the current Medicare program.

MEDICAID

The largest portion of ongoing long-term care expenses in this country are paid for by the federally enacted, federal/state **Medicaid** program (see Table 9–5). Although there are some variations among individual states, the percentage of nursing home residents qualifying for Medicaid hovers near 80 percent.

TABLE 9–5. Medicaid Payments to Nursing Facilities (excluding homes for people with mental retardation) 1980–1995

Year	Expenditures in Millions of Dollars
1980	7,887
1985	11,587
1990	17,693
1995	29,052

Source: Statistical Abstract of the United States, 1997, ed. 17. U.S. Department of Commerce, Washington, DC, 1997, p 118.

The Medicaid program was initially enacted as a part of President Johnson's "War on Poverty" in 1969. The program's initial focus was to provide medical care for poor Americans. The Medicaid program pays health care costs for individuals with very low incomes and very limited assets. The program was expanded in the early 1970s to include nursing home cost coverage for poor, primarily elderly, people. Current figures indicate that while the majority of Medicaid recipients fall into the "community-based" Medicaid program, (i.e., low income and limited assets), the program expenditures have evolved so that a greater proportion of Medicaid funds are now spent on long-term care expenses for elderly Medicaid recipients rather than on regular health care costs. The growth of the program can, in part, be traced back to 1980 legislation that expanded the long-term care Medicaid coverage from relatively poor elderly individuals to include many middle-class elders with limited assets.

Initial Medicaid rules governing eligibility for long-term care coverage allowed an individual to retain only $2000 in assets. A couple together was allowed to retain $3000 in assets. Because women tend to outlive their spouses by several years, the result was the forced impoverishment of elderly women after being widowed. What typically happened was that the male spouse had a catastrophic health event requiring nursing home care. In taking care of him, the couple "spent down" their funds to $3000. Once the husband died, his surviving widow had only $3000 to live on for the rest of her life. Congress viewed this as an unintended and inequitable result from the earlier expansion of Medicaid benefits.

Legislation created the concept of a **community spouse resource allowance (CSRA).** This allowed a noninstitutionalized spouse, i.e., the one living in the community or so-called community spouse, to retain enough assets to continue to conduct his or her life relatively independently. The figure is neither incredibly generous nor unduly harsh. The CSRA amount is set by the federal government. In 1997, the CSRA amount was $79,020.[3]

There is an immense amount of misinformation and rumor regarding the

Medicaid program. Dated or incorrect information can be financially damaging to individuals or couples. Anyone who is facing the prospect of having a loved one institutionalized in a nursing home or residential care facility is advised to seek out a professional whose practice focuses on the financial aspects of Medicaid eligibility and/or cost reimbursement for medical services. Many social workers are specifically trained in this area. There are also attorneys who focus their practice on elder law. The National Academy of Elder Law Attorneys (NAELA) is a national organization of attorneys who focus their practice on elder law. Most states now have an elder law chapter or subcommittee of the state bar association.

There are several reasons for lack of good information regarding Medicaid eligibility. One of the primary sources of confusion stems from the fact that Medicaid law is a complicated combination of federal and state law. The Medicaid benefits package was established and is updated by federal law. The program is administered and enforced, in part, through the federal Health Care Financing Administration (HCFA). Most of the program's financial guidelines are created by federal statute and regulation. However, the program does give individual states significant latitude in writing their own specific rules of Medicaid eligibility, which has resulted in substantial differences among the states. What is true in one state may not be accurate or relevant in another state.

There are two primary criteria for individuals to become eligible for long-term care benefits under the Medicaid program:

• Medical eligibility
• Financial need

Long-term care Medicaid benefits are not paid for an individual who seeks to be placed in a nursing home as a matter of convenience. Although such cases are relatively rare, there are instances in which people are isolated and have little or no contact with either family members or a support community. For these people the structured environment of a nursing home may be appealing. Generally, medical eligibility for nursing home care is determined by an individual's attending physician. When a physician is of the opinion that it is no longer safe for a person to remain either at home or in a residential care environment, then he or she makes the recommendation to have that individual placed in a nursing home. This fulfills the medical need criterion. However, a trend seems to be developing in some states that are seeking to reduce the state's costs under the Medicaid program, or are encouraging a focus of "deinstitutionalization," to promote more home-based care and/or assistance in residential care facility settings. These states use a screening tool with objective criteria, administered by a representative of the state rather than by an individual's attending physician, to attempt to determine what level of care is absolutely necessary for the Medicaid recipient.

Unlike Medicare, Medicaid is not an entitlement program, and therefore individuals do not automatically receive benefits. A person must financially qualify for the program. Medicaid rules describe ownership of several types of assets that are exempt from consideration when seeking Medicaid eligibility. While specific rules regarding exempt assets vary from state to state, there are several items that are exempt assets in every state:

- Homestead and personal property
- Prepaid funeral and burial expenses, including funds put into a mortuary trust, and funds paid for a burial plot and headstone
- The value of a vehicle
- Liquid assets of $2000 for a single person or $79,020 for a couple (CSRA amount)[3]

Many states have additional items that are considered exempt assets. Individuals and their families are encouraged to seek out accurate and current information regarding local rules.

In addition to exempt assets, there are local rules that allow the community spouse to receive a certain level of income in order to manage his or her affairs. Nationally the amount of income that a community spouse is allowed to receive is not consistent. This becomes a pertinent issue, for example, when a husband who has worked outside of the home is entitled to higher Social Security and/or pension benefits, while his wife, who has primarily worked in the home, receives meager Social Security benefits and no pension. In such a case, the spouse at home is often entitled to receive a portion of her husband's check in addition to her CSRA.

There is considerable confusion regarding the ability of an individual or couple to transfer assets prior to applying for Medicaid benefits. Couples need to know that there are no transfer penalties incurred on transfers between spouses. If one spouse is entering a nursing home, it is permissible to place the assets of the couple in the name of the community spouse. The institutionalized spouse is allowed to have only $2000 in his or her name. Most states generally allow a period of time to effect the transfer of jointly held assets into the name of the community spouse.

There are restrictions, however, both at the federal and state level, on the transfer of assets to other third parties such as children. Often the transfer of assets is permissible but entails an asset transfer penalty during which a period of ineligibility for Medicaid benefits is imposed as the result of transferring assets. An individual, couple, or fiduciary acting on behalf of an individual or couple should always seek financial or legal advice to ensure that asset transfers comply with federal and state laws and regulations. Currently, federal law provides that states may "look back" for a period of 36 months at all financial records (including transfers) made by an individual or couple prior to applying for Medicaid benefits. One must always ensure that adequate funds are available to pay privately for the needs of an individual for the entire duration of any imposed transfer penalty period.

A key distinction is that funds spent on exempt assets are not subject to transfer penalties. For example, an individual or couple has "aged in place." They may have become relatively isolated over time and probably have not kept their home as safe or as well maintained as it should be. Funds spent on necessary home improvements or maintenance, such as the replacing of a roof, a furnace, or windows, are permissible transfers. Medicaid regulations also permit and even encourage people to expend funds in order to adapt the home to make it a safer environment (e.g., adding a ramp, lighting, grab bars or transfer benches in bathrooms, or amenities at ground level in order to avoid dangerous climbs on staircases).

Often, the fear of not having enough money to cover the cost of long-term care in the future has prevented people from spending the necessary funds for crucial medical attention or for items such as eyeglasses, hearing aids, and dental work, even though such expenditures are also permissible and encouraged. If an individual or couple has not made funeral arrangements, prepaying for those arrangements is appropriate. If a couple does not have safe and reliable transportation, they should consider purchasing a new or used car. Having a safe, reliable vehicle, which is large enough to be able to carry a wheelchair, is often a key to providing an enhanced quality of life for both the institutionalized spouse and the community spouse. The primary concept here is to "not spend the same money twice." Individuals and couples should make use of the opportunities to spend their funds on exempt assets prior to applying for Medicaid assistance, because it does not make sense for them to pay for exempt items out of funds that are also exempt.

VETERANS ADMINISTRATION BENEFITS

Veterans' benefits are federal entitlement benefits administered by the federal Department of Veterans Affairs. The general requirements for eligibility for Veterans Administration (VA) benefits include active duty service in the armed forces with no dishonorable discharge. Medical benefits available to eligible veterans may include hospital, nursing home, and home health care, as well as outpatient medical treatment, home health services, and community residential care. In certain cases, the spouse and children of disabled or deceased veterans may also be entitled to care.[3]

In order to qualify for VA medical benefits, the veteran must usually have a service-connected condition, a non-service-connected disability with the inability to pay for care, or a disability that was incurred or aggravated in the line of duty and led to discharge from the armed forces. Veterans who have a service-connected disability are entitled to free hospital, nursing home, and/or outpatient care. A veteran with non-service-connected disabilities receives free hospital and nursing care if he or she is eligible for Medicaid, receives a VA pension or meets certain income criteria. Veterans with non-service-connected disabilities may receive institutional care on a space-available basis. This care is not cost free, but is subsidized by the government. Individuals are encouraged to contact their local Department of Veterans Affairs in order to determine what benefits they might be entitled to.

STATE PROGRAMS

Although still a relatively small part of the funding of long-term care services for the elderly, funding for many state programs is growing considerably. Several states, faced with drastically increasing Medicaid costs as a result of nursing home bills for elderly Medicaid recipients, have begun to develop programs that seek to assist elderly individuals in remaining in their homes or communities. Funding for community-based care, when coupled with certain Medicare and Medicaid benefits and an individual's private resources, enables the establishment of an adequate plan of care that allows seniors to remain safely in their homes for a longer period of time.

The cost of keeping frail but competent individuals in their own homes is often far less than institutionalizing those individuals in a nursing home setting. These state programs may provide funding for direct medical services such as nursing visits and also the services of a home health aide who is able to help the elderly individual or couple with practical day-to-day tasks such as cleaning, cooking, shopping, and laundry. State programs may also provide assistance to make the home physically safe by adding practical safety features such as ramps or first floor bathroom facilities.

Inconsistencies exist among state programs, and many of these programs have long waiting lists. Individuals and their fiduciaries are strongly encouraged to assertively seek out information from state agencies (area agencies on aging) and local nonprofit agencies regarding assistance for extended care expenses that might be available at the state level.

PRIVATE SECTOR FUNDING

There are two primary sources of private sector funds available to pay for long-term care expenses: individual payments and long-term care insurance. Payments for long-term care that individuals make from their accumulated savings and current income account for approximately one third of all chronic long-term care expenses.[5] Long-term care insurance or variants such as nursing home insurance or home health care insurance pays for less than 5 percent of long-term care costs. However, the use of long-term care insurance is growing dramatically. Because it is unlikely that public sector resources and benefits will be expanding to cover additional long-term care costs, all insurable individuals with moderate or substantial assets may want to consider purchasing long-term care insurance. This product is becoming a standard part of prudent financial and estate planning.

PERSONAL SAVINGS, PERSONAL CHOICES

For those individuals who have failed to develop a plan for long-term care expenses, the moment they become aware that their benefits under the Medicare program (and consequently, their Medicare supplement) have ended (or will end shortly) can be traumatic. To discover that they will be required to begin using a portion of their life savings to pay for these costs is often devastating and terrifying. Individuals may become angry, overwhelmed, and disoriented when squarely faced with the reality of the situation. Once the necessity of paying for long-term care costs actually arrives, there is no more opportunity to believe "this won't happen to me." Services are rendered, and the bills must be paid. The situation can lead to great bitterness in one's final years.

One of the initial choices individuals and families are faced with is whether or not to set up a formal or informal plan. If the elderly individual requires institutionalization because it is not possible for him or her to be safe at home, the individual or family will be limited to those facilities located in his or her local area. Factors such as availability, cost, affiliation with physicians, and eventual possibility of the available slot to be converted to public sector funding (Medicaid) are all factors that must be taken into consideration. Families are well advised to do serious comparison shopping prior to signing a contract with any facility.

In many areas of the country, private **geriatric care managers** (GCMs) are available for consultation regarding the various aspects of local facilities. Also many public sector and nonprofit agencies act as consultants or as clearing houses for information on local facilities. Obtaining the best objective information available is critical to a successful transition, because the placement of individuals in facilities and the arrangement for payment of those costs can be a complicated, confusing, and highly emotional process. Seeking out and relying on the experience of individuals who have helped others through the placement process can be especially helpful at this juncture.

Professionals may need to advocate on behalf of the individual to ensure successful placements. Hiring someone with experience (e.g., a geriatric care manager, medical social worker, or attorney) who is independent and unaffiliated with any particular institution will give the consumer of long-term care services a better opportunity to make informed choices.

HOME CARE SERVICES

An elder who requires extensive assistance in order to continue living in his or her own home presents another set of issues. Older people and their significant others may have difficulty fully comprehending how dramatically their lives will change following a catastrophic health event such as a stroke, heart attack, or broken hip. Partners or family members who have been caregivers for an elderly person experiencing a progressive, cognitive decline due to dementia or Alzheimer's disease are often unable to detect how progressive the assistance provided has been. The need for care in one's home, by its nature, requires that an individual's privacy and well-established daily routines are severely interrupted.

Assistance may be needed besides traditional health care. For example, people may need help with tasks such as housework, grocery shopping, laundry, transportation, and home maintenance. For individuals who have grown up and come of age in the Depression, and generally have a history of frugal handling of their finances, it can be mortifying to pay other people to do what they have done for themselves all their lives. Individuals in this situation will often make decisions regarding their care, not based on their needs, but based exclusively on the cost of those services.

When faced with the reality of privately paying for home health care expenses, families may explore the potential costs of extensive home health care provided by an agency and panic. Families commonly try to set up informal relationships and muddle through as well as possible for as long as possible. Incredulously, some people who have been cautious and meticulous in the handling of their personal and financial affairs will suddenly rely on "the friend of a friend of a friend" to provide assistance for the most intimate details of their lives.

Caution in this situation is well advised. An elder person requiring significant home health care is, by definition, vulnerable and dependent. Often, these elders are living on the verge of competency. Cognition (including memory, problem solving, and judgment) is often mildly, inconsistently, or globally impaired. If a problem arises, with either the level of care or finances, these individuals are often unlikely to be able to provide valid information to substantiate a case of improper care or other wrongdoing.

Often the payments made under informal arrangements are also made informally. Many informal care providers request that they be paid without the benefit of a payroll system. This should always be a red flag to the family or fiduciary who is responsible for the elder. In the event that any disagreement or dispute arises, the elder person or his or her fiduciary potentially could be placed in the defensive position of failing to properly withhold taxes and other assessments due federal or state governmental entities.

Informal arrangements involve other significant risks as well. Caregivers in such situations are rarely bonded or insured. Workers compensation usually does not cover those individuals. In the event that a caregiver becomes injured in the course of his or her employment (which can happen frequently when physical assistance is being provided), a potential claim easily could be asserted against an elderly individual who may own a home and other significant assets. Personal injury claims are commonly litigated by personal injury attorneys on a contingency fee basis. One cannot reasonably expect that an injured worker will refrain from making a claim against an elderly care recipient merely because it is distasteful to do so.

There is also risk from the reverse perspective. If the elderly person becomes injured because of improper care or inattention of an informal caregiver, rarely will there be adequate assets from which to recover damages from that individual unless he or she is bonded and insured. The best course of action for family members needing to piece together an adequate plan of care for an elder in his or her home is to use the services of a reputable, certified, bonded, and insured home health care provider. Using the services of a geriatric care manager or elder law attorney to oversee and/or review the plan of care also ensures that an independent, objective advocate for the elder will be there if the need arises.

SOURCES OF FUNDS

People's assets are held in a myriad of different investment vehicles. When putting together a plan of care for private payment of long term-care expenses, it will be necessary to complete a full inventory of the individual's assets. Both liquid and nonliquid assets need to be reviewed.

Obvious sources of assets accumulated by individuals include savings accounts, checking accounts, certificates of deposit in banks, credit unions, and other thrift institution accounts, and mutual fund or money market accounts, which are reported either individually by the different fund sources or as part of an umbrella account at a brokerage house or at a financial institution.

A thorough search through an individual's financial records often will yield several life insurance policies, some current and some much older. Especially considering the older policies, the cash value of the policies may be greater than their face value. One will need to contact the home office of each of the companies to determine the current cash value.

Another contract sold by life insurance companies is an annuity contract. Some annuities are currently in a payment status in which monthly payments are being made to the annuitant. Other annuities, known as deferred annuities, have not begun to pay out funds. These contracts continue to build funds on a tax-deferred status.

Individuals may have several retirement accounts. Some retirement funds come in the form of pension payments from places where the elderly person was employed for long periods of time. However, in the 1980s and 1990s, tax incentives at the federal level have provided the impetus for several retirement savings programs. These funds are not required to be managed by one institution. One person may have several different retirement accounts, including **individual retirement accounts** such as **(IRAs), Keogh plans, 401(k) plans,** and Teachers Insurance Annuity Association (TIAA) and **Teachers Supplemental Annuity (TSA) plans.** Individual vendors or institutions can provide current information regarding assets held in the different accounts. Many older persons also hold U.S. savings bonds. The actual value of savings bonds may be much greater than the face value of those bonds, depending on when they were purchased and whether or not the bonds have been accumulating or paying out interest.

It is advisable to ask individuals whether or not anyone owes them money. Older persons often have sold a home or another piece of real estate and have taken back a mortgage as part of that sale. One will want to ascertain whether that mortgage was validly executed and whether or not it has been recorded. Further, it is necessary to ascertain whether or not payments are current on the mortgage note and whether or not an amortization schedule (a chart showing how much of the loan has been paid and how much remains to be paid) exists. Individuals often have loaned money to friends or family members. Sometimes these notes have been properly memorialized with a promissory note, but many times this is not the case. It is important to determine how all the parties to such a transaction currently view the situation. Is this, in fact, a loan which has been made with the expectation of repayment, or was it actually made as a gift? The perception of the transaction between the elder loaning the money and an individual (often one of his or her children) who has received the money sometimes can be very different. It is much better to sort out these questions prior to having to submit information to a state agency for a Medicaid application or as part of an investigation by a personal representative of an individual's estate.

A thorough review of all real estate held by the individual is necessary. It is wise to try to find realistic valuations of property, either by securing a real estate appraisal or through a thorough market analysis. An appraisal is usually done by an individual certified in his or her state by training and experience to give accurate values to real property. The fees for appraisals can range between $250 and $500 per parcel (and are much higher in the case of commercial real estate). A market analysis does not carry the same weight as a certified appraisal, but it also can be a useful tool in developing a general understanding of the value of real estate. Market analyses are usually done for a nominal fee by a local real estate broker familiar with the area and type of property.

During the inventory of real estate, it often becomes clear that a particular parcel or two is no longer much used or needed by the elder individual. Serious consideration should be given to selling any parcel that no longer retains any real utility. This may have a triple benefit effect. Not only will the sale provide additional liquid cash to an individual's portfolio, but it removes the expense of taxes and maintaining the property as a financial drain from the individual's resources as well. It also can remove the physical and emotional burden of maintaining and caring for a little-used piece of property.

Finally, it is often worthwhile to do an extensive review of an individual's personal property, including vehicles. Many times, individuals are surprised to discover the magnitude of possessions that they have accumulated over a lifetime. Individuals may have many items that they are either willing to give away or to sell in order to raise additional cash. The selling of any "extra vehicles," again, has the dual benefit of raising funds and removing the costs of insuring, registering, and maintaining that vehicle.

LONG-TERM CARE INSURANCE

The magnitude of the changing demographics in the United States, in which the number of elders will continue to grow year after year until the year 2020, will require an additional private sector response for providing long-term care benefits if we are to avoid a massive crisis.

Long-term care insurance will be one of the pillars on which our evolving system of providing financing for extended care expenses will be built. Middle-class Americans who are between the ages of 55 and 70, who are still healthy and insurable, need, as a matter of course, to begin considering the purchase of long-term care insurance as part of their standard financial and estate planning strategies. While the cost of long-term care insurance varies greatly, a few examples are provided here,

- Man, aged 50, approximate range $100 to 200 per month
- Woman, aged 30, approximate range $75 to 150 per month
- Either one, aged 60, approximate range $150 to 300 per month6

Long-term care insurance is a product that pays for long-term care expenses when benefits under a Medicare and Medicare supplement program are terminated, and/or when an individual or couple is ineligible for Medicaid benefits, either because they do not qualify medically for such a program or because the individual or couple has assets greater than allowed by law.

Long-term care insurance usually pays for the costs of care no matter where an individual is residing (e.g., at a nursing home, a residential care facility, or at home), although there are some derivative policies that provide benefits only for nursing home care or only for home health care. Currently, long-term care insurance policies and their derivatives pay approximately 5 percent of long-term care expenses. However, because of tightening standards for both Medicare benefits and Medicaid eligibility, the need for individuals to self-fund their long-term care expenses will only increase.

The benefits of including long-term care insurance into a financial plan are several. For one, policies are portable. The benefits travel with the elderly person. Individuals and couples are able to make life decisions as to where they would like to live independent of the particular Medicaid eligibility rules of a given state. Many of the high-quality long-term care vendors also have working arrangements with the major home health care insurance providers to offer a substantial discount for the home health care services they provide as long as the individual or couple receiving services is a policyholder with the insurance vendor.

The payment of benefits by vendors is usually triggered by the inability of an individual or couple to perform two of five or two of six of the activities of daily living (ADLs). The most common ADLs used by the insurance industry are continence, dressing, eating, toileting and transferring. Several vendors also include bathing as one of the covered ADLs.

Most vendors have specific language that addresses cognitive impairment. This provision can act as a trigger to secure benefits for an individual who is unable to pass certain tests assessing his or her cognitive ability. This is important because an individual with Alzheimer's disease or some other form of dementia may be physically capable of completing the movements necessary to do the stated ADL, but may have a cognitive impairment that renders him or her incapable of performing the ADL tasks without physical or verbal assistance. Most states prohibit companies from containing an exclusion for Alzheimer's disease, but the standard is not uniform. Typically, long-term care insurance will pay benefits for a selected period of time—2 years, 3 years, 5 years, or for the lifetime of the insured. Elimination periods (specific waiting times in which no benefits are paid) vary. These time frames generally run 20, 30, 60, 90, or 100 days. Long-term care policies are designed to pay a certain daily benefit. Usually, that figure should be pegged to the average cost of nursing home care in the individual's area.

The benefit, whether payable for nursing home care or for home health care, provides a "backstop" that allows individuals the freedom to receive the care they need while still preserving a major portion of their assets. Individuals who have secured long-term care insurance are more willing to seek and receive care for services that allow them to stay in their home longer. Many times, individuals simply refuse to seek the care they need if they think they will have to pay for it dollar-for-dollar out of their savings. This can lead to additional health care crises, which in turn can push people from their homes prior to the time that would otherwise be necessary.

Purchasing long-term care or home health care insurance can also buy time for an individual and his or her family to provide immediately needed services that keep them safe while they make other appropriate arrangements. Organizing and disposing of assets and putting together an effective long-term plan of care all require a lot of time. Knowing that there are funds to pay for necessary services after this initial time period reduces the stress of the situation and enables individuals and their families to make more informed and reasonable judgments and decisions. Most state insurance commissions have useful information regarding the vendors in their state. In addition, the National Association of Insurance Commissioners (NAIC, 120 West 12th Street, Suite 1100, Kansas City, MO 64105-1925) publishes a useful and informative shoppers' guide to long-term care insurance.

▨ COST CONTAINMENT

As health care expenditures continue not only to increase but also to take an ever greater portion of our gross national spending pie, it would be remiss not to mention **cost containment.** Several ideas have surfaced, but a clear path for the next century has not made itself clear. Proposals include the following:

- A national health care plan that provides basic health care benefits for all citizens or residents
- Continuing with the managed care philosophy, which pledges cost effectiveness in health care spending
- Rationing health care based on need, age, or some other defining characteristic (such as the existence of living wills)
- Furthering the idea of health promotion (which is sometimes included under managed care, although not always emphasized)

The first two ideas have had entire volumes devoted to them; interested readers are encouraged to explore these options on their own. Rationing health care and health promotion are explored briefly here.

The rationing of health care services already exists. Those who have the funds seek out the best specialists and pay for the most advanced technology, although even these measures do not always stave off death. Since these services are available for some, many others think they should be available for all (or at least themselves) in time of need as well. However, our health care system cannot sustain such spending. Most agree that allocation of resources is something which will need to be done in the future. Arcangelo[1] states that the problem is that the sickest patients (often elderly) account for the greatest health care expenditures (the sickest 5% incur 58% of the costs [p. 26]). In the section supporting rationing she states: "unless health care for the elderly is limited, future generations will be cheated." On the other hand, she unequivocally states that age should not be the only factor to consider in rationing health care, but that quality of life issues and cost benefits should be important considerations too, especially considering that the elderly are hardly a homogeneous group by almost any standards except chronological age.

The opponents to age-based rationing see it as yet another example of ageism, demonstrating once again that elders are not valued. Rationing health care presents a difficult ethical debate that is far from over. Self-rationing health care measures such as living wills, if followed as intended, may provide our best answer, because they will avoid one group making life and death decisions for another group.

According to Gillis,[7] residents of the United States have traditionally decided that whatever could be done to save someone or to prolong his or her life should be done no matter the cost. This has led to an individualistic, flawed system that spends too much for too little gain. People have longer lives, but the quality of their lives is not necessarily good. In addition, some of our uninsured residents are not given even the benefits of basic health care. High-technology medical care for some has been favored over basic care for all.

Health promotion is an idea that espouses the old adage "An ounce of prevention is worth a pound of cure." It promotes the idea that if we take good care of ourselves during our entire lives, less will have to be spent on the heroic measures toward the end. Gillis[7] proposes that preventive measures, such as regular exercise, regular checkups, good diet, enough rest, and healthy lifestyles, would provide the "greatest good for the greatest number" and that we would find an overall decreased use of the health care system. On the opposing side, it must be stated that research that definitively demonstrates the value of these preventive measures is not that common. Unfortunately, this makes sense, because it is difficult to measure something that does not happen (perhaps because of the health promoting activities).

Fowler[8] states that the vast majority (86%) of older Americans are living with at least one chronic disease. She proposes that health care measures with these elders should not have the goal of curing these chronic conditions but rather should aim at decreasing their symptoms, limiting the progression of the condition, and improving the person's ability to function in daily life. She reports that, generally, older adults are willing to participate in exercise and other health promoting activities and that through these measures they can increase the likelihood of successful aging even within the relative confines of one or more chronic conditions.

The agenda of the federal government, Healthy People 2000, which is funding research in the area of health promotion, states these objectives:

- To increase the healthy life span of people living in the United States
- To decrease health disparities among those people
- To provide access to preventive services for all
- To decrease difficulty in performing daily tasks, especially for elderly people

Health promotion, if made an essential way of life rather than just a nice idea, may indeed provide our best chance for improving health care while keeping costs manageable.

SUMMARY

Health care costs for the elderly primarily are covered through three programs: Medicare, Medicaid, and other insurance packages (e.g., Veterans' benefit plans, and private long-term care plans). Long-term care is the largest single expenditure, primarily for elderly people, costing approximately $80 billion in the United States in 1997. This chapter has attempted to give an overview of the long-term care system as well as an introduction to the Medicare and Medicaid programs. Considerations for health care spending decisions were outlined. These decisions are obviously best made while one is competent and healthy. Preplanning can often avoid excessive cost and family disagreements. Health care financing is becoming a great burden on our society as we gain access to ever more complex and expensive technologies that can delay the moment of death (although not necessarily sustain the quality of life). Therefore, it is increasingly important to make rational, well-thought-out decisions about the use of health care dollars, especially, although certainly not exclusively, for the elderly people of our country. Through their own involvement in these difficult choices, they can ensure fairness and dignity for themselves and for future generations.

▣ REVIEW QUESTIONS

1. Which of the following expenditures is not an exempt purchase before applying for Medicaid?
   A. Roof replacement
   B. Hearing aid
   C. Ramp to enter home
   D. New furniture
   E. Prepaid funeral expenses

2. The cost of nursing home care:
   A. Is approximately $2000 per month.
   B. Is approximately $8000 per month.
   C. Is funded largely by Medicare.
   D. Is funded largely by Medicaid.

3. The Medicare program pays for all of the following EXCEPT:
   A. Hospital stays
   B. Custodial care
   C. Outpatient visits
   D. Home health care

4. A living will is established to:
   A. Give instructions regarding health care measures in the event of a catastrophic injury or illness.
   B. Provide death care instructions.
   C. Provide definitive approval for a DNR (do not resuscitate) order.
   D. Provide guidance on needed institutional placement in the event of a catastrophic injury or illness.

5. Private sector insurance pays for approximately what percentage of long-term care costs?
   A. 17%
   B. 3%
   C. 10%
   D. 20%

6. Informal caregivers of the elderly:

    A. Are covered by workers compensation.

    B. Are usually bonded and insured.

    C. Are a liability for the elderly person.

    D. Are always paid through a payroll system.

7. Health promotion includes all of the following EXCEPT:

    A. Seeing a physician monthly.

    B. A healthy diet.

    C. Getting enough rest.

    D. Avoiding alcohol/drug abuse.

8. Medicaid:

    A. Has always paid for long-term care.

    B. Is a joint program between the federal government and individual states.

    C. Pays for a smaller proportion of long-term care expenses than Medicare.

    D. Allows a person to maintain $40,000 in assets without affecting eligibility.

9. Transferring assets to hasten Medicaid eligibility:

    A. Is against the law.

    B. Is allowed as long as the transfer is to one's children.

    C. Is allowed between spouses.

    D. Is not allowed for a period of 10 years.

10. State programs to supplement funding for an adequate plan of care for elderly persons:

    A. Are consistent from state to state.

    B. Are decreasing in scope and number.

    C. Provide only hospital-based care.

    D. Often have long waiting lists.

▨ LEARNING ACTIVITIES

1. Conduct a debate on the rationing of health care (see reference 1). Try to reach consensus on some issues with the entire group.

2. Discuss the issues surrounding advanced directives, including personal choices, compliance, and the consequences of noncompliance. Write simplified advance directive for yourself. Share these with a partner.

3. Hold a brainstorming session listing all the possible solutions to our current health care dilemma. (Remember, during brainstorming there are no wrong answers.) Pick a few from the list that have realistic possibilities. Discuss how your class could have an impact on the future of health care in this country.

4. For a semester project, explore health care programs (including financing care for the elderly) in other countries such as Canada, Finland, Russia, Iraq, Brazil, Aus-

tralia, China, and Nigeria. Answer questions such as: How do these health care programs compare with our own? What could we learn from this country's system? How are the elderly cared for in this country?

▥ REFERENCES

1. Arcangelo, V: Should age be a criterion for rationing health care? Nursing Forum 29 (1):25–29, 1994.
2. Health Insurance Association of America: Guide to Long Term Care. HIAA, Washington, DC, 1996.
3. Regan, JJ, et al: Tax, Estate and Financial Planning for the Elderly. Matthew Bender, New York, NY, 1997.
4. 1997 Guide to Health Insurance for People with Medicare. Developed jointly by the National Association of Insurance Commissioners and the Health Care Financing Administration of the U.S. Department of Health and Human Services, NAIC, Kansas City, MO, 1997.
5. Health Insurance Association of America. Guide to Long Term Care. HIAA, Washington, DC, 1997.
6. UNUM Representative: Personal communication, June 24, 1998
7. Gillis, AJ: Allocation of healthcare resources: The case for health promotion. Nursing Forum 27(4):21–26, 1992.
8. Fowler, SB: Health promotion in chronically ill older adults. Journal of Neuroscience Nursing 28(5):39–43, 1996.

We hope that prevention and health
promotion, rather than
care for illness, will prevail.
Dr. Mimi Fields, Pew Commission

Health Care Providers Working with the Elderly

Regula H. Robnett and Walter C. Chop

CHAPTER OUTLINE

BEHAVIORAL OBJECTIVES

Upon completion of this chapter, the reader will be able to:

1. List the possible members of a health care team.
2. Describe multidisciplinary, transdisciplinary, and interdisciplinary health care teams.
3. Briefly describe each of the following health care professions:
- Case Manager
- Dietician
- Emergency medical services
- Nursing
- Occupational therapy
- Physical therapy
- Radiography
- Respiratory care
- Social work
- Speech-language pathologist
- Therapeutic recreation
4. Describe how the health care professionals in the fields listed work specifically with elderly people.
5. Define the Pew Commission and give a brief summary of their third report.

KEY TERMS

Case management
Emergency medical services (EMS)
Emergency medical technician (EMT)
Gerontological nursing
Interdisciplinary team
Multidisciplinary team
Occupational therapy (OT)
Physical therapy (PT)
Pew Health Professions Commission

Radiologic technology (RT)
Registered dietician (RD)
Respiratory care practitioner (RCP)
Social work
Speech-language pathologist (SLP)
Therapeutic recreation specialist (TRS)
Transdisciplinary team

INTRODUCTION

This chapter is designed to give the reader an overview of different types of professionals who provide health care services for the elderly. Most segments describing different professions were written by an expert in that field. The disciplines are described alphabetically to avoid giving the impression that one profession in any way provides a more essential service than any other. All are valuable members of the health care team; each one provides a vital link in the continuum of care.

Since health care is most often provided in the context of a health care team, a summary of different kinds of health teams is also provided in this chapter. Not all the professionals described are represented in every health care team. A team is formed to coordinate health care services for a particular patient and will only include the members who provide the services needed for that person. Nor are all professions who interact with the elderly described; the list would be overwhelming.

Finally, a summary of the Pew Health Professions Commission's third report is provided. The Pew Commission is a national commission established by the Pew Charitable Trusts in Philadelphia and administered through the Center of Health Professions at the University of California, San Francisco. The commission's reports speak to the changing needs of health care consumers and the demand to reduce the number of health care workers overall. In preparing for the next century, the commission seeks to find the best way to adapt the system to fit our changing health care needs and to ensure accountability and competence of all health care providers.[1]

HEALTH CARE TEAMS

Health care is most often provided in the framework of a team. The team consists of at least the health care provider and the patient or client, whose life is directly affected by the care given. Often, more than one professional and other patient support persons (such as family members and friends) are team players as well. Providers can include

- Physicians and their assistants
- Nurses and their assistants
- Occupational, physical, respiratory, and speech therapists (assistants and aides as well)
- Case managers
- Psychologists and psychiatrists
- Nutritionists or dieticians
- Laboratory/medical technicians
- Medical equipment vendors
- Therapeutic recreation specialists
- Social workers

The three basic types of teams in today's health care arena are

- Multidisciplinary
- Interdisciplinary
- Transdisciplinary

Each provides a different perspective on the roles of the providers and how they should interact with one another. Each provider in a **multidisciplinary team** has his or her own role, which is carried out without interference. For example, the physical therapist will work on gait training, the nurse on medication management, and the dietician on caloric intake. They then share any pertinent information about the patient and events that have occurred on an as-needed basis or during a regularly scheduled team meeting. In an **interdisciplinary team,** patient goals are shared by members of the team; each provider works with the patient to promote the overriding goals of health care intervention. The goal may be broad, such as returning the patient to an independent living situation. Within this overarching goal, each provider would then have related, more discipline-specific, goals for the patient intended to reach the anticipated outcome. (For example, the occupational therapist might have goals related to activities of daily living [ADLs], while the speech therapist might have communication goals.) In a **transdisciplinary team,** members also share their expertise with one another, and their individual disciplinary roles are not always clear-cut. Available resources are used to their maximal potential, and carryover from one discipline to another is common. The therapists and nurses work together to support one another's goals for the patient (and may even seem to be doing the other's job).

The interdisciplinary team is often viewed as the ideal to strive for in providing services. While it promotes the sharing of all pertinent information, it does not cross role boundaries during the health care intervention process.

More likely than not, as a health care professional, you will become the member of a health care team. As a team member you will need to take on certain responsibilities, including speaking up in the group and advocating for the welfare of the patient. To be effective, team members need to have good communication skills, respect for other members, confidence in their own professional skills, and a commitment to the team process. The assumptions of the team process include a belief in both interdependency and the superiority of group versus individual problem solving.

⬚ HEALTH CARE PROFESSIONALS

- Case managers
- Dietician (registered dietician [RD])

- Emergency medical services provider
- Nursing professionals
- Occupational therapy practitioner (OTR or COTA)
- Physical therapist (PT) and physical therapist assistant (PTA)
- Radiographer
- Respiratory care practitioner (RCP)
- Social worker
- Speech-language pathologist (SLP)
- Therapeutic recreation specialist (TRS)

🔳 CASE MANAGERS

A case manager often works as part of a health care team to ensure effective coordination of services. In this time of increasing managed care, **case management** is seen as a tool to promote cost-effective outcomes, although the concept of case management is not new, having been introduced in the 1960s with the workers' compensation and rehabilitation legislation. Currently the Case Management Society of America (CSMA) estimates that there are approximately 100,000 case managers in the United States, 16,000 of whom are certified.[2]

The CSMA has established standards of practice for case management. Certified case managers, who often have training in nursing, but may come from other clinical health care disciplines such as medical social work or rehabilitation, follow these standards. Because of their ability to work collaboratively, their knowledge of resources in the health care arena (including funding sources), and their ability to monitor and evaluate health care services, case managers often play a primary role in many health care teams that work with the elderly. It is especially important to have a case manager involved for "high end health care users" (the 10% of the patients whose health care expenses equal 70% to 80% of the total health care costs),[2] as these tend to present the most complex health care needs. Case management involves trouble shooting and problem solving, patient advocacy, and effectively determining realistic outcomes of service provision. Case managers work with the elderly primarily in general hospitals, long-term care facilities, home health care, and rehabilitation centers.

For more information, contact the Case Management Society of America, 8201 Cantrell, Suite 230, Little Rock, AR 72227–2448, (501) 225-2229.

🔳 DIETICIAN *Louise D. Whitney*

Clinical dieticians are a vital part of the medical team in hospitals, nursing homes, health maintenance organizations, and other health care facilities.

They work with doctors, nurses, and therapists to help speed patients' recovery and lay the groundwork for long-term health care.

Dieticians also work in public and home health agencies, day care centers, health and recreation clubs, and in government-funded programs that feed and counsel the elderly. Whenever proper nutrition could help improve someone's quality of life, they reach out to the public to teach, monitor, and advise.

Dieticians have many opportunities to work with the elderly in improving their nutritional well-being in a variety of settings. The **registered dietician (RD)** might visit elderly patients in long-term care facilities, during routine doctor's office visits, in health department settings, and other community health and education programs.

Crucial to the work that dieticians do in improving nutrition in the elderly is the personal interview. Vital information about the patient's health history and socioeconomic background is gathered during this conversation. If the patient is not in a position to discuss this information directly with the dietician, then communication with the medical team might assist the RD in developing a nutrition care plan.

Dieticians also come in contact with the elderly in community health education settings. These might include informal workshops where the RD gives advice for preparing meals for one, shopping and meal planning on a limited income, and how to meet the changing nutrition needs that accompany aging.

For more information, contact the American Dietetic Association (ADA), 216 West Jackson Boulevard, Chicago, IL 60606, (312) 899-0040.

EMERGENCY MEDICAL SERVICES   *Liz Delano*

A major problem in the United States is the sudden loss of life and disability that occurs with severe accidents and illnesses. The field of **emergency medical services (EMS)** responds to these events with a variety of trained personnel including basic **emergency medical technicians (EMTs)**, intermediates, and paramedics. They perform patient assessment, provide basic and advanced life support, and complete needed interventions prior to arriving at the hospital. Patients of all ages and with various medical problems are treated, but some types of people need more specialized care. One of these types is the geriatric patient.

As in any area of geriatrics, preconceived notions or ideas about aging and what the older population is like can alter the way a person is treated. In the field of EMS the attitude of the caregiver can literally make the difference between life and death for a sick or injured older person.

All of us like to believe that we have no biases or prejudices about the elderly, but in fact most of us do. Some of these views may seem benign, but if EMS providers believe that all old people eventually get senile, they could miss a serious illness that presents itself with altered mental status as its only sign. EMS personnel may be the only people to see the patient in his or her own environment, and those observations can be extremely important in the final medical evaluation. EMS providers need to become aware of their own feelings before evaluating patients. They need to base their evaluations on objective, valid, and reliable assessments and a working knowledge of emergency medicine.

As mentioned previously, EMS providers may be the first or only people to enter the patient's home. As they enter the home, what they observe helps with their patient assessment. They note whether or not the house is being maintained. Are all the windows intact or are some broken? Are there light bulbs in all the sockets and do they work? Is the walkway shoveled or the lawn mowed? Are there old papers piled up on the porch or mail in the box? Answers to these questions help determine whether there is a reduced ability of the patient to ambulate well or move around.

When EMS providers are in the house they pay attention to the temperature. Even if the room is warm enough for younger people, it still may be too cool for the patient. Hypothermia for the general population is usually the result of acute exposure to cold temperatures, but in the elderly, chronic exposure to even mildly cooler temperatures can lead to serious medical problems.

EMS providers often look in the cupboards or the refrigerator for medications. This is a good opportunity for them to determine whether nutritional needs are being met by quickly checking to see what food is available. Is there a variety of fresh foods, or does the food appear to be old or moldy? Nutritional problems in the elderly can be a cause of certain medical problems and can contribute to others (see Chapter 5).

Another important factor noted by EMS providers is whether or not the patient is still active and socializing. Clinical depression is often missed in this age group (see Chapter 4). Neighbors or family may report that the patient's lifestyle has changed recently or that he or she no longer goes out. A physical problem could have limited his or her activity level, leading to isolation, loneliness, or a feeling of helplessness.

Unfortunately geriatric abuse is on the rise in this country, and once again the EMS provider may be the first person in the house who is able to see the signs of abuse. The provider can look for obvious as well as subtle indications of abuse. Some of the less obvious signs might include inadequate clothing, broken eyeglasses or medical devices that do not work, numerous bruises, untreated cuts or injuries, or signs that medications are being administered incorrectly or being withheld. Not having a family physician or giving a medical history inconsistent with observed injuries are also potential signs of abuse or neglect.

Those in the field of EMS are taught to rely on the patient's pain response when performing the assessment. However, some older patients have a diminished pain response secondary to a variety of physiological changes. As a result, it is easy to miss a serious injury because the patient does not complain of pain. Therefore, the EMS provider would also consider the mechanism of injury or the nature of the illness. When evaluating vital signs, the EMS provider tries to consider what is normal for a particular patient, not only the average ranges used in traditional medicine.

Documentation of any medical or social problems should be included on the ambulance run report. While important for any patient, this may be even more critical for the geriatric patient to attain the appropriate follow-up care.

EMS providers are trained to provide emergency medical care in a wide variety of settings. They need to be kind, objective, and extremely observant. The EMS professional helps the patient relax, while at the same time providing immediate medical care and noting important environmental and physical conditions. EMS providers are trained to provide emergency medical care in a wide variety of settings. EMS professionals are an extremely important link in the health care system, especially for the elderly. For more information contact your local EMS office.

⬚ GERONTOLOGICAL NURSING *Nancy Smith*

The health care system is in a state of continuous change. These changes have had an impact on all aspects of health care delivery, including nursing, which has evolved into a respected profession in the last few decades. Not only do nurses provide direct patient care, but they also plan and manage care for individuals, families, and communities. Nurse practice acts have defined nursing in terms of diagnosing and treating human responses to actual or potential health care problems. This framework has necessitated that nurses possess greater knowledge and technical skills than ever before when caring for patients.

Gerontological nursing practice reflects these changes in health care and in nursing. The most significant demographic impact on health care has been the aging society. Although nurses have always cared for the elderly, gerontological nursing practice has only recently developed into a respected specialty. The American Nurses Association (ANA) created Standards of Practice for Gerontological Nursing in 1976. A major revision of the scope and standards of gerontological nursing practice occurred in 1994. This document provides a framework for nurses involved in the care of the elderly. Box 10–1 provides a brief description of basic gerontological nursing practice.

There are few health care settings that do not include elders. Generally speaking, most health care settings also include nurses working in various capacities. Nurses are involved in direct elder care in hospitals, long-term

---

BOX 10–1. BASIC GERONTOLOGICAL NURSING PRACTICE

The responsibilities of the gerontological nurse include direct care, management, and development of professional and other nursing personnel and evaluation of care and services for aging persons. All professional nurses practicing gerontological nursing have the basic knowledge and skills to do the following:

1. Use the nursing process to develop the aging person's care plan.
2. Establish a therapeutic relationship with the aging person and family to facilitate their cooperation in developing the care plan.
3. Recognize age-related changes based on an understanding of physiological, emotional, cultural, social, psychological, economic, and spiritual functioning.
4. Collect data to determine health status and functional abilities in order to plan, implement, and evaluate care.
5. Participate as a member of the interdisciplinary team.
6. Participate with aging persons, families, and other health professionals in ethical decision making that is client-centered, empathetic, and humane.
7. Serve as an advocate for aging persons and their families.
8. Teach aging persons and families about measures that promote, maintain, and restore health to promote comfort.
9. Refer the aging person to other professionals or community resources for assistance as necessary.
10. Apply the existing body of knowledge in gerontology to nursing practice and interventions.
11. Exercise accountability to the aging person by protecting his or her rights and autonomy.
12. Engage in continuing professional development through participation in continuing education, involvement in state and national professional organizations, and certification.
13. Use the standards of gerontological nursing practice to increase the quality of care and quality of life of the aging person.

Source: Scope and Standards of Gerontological Nursing Practice. American Nurses Association, Washington, DC, 1994. Reprinted with permission.

care centers, and in home care. Nurses frequently work with elderly patients in respite programs, geropsychiatric programs, assisted living and congregate housing centers, and in adult day care programs. Many elders enjoy a high level of health, in part as a result of health promotion activities conducted by nurses and other health care professionals. Health protection behaviors are also taught, so that an older individual is able to direct his or her behaviors at decreasing the risk for a specific disease.[3] There is a greater incidence of acute and chronic physical and mental illnesses in the elderly population. This requires that nurses have a high level of knowledge and technical competence when caring for elderly patients. Nurses work closely with other health care professionals to provide appropriate and comprehensive care to geriatric patients.

Gerontological nurses are strong advocates for elders and recognize the unique needs of the elder population. A registered nurse who works daily with elderly people is recognized as an expert in this area of patient care. It is possible for registered nurses (RNs) to be certified as gerontological nurses through the ANA. In addition, master of science in nursing programs prepare nurses to be gerontological clinical nurse specialists or ANA certified gerontological nurse practitioners. Nurses also engage in research about the physical and psychosocial needs of the elderly. As Rempusheski[4] has written:

> Gerontological nursing encompasses the definitions of gerontology . . ., geriatrics . . ., geriatric nursing (care of an elder during wellness and illness, including promotion and maintenance of health, prevention of illness and disability, care of the ill leading to restoration, rehabilitation, or a peaceful death), and geriatric nursing research (systematic study of nursing action and theory in relation to elder care and responses by elders to care received). (p. 4)

Gerontological nursing has a challenging future. Community planning for care of elders will require multidisciplinary and interdisciplinary approaches. Nurses will continue to provide and plan for care, manage patient care, and engage in health promotion/health protection activities for the elderly. They will work with other health care professionals to meet the needs of the aging population.

For more information contact the American Nurses Association, 600 Maryland Avenue, S.W., Suite 100 West, Washington, DC 20024-2571, (202) 651-7000.

OCCUPATIONAL THERAPY   *Regula H. Robnett*

Occupational therapy (OT) is perhaps the least understood of the health professions. One hears the name "occupational therapist" and conjures up an image of someone who will help them to get a job. To many people the word *occupation* means simply "work." More than a few elderly people have stated to their occupational therapy practitioner that they did not need OT services because they were already retired. It takes a bit of explaining to convince the person that the OT view of occupation encompasses much more than a job.

Someone's occupation includes everything purposeful that he or she does during the course of a day or waking period. This includes work or learning activities, ADLs (e.g., bathing, dressing, grooming, and sexual expression), leisure pursuits, and instrumental activities of daily living (IADLs) (e.g., tasks such as home management, caring for others, and money management). Occupational therapy clinicians work with people of all ages to help them in gaining or regaining function in the activities that have importance to them. Occupational therapy is patient or client-centered in that the patient's goals must be considered and respected as part of the rehabilitation process. If the person is unable to express his or her goals, then the family or guardian is consulted to make sure the client's wishes are known.

As a member of the health care team, the occupational therapy practitioner works with elderly people primarily to restore function so that they can return to completing the tasks they were able to do prior to an injury or a decline. Full return to former level of functioning may not always be possible, but the goal is usually to come as close as possible, as well as to ensure safety.

Occupational therapy practitioners believe that engaging in purposeful activities is a worthwhile endeavor in helping to restore function. They are experts in task analysis, that is, they are able to break down almost any activity into its component parts in order to understand what skills a person needs in order to be successful at it. For example, even a seemingly simple task like putting on a shirt is quite complex when all the specific skills a person needs in order to be able to put it on correctly are considered. Adults usually complete dressing tasks without much conscious effort. However, to normally and easily complete the task of putting on a shirt, one needs adequate range of motion and strength of the shoulders, elbows, wrists, and fingers, sight, proprioception (body awareness), fine and gross motor coordination, and cognition (for sequencing, choosing the proper clothing, etc.).

Strokes (cerebrovascular accidents [CVAs]), and other ailments that become increasingly more common with age, tend to cause impairments in one or more of the individual skills older people need to complete their "occupations" successfully. The occupational therapist determines what the person's strengths and weaknesses are through an interview and evaluation process. Clinicians use the results of the evaluation as well as a variety of theories from both within and beyond the profession to guide their intervention. They use their expertise in order to help the person complete the tasks he or she needs and wants to be able to do.

Besides the therapeutic approach, which emphasizes prevention and protection (e.g., educating people about how to maintain or improve functioning or to protect themselves from potential harm), the occupational therapy practitioner basically uses two approaches:

- Remedial approach
- Adaptive approach[5]

The remedial approach in occupational therapy seeks to restore functioning by improving specific component skills such as strength, fine and gross motor coordination, range of motion, and cognitive skills such as attention span or ability to follow directions. Through involvement in pertinent activities, patients are able to practice and improve their functional level. This may involve the therapist grading (or changing) the task in various ways so that it is at a level that will foster success and improve the component skills described.

Rehabilitation following a stroke provides an example of this approach. If the person who has had a stroke has a weak right arm and is unable to feed himself or herself, the occupational therapy practitioner may help the person to use the arm more functionally by stimulating or facilitating the muscles, guiding the arm, reminding the person to use the hemiplegic arm, and encouraging and coaching him or her to practice feeding or to complete similar functional tasks. This approach works best when the person still has some use of the extremity. (One cannot remediate any portion of the body that has lost complete innervation from the brain.)

The adaptive approach involves the occupational therapist's adapting the task and/or environment in order to compensate for the loss of skills. Many OT practitioners pride themselves on their creativity in this area. What may seem to be an impossible task due to the level of impairment can at times be accomplished through the creative problem solving process involving the client as well as the clinician. The use of the adaptive approach is accomplished in four primary ways:

1. Teaching the person new compensatory skills that will still allow him or her to function as normally as possible (e.g., learning to eat and write with the left hand if right-handed, or learning to type if writing is no longer possible).
2. Changing the task to make it easier (e.g., learning a new way to dress using only one arm). In the case of dressing mentioned earlier, the patient may find it easier to get dressed if the clothing used is simpler (e.g., a sweat suit instead of a three-piece suit).
3. Using adaptive technology to help the person be more functional (e.g., for someone unable to reach their feet, learning to put on socks with a special device called a sock aid). Many gadgets are available that can be useful in assisting people to be able to complete nearly all activities—from assembling a kit to zipping a coat. Occupational therapy practitioners are often skilled at finding or designing helpful, low-cost adaptive equipment.
4. Adapting the environment to make it safer or more accommodating for the person (e.g., environmental adaptations to make buildings more accessible for people with disabilities). This approach of milieu enhancement can also be helpful for those with dementia or psychiatric illnesses.

Occupational therapy is a holistic profession, seeking to help the person, not only physically, but cognitively and emotionally as well. Occupational therapy practitioners may obtain degrees at the associate level (certified occupational therapy assistants [COTAs]) or at the bachelor's or master's level occupational therapist, registered (OTRs). They are regulated in every state (through licensure, certification, or trademark laws) and are required to take a national certification examination before practicing. Occupational therapists with enough experience and knowledge can take an examination to obtain specialty certification as experts in pediatrics and neurorehabilitation through the American Occupational Therapy Association, Inc. (AOTA). A specialty certification in geriatrics may be available soon. Common sites for occupational therapy practitioners working with the elderly include long-term care facilities, acute care and rehabilitation hospitals, home health care agencies, and assisted living centers.

For more information, the interested reader should contact the American Occupational Therapy Association, Inc., 4720 Montgomery Lane, Bethesda, MD 20814, (301) 652-AOTA.

PHYSICAL THERAPY *Joyce L. MacKinnon*

Physical therapists (PTs) are health care professionals who are educated at either the baccalaureate or master's degree level and who have completed a course of study from a program approved by the Commission on Accreditation in Physical Therapy Education (CAPTE). They have passed a national examination and are licensed by the state in which they practice. They are supported by physical therapist assistants (PTAs) who have been educated at CAPTE-approved, 2-year college level programs. Physical therapist assistants have passed a national examination and are licensed in the states that require licensure. Physical therapy aides are people who are trained on the job to perform tasks under the direction and supervision of physical therapists and assistants.

The Board of Directors of the American Physical Therapy Association (APTA) developed a definition of **physical therapy** (**PT**) that has been accepted by APTA members. Physical therapy occurs either by, or under the direction of, a physical therapist. It includes "examining patients with impairments, functional limitations, and disability or other health-related conditions in order to determine a diagnosis, prognosis, and intervention."[6] Physical therapists and assistants alleviate these impairments and functional limitations through a variety of methods, and prevent them from occurring in the first place through health promotion activities. Physical therapists also engage in consultation, education, and research.

Many physical therapists, assistants, and aides work with older adults. Those physical therapists whose skills and expertise with this population have been recognized through a rigorous testing and review process are credentialed as certified clinical specialists in geriatrics. However, whatever the background and credentials of those physical therapists who work with older adults, the focus of prevention, evaluation, and treatment is always on function. Interestingly, many of the physiological changes that are observed in older adults parallel those observed in younger, sedentary adults. Through research studies and clinical observations, it appears as though many of these changes can be slowed through the use of exercise. Not only does exercise have a favorable impact on bones, muscles, ligaments, lungs, and the heart, but it can also influence sleep patterns and moods.

In reviewing biological, physiological, and anatomical changes that accompany aging, there are some aspects of the aging process that physical therapists can positively affect, and others that therapists must merely recognize as having an impact on treatment outcomes. For instance, aging is usually accompanied by an increased density and thickening of collagen fibers. In some cases, elastin fibers are replaced with collagen. What this means to physical therapists is that they must realize that tissue is becoming less elastic and flexible. Therefore, an older adult may not be able to achieve as much flexibility as a younger adult. However, it must also be kept in mind that changes related to aging occur at different rates among individuals and even among systems within the same individual. Conversely, although muscle strength does decrease with age, people can be placed on exercise programs to include weight training that will slow down the rate of decline. The older adult usually needs to start out with lower weights and few repetitions and will progress to increased weight and repetitions more slowly than a younger adult. Besides muscle strength, body composition (the ratio of lean muscle tissue to fat concentration), cardiopulmonary function, and endurance can be positively affected with exercise.

One disease process that is receiving increased attention is osteoporosis. Physical therapists can work with other members of the health care team to prevent or retard osteoporosis by prescribing an exercise program of weight-bearing and resistive exercises, postural training and back extension exercises, and flexibility activities. They can also treat patients who develop this condition by providing pain relief, general conditioning activities, back extension and abdominal strengthening exercises, and a complete graded exercise program. Therapists can work with other health care professionals to address psychosocial components of the condition as well, alleviating unwarranted fears of movement or diminution of social roles.

Physical therapists can have an impact on the aging process at three distinct levels:

1. They can focus on health promotion and disease prevention activities, such as encouraging older adults to remain current for immunizations or receive vaccinations for diseases such as influenza. They can encourage older adults to avoid injurious behaviors such as excessive smoking and alcohol consumption, maintain good nutritional habits, maintain and improve fitness levels, and reduce stress.

2. Therapists can focus on secondary prevention measurements such as encouraging older adults to get mammogram, bone density, and blood pressure screenings and have cholesterol levels checked.
3. Finally, therapists can urge older adults to engage in health protective behaviors, such as wearing seat belts, having smoke detectors installed in the home, and having adequate lighting and guard rails when necessary.

Since the focus of disease prevention or rehabilitation after accident or illness is on function, the physical therapy assessment of an older adult is based on a functional assessment. The therapists may take discrete measures of muscle strength, joint range of motion, and cardiopulmonary function but will be more interested in how these measures translate into functional activity. For instance, does the patient have enough strength, motion, and endurance to bathe and dress himself? Can he or she perform light housekeeping tasks and go up and down stairs? Can the patient get out of the house, go to the bus stop, get on the bus, go to the grocery store, shop, and return home?

Physical therapists have much to offer older adults to assist them in maintaining their independence and function. Physical therapists work with older adults in a variety of settings, from acute care hospital to rehabilitation center to home. They use skills and techniques to increase functional abilities modifying these skills to address the sequelae of usual aging. They interact with other health care professionals and with the patient's family to develop and meet patient-centered goals so as to encourage optimum patient functioning.

For more information contact the American Physical Therapy Association, 1111 N. Fairfax Street, Alexandria, VA 22314, 1-800-999-2782.

☒ **RADIOGRAPHY** *Sally Doe*

Radiologic technology (RT) is the health profession that involves imaging various anatomical regions of the body for diagnostic purposes, generally utilizing radiation (x-rays) as the source of energy. Radiographers must use a variety of equipment and imaging systems depending on the complexity of the anatomical region or organs. Radiographic procedures vary from those that are relatively commonplace, such as radiographs of the chests or extremities, to those that are very sophisticated technologically, such as angiography. Diagnosis through a radiographic procedure is often one of the first areas of investigation on the patient's behalf. Consequently, radiographers often see very ill and traumatized patients as well as perform radiographs during surgery. Radiographers must, therefore, be able to adapt procedural standards and equipment limitations to the needs of a patient.

In addition to possessing excellent patient care skills and having empathy and compassion for patients, radiographers must consider several important aspects for the geriatric patient. X-ray tables are, by necessity, hard, and some radiographic procedures require the patient to remain lying on the table for perhaps as long as 1 hour. Radiographers make use of special cushioning devices designed for the x-ray table to minimize patient discomfort and must pay particular attention to the physical warmth of the patient during his or her time of relative immobilization. Excellent communication skills are of particular importance in terms of explaining not only the procedure completely to the patient but also in giving clear and concise instructions to enlist the patient's cooperation.

Other imaging modalities closely aligned with radiography include computed tomography (CT scanning), magnetic resonance imaging (MRI), sonography (formerly ultrasound), and nuclear medicine. Computed tomography and nuclear medicine utilize radiation as the source of energy for imaging; while magnetic resonance imaging utilizes a very strong magnetic field, and sonography utilizes sound waves. Regardless of the type of energy used, imaging requires specific orientation of the part being examined to the image receptor and requires some period of immobilization for the patient. Consequently, radiographers are ever mindful of the patient's condition and comfort.

Radiographers may obtain degrees at the associate, bachelor's, or master's level. They are licensed in the majority of states. The American Registry of Radiologic Technologists offers a national certification examination to those who have the educational qualifications. Employment sites include hospitals, outpatient facilities, physicians' offices, and home health care agencies.

For more information contact the American Society of Radiologic Technologists, 15000 Central Avenue, S.E., Albuquerque, NM 87123, (505) 298-4500.

⬚ RESPIRATORY CARE *Walter Chop*

Respiratory care practitioners (RCPs) work with patients of all ages; however, it is the elderly who occupy the majority of their time. The need for RCPs will continue to rise with the concurrent increase in this segment of the population.

One of the most common symptoms associated with cardiopulmonary disease is dyspnea (difficulty breathing). An estimated 45 percent of those older than the age of 70 exhibit dyspnea on exertion, while 65 percent of men and 48 percent of women in this age bracket have a cardiopulmonary disorder.[7] RCPs administer aerosolized medications to relieve symptoms of cardiopulmonary disease. They also monitor life support systems in intensive care units and function as vital members of the hospital cardiac arrest team. In addition to this, they perform diagnostic pulmonary function testing and arterial blood gas measurements. They also assist physicians during bronchoscopic examination to the lungs. Chest physiotherapy, breathing retraining, and patient education are also an integral part of an RCP's duties.

Although healthy older individuals can usually compensate for age-related changes to the pulmonary system, they do, however, remain vulnerable to environmental insults such as air pollution and second-hand smoke. Elderly persons are also at increased risk of developing pneumonia, especially if they are residents of long-term care facilities. RCPs are in the "front line" treating these conditions with medication, chest physiotherapy, oxygen, and, if need be, mechanical ventilation.

As the trend to discharge patients from acute care facilities as quickly as possible continues, both long-term care and home care will experience continued growth. RCPs work in both these settings providing and monitoring oxygen delivery and life support systems. Assessment and evaluation for the patient from a cardiopulmonary perspective is also performed by respiratory therapists. This information is then relayed to the physician.

RCPs are required to become licensed in all but a few states. This helps ensure patient protection as well as establishment of standards for the safe practice of respiratory care. For more information on a career in respiratory care, contact the respiratory care department in your local hospital, career counselors at a school or college in your area, or the American Association for Respiratory Care, 11030 Ables Lane, Dallas, TX, 75229, (972) 243-2272.

SOCIAL WORK *Betsey Gray*

In response to society's increasing awareness of our older population as a heterogeneous group with special and diverse needs, social work practice with the elderly is emerging as a new and valuable specialty within the profession.

The National Association of Social Workers[8] defines **social work** as "the professional activity of helping individuals, groups or communities enhance or restore their capacity for social functioning and creating societal conditions favorable to this goal."

Social workers are particularly sensitive to the social, cultural, biological, and psychological factors that impact on a person's life. They perform many functions and are often asked to act as evaluators, facilitators, advocates, community organizers, and program planners. A code of ethics for the profession emphasizes the importance of treating people with dignity and respect. Social workers view themselves as agents of change and are seen as a voice of the oppressed in our society.

Those social workers with an interest and expertise in working with the elderly are becoming more common in settings that provide services to this age group, including hospitals, mental health centers, residential settings, home health care agencies, and community programs. The following is a description of some of the responsibilities a social worker encounters in these settings.

The primary responsibility of a hospital or medical social worker is to work with the elderly patient in determining a plan following discharge from the hospital. This involves doing a thorough assessment of the needs of the patient, speaking with family members, and locating resources in the community. The social worker collaborates with the other professionals involved in the patient's care and at times acts as an advocate in ensuring that the patient's wishes are followed. It is important for the social worker to be familiar with community resources as well as federal and state programs that may be available to the elderly person.

Mental health centers are now developing specialized units for treating older people with mental health issues. Depression resulting from loss and isolation, dementia, substance abuse, and elder abuse are some of the problems that a social worker might encounter in an elderly person seeking services. The social worker trained in working with the elderly begins with a comprehensive biopsychosocial assessment, being sensitive to all factors that may be contributing to the problem. He or she is particularly attentive to the supports that the person has and areas where these may be able to be increased. A treatment plan, which often involves other professional services and resources in the community, is then developed by the social worker in collaboration with the elderly person. The social worker can act as the case manager in accessing these resources and monitoring the delivery of services and can also provide individual, group, and family counseling, if appropriate. Integral to all the work that the social worker does is the importance of treating the elderly patient with respect and dignity and acknowledging his or her right to self-determination.

For elderly people in residential settings such as a nursing home or assisted living facility, the social worker plays a key role. Most often the social worker is the first person to meet with residents and their family members, explain the procedure for admission, and answer questions about Medicare and Medicaid. At intake time, the social worker is a member of the team that does the initial assessment. Being cognizant of the losses people experience when leaving their homes, the social worker offers support and empathy as a way of helping them adjust to their new surroundings.

Residential settings vary in the social work services offered to their residents. Many are beginning to see the need for supportive services and will ask the social worker to facilitate groups for the residents. Individual counseling can also be offered to a resident when needed. In addition, groups to aid family members may be provided for the resident's family. Lastly, social workers lead in-service training for staff on various subjects relative to the work they do.

With the emergence of managed care, people are being discharged from hospitals much sooner and often return to their homes with a need for ongoing services. Through a team approach, the home health care agency provides those medical and related health care interventions that will allow the elderly persons to remain at home for as long as possible. Social workers are a fairly recent addition to the service providers available through home health care agencies. When it is determined by a member of the team that social work services are needed by the patient or family, a social worker will make a home visit and do a psychosocial assessment. The social worker will meet with family members as well as the patient and together work out a plan to address the problems presented. Typical problems may include financial issues, adjustment to a terminal or other severe illness, living arrangements, and family relationships. As in other settings, the social worker needs to have a working knowledge of community resources and the way to access services.[9]

Social workers, because of their training, are often found helping communities and groups develop new programs to assist the elderly. The National Association of Social Workers is very involved in the legislative process on the state and national level. All social workers are encouraged to be politically active so as to have a strong voice in decisions that are being made that affect the people they are serving. As our population continues to age and legislation focuses on the elderly population, the voice of the social worker will be heard on many different levels in our society.

For more information contact the National Association of Social Workers, 750 First Street, NE, Suite 700, Washington, DC 20002-4241, 1-800-742-4089, e-mail: info@naswdc.org.

▨ SPEECH-LANGUAGE PATHOLOGIST
Susan Claybrook

A **speech-language pathologist (SLP)** is a professional who provides evaluation and intervention to persons with speech, language, voice, fluency, cognition, hearing, and swallowing (dysphagia) deficits. SLPs may work with the elderly in a number of settings, including nursing homes, hospitals, acute inpatient and outpatient rehabilitation centers, and home care (in patients' homes).

The role of the SLP is to provide a thorough evaluation in order to determine the strengths and weaknesses of the patient. To get started with this process, the therapist reviews available documentation that was written by any medical or therapeutic staff members who have worked with the patient. The SLP also interviews family members for their perceptions on the abilities of the patient.

It is the SLP's responsibility to rehabilitate patients to their previous level of functioning, or as close to it as possible, so that they may return to or remain at home. The goal is for patients to become as functional in society as they were prior to the disability. However, as a result of their diagnosis, there are persons who continue to decline over time. In this instance, it is the SLP's job to determine the skills they have remaining and build on those, so that they can continue to do as much for themselves as possible. This is known as functional maintenance and is often the purpose of treatment in a long-term care setting. The SLP also provides inservice and hands-on training on topics and techniques that will allow staff, family, care givers, and the patients themselves to best communicate with one another.

AREAS ADDRESSED BY THE SPEECH-LANGUAGE PATHOLOGIST

- **Speech:** Slurring, articulation, apraxia, inability to speak, rapid rate of speech, unintelligibility, dysarthria
- **Voice:** Whispering, loudness, hoarseness, fading of voice, loss of voice, gurgliness
- **Fluency:** Stuttering
- **Cognition:** Verbal memory, verbal orientation and sequencing, verbal reasoning and problem solving, math, spelling, oral reading, word recall, telling time, processing information, attention skills
- **Language:** Ability to communicate all wants and needs, comprehension, nonverbal or body language, vocabulary, sentence structure, turn taking, following directions, inappropriate language
- **Hearing:** Hearing screenings, aural rehabilitation, assisting with maintaining functional hearing aids (cleaning ear molds, checking batteries, determining whether aids are being put on and removed properly)
- **Dysphagia:** Difficulty swallowing (liquids, solids, pills, etc.), drooling, weight loss, trouble chewing and clearing mouth, pocketing food, choking, spitting out food, refusal to eat, poor safety while eating, hiccuping or burping after meals, removal of feeding tubes, establishing safe liquid and solids intake, determining safe food and liquid consistency levels, teaching caregivers and/or staff to apply adhesive and insertion and removal and care of dentures, doing bedside swallow evaluations and modified barium swallows

The SLP works as a member of a health care team to enhance the quality of life for each patient. The interested reader can obtain more information about speech-language pathology by contacting the American Speech, Language and Hearing Association, 10801 Rockville Pike, Rockville, MD 20852, (301) 897-5700.

THERAPEUTIC RECREATION *Nancy Richeson*

The fastest growing segment of the American population is the age group older than 65 years old. Currently, there are more than 25 million people older than 65, and as the baby boom generation matures, it is projected to grow to more than 65 million, encompassing more than 29 percent of the population.[10] As Americans age, their health care needs will also increase, and this will prove to be challenging for our society. The long-term health care needs of this group are estimated to double by the year 2030. One consequence of societal aging is that the demand for services that help to maintain and/or improve the health of seniors will continue to grow.[11]

According to Teaque and MacNeil,[12] one form of health service that has increasingly received attention for its preventive as well as therapeutic qualities is therapeutic recreation services. Therapeutic recreation programs at facilities should be among the most important factors evaluated by consumers before selecting a long-term care facility. The Omnibus Budget Reconciliation Act (OBRA)[13] of 1987 sets forth standards for long-term care facilities (see also Chapter 8). Included in the law is the following provision:

> The skilled nursing facility . . . must provide . . . an ongoing program, directed by a qualified professional, of activities designed to meet the interests and the physical, mental, and psychosocial well-being of each resident.

Currently only 5 percent of the U.S. population age 65 and older live in long-term care facilities. This represents less than 2 million people. However, as more people live longer, the percentage of elderly people in long-term care is expected to rise to more than 20 percent. By 2040, 5.5 million people are likely to live in long-term care facilities.[14] Quality therapeutic recreation services are a necessity in long-term care.

The literature in therapeutic recreation describes the therapeutic approach as one that is intended to stimulate a change in behavior directed by one or more goals in different areas of functioning (e.g., physical, emotional, mental, social).[10] Therapeutic recreation specialists in long-term care use activities to

- Promote health
- Prevent impairment and dependence
- Maintain optimal functional capabilities
- Remediate disabilities

As stated by the American Therapeutic Recreation Association (ATRA), **therapeutic recreation specialists (TRSs)** are those professionals who have completed a degree in therapeutic recreation (or recreation with an emphasis in therapeutic recreation). National certification is available through the National Council for Therapeutic Recreation Certification (NCTRC). A few states regulate this profession through licensure, certification, or regulation of titles.

Therapeutic recreation specialists work as part of the initial health care team whose members gather pertinent information about a long-term care resident through the administration of a standardized assessment, also referred to as the minimum data set (MDS). A completed MDS on each resident is required for long-term care facilities that participate in Medicare and Medicaid programs. Therapeutic recreation specialists also collect information about leisure needs and interests from other sources such as medical records, medical staff, and family members. Based on the results of the assessments, the therapeutic recreation specialist writes an individual treatment plan. Activity programs are developed based on the residents' needs, abilities, and interests. Other documentation tasks the therapeutic recreation specialist must complete include writing progress notes, charting attendance records, developing a monthly calendar, and updating resident's records as required.[15]

The therapeutic recreation specialist is responsible for the development of a comprehensive therapeutic recreation program. Often therapeutic recreation programs are provided on a continuum, with diversional activities provided simply to fill time in the resident's day on one end to treatment-oriented activities focusing on maintaining or improving functional abilities on the other. A balanced program provides treatment, education, and diversional opportunities to meet the residents' individual needs as determined by the therapeutic recreation assessment.[15]

An example of a therapeutic recreation treatment intervention in a long-term care facility could be a sensory stimulation program designed to maintain or improve sensory function. This program could be administered on a one-to-one basis or in a small group with other residents who have similar needs. Other therapeutic recreation treatment interventions could include validation therapy, reminiscence/life review, animal facilitated therapy, community outings, therapeutic activities, leisure education, physical activity, social opportunities, one-to-one treatment, and adult education opportunities. Additional responsibilities of the therapeutic recreation personnel could include coordinating volunteers, determining staffing needs, developing an operating manual, evaluating the program, and monitoring quality improvement measures.

In conclusion, therapeutic recreation specialists are important members of the treatment team. Therapeutic recreation programs assist residents in increasing or maintaining their functional abilities and in developing their leisure skills. In addition, therapeutic recreation programs educate individuals about the value of leisure and provide recreational opportunities. The ultimate goal of any therapeutic recreation program, is to help restore the individual to optimal health and well being.

For further information on therapeutic recreation call either the American Therapeutic Recreation Association (ATRA) at (601) 264-3413, Internet address: http://www.atra-tr.org, or the National Therapeutic Recreation Society at (703) 858-2151, e-mail: NTRSNRPA@aol.com.

⬚ PEW HEALTH PROFESSIONS COMMISSION REPORT

The **Pew Health Professions Commission**[16] cites a rising geriatric population with increasingly unmet health care needs. This fact, the group states, strongly suggests the necessity for better educational preparation for those allied health professionals who are currently, or will be, serving older people. Lack of such preparation may only foster negative attitudes and stereotypes toward the aging population.

The allied health professions constitute more than 60 percent of the entire health care work force and represent more than 200 individual professions. For practical purposes, the allied health professions include all the diverse health professions requiring postsecondary education with the exception of nurses, physicians, and dentists. Data suggest that allied health education programs, especially at the associate degree level, pay scant attention to educating the student in the field of geriatrics. This is due in part to lack of geriatric education requirements for program accreditation.

As the impact of a rapidly aging society begins to make itself evident, allied health educational programs need to establish their objectives accordingly. These should include the acquisition of specific assessment, treatment, and evaluation skills relevant to the needs of elderly persons. Student level clinical involvement with older persons will be of the utmost importance in ensuring that these objectives are achieved. The American Society of Allied Health Professions (ASAHP), in a task force report on gerontology and pediatric care education, states the following in this regard:

> In general, an increasing percentage of clinical contact for allied health students will be with older patients. Similarly, more and more allied health professionals will carry patient loads predominantly or exclusively geriatric. In recognition of this, all allied health educational programs must provide comprehensive yet well-defined geriatric curricula and ample opportunity for high quality geriatric clinical experience.[17]

Also recommended by the task force is the need for more interdisciplinary education and practice. Collaboration among health care providers will be essential for providing high-quality, cost-effective care to older adults. Communication skills, team building, and concepts of coordinating care must be essential components of educational programs. Allied health students should have early clinical orientations to facilities that have interdisciplinary geriatric services.[18]

The gerontological portion of a model allied health curriculum should include the following content areas:

- Demographics of aging
- Biological, social, and psychological aspects of aging
- Pathological problems of elderly people
- Ageism and the stereotypes of aging
- Legal and ethical dimensions of treating the elderly
- Death and dying
- Public policy and models of health care delivery
- Health promotion and disease prevention for the elderly

- Health care team development
- Roles of other health professionals
- Planning and operations
- Patient advocacy
- Interpersonal management
- Research skill development[17]

Clinical training should take place in as wide a variety of settings as possible, including hospitals, long-term care facilities, rehabilitation centers, independent living centers, and home-based care agencies. Teaching skills will need to be emphasized and sharpened as allied health professionals will be expected to teach family members, other informal caregivers, and paraprofessionals techniques to help with patient care and intervention.

SUMMARY

The authors hope that this chapter has provided readers valuable information related to the original learning objectives. The reader should now have adequate knowledge about the various health care professionals who work with the elderly, or at least know where to seek this information in the future. Sources for additional details are usually included at the end of each segment and can be accessed as needed.

The various health care providers do have certain traits in common. All seek to promote caring and respect for the elderly (as well as all their other clients). All the professions described are founded on a solid knowledge base related to their specific scopes of practice, and most provide treatment in the context of a health care team. The team concept predominates in health care today as a way to ensure efficacy and cost-effectiveness in health care delivery. Perhaps the reader is now more convinced about the necessity of the team approach and may be more willing to join as a health care team player.

Finally, because of the probable impact that the current and future Pew Commission reports will have on both health care education and service provision, the authors believe it is essential for the students of various health care professions to be aware of this influential group and its various expert recommendations, all of which are aimed at improving health care in the United States.

REVIEW QUESTIONS

1. The Pew Commission:
    A. Regulates health care workers in long-term care.
    B. Advocates for better educational preparation for health care professionals working with the elderly.

C. Advises allied health professionals to do some of the work of physicians.

    D. Advocates for less clinical training and more classroom education for health care professionals.

2. A health care team in which broad patient goals are shared by members of the team is called a(n):

    A. Interdisciplinary team

    B. Transdisciplinary team

    C. Multidisciplinary team

    D. Medical care team

3. EMS professionals do all of the following EXCEPT:

    A. Plan for the person's discharge from the hospital.

    B. Enter a person's home to begin treatment.

    C. Take note of the patient's surroundings.

    D. Evaluate vital signs and provide emergency medical care.

4. Task analysis and the remedial and adaptive approaches are skills used by a(n):

    A. Gerontological nurse

    B. Nutritionist

    C. Radiologist

    D. Occupational therapist

5. One who minimizes patient discomfort during periods of immobilization for a medical test is titled a(n):

    A. Occupational therapist

    B. Radiologist

    C. Physical therapist

    D. Social worker

6. RCPs complete all of the following tasks EXCEPT:

    A. Mechanical ventilation

    B. Monitoring life support systems

    C. Range of motion exercises

    D. Pulmonary function testing

7. The professional most likely to have the primary role of determining the plan for a person being discharged from the hospital is a(n):

    A. Social worker

    B. EMS professional

    C. Therapeutic recreation specialist

    D. Radiologist

8. If you notice your patient is having difficulty swallowing and coughs after every sip of water, the most appropriate referral for a consultation may be to a:

    A. Social worker

    B. Physical therapist

C. Speech-language pathologist
D. Dietician

▓ LEARNING ACTIVITIES

These are appropriate for small group discussions.

1. Sam, an elderly man, has had a stroke (CVA) and has been admitted to a rehabilitation hospital. Who are likely to be members of his health care team and what roles are each of them likely to take?

2. How might the responsibilities of these team members change in the different kinds of health care teams: multidisciplinary, interdisciplinary, and trandisciplinary.

3. If you were going to start a commission with the purpose of improving health care specifically for the elderly, whom would you invite to be participants (individual people *or* representatives of certain professions)? What major issues will they need to confront? Would you personally want to be a member of this commission? Why or why not?

▓ REFERENCES

1. Pew Health Professions Commission: Third Report: Critical Challenges: Revitalizing the Health Professions for the 21st Century. University of California, San Francisco, December, 1995.
2. Case Management Society of America: Updated Brochure, distributed in 1997.
3. Stanley, M, and Beare, PG: Gerontological Nursing. FA Davis, Philadelphia, 1998.
4. Rempusheski, VF: Historical and futuristic perspectives in aging and the gerontological nurse. In Baines, EM (ed): Perspectives on Gerontological Nursing. Sage Publications, Newbury Park, CA, 1991.
5. Zoltan, B: Vision, Perception and Cognition, ed 3. Slack, Thorofare, NJ, 1996.
6. A Guide to Physical Therapy Practice, Vol 1. Phys Ther. 75:707–764, 1995.
7. Matteson, MA, and McConnell, E: Gerontological Nursing: Concepts and Practice. WB Saunders, Philadelphia, 1988.
8. Barker, RL: The Social Work Dictionary, ed 3. National Association of Social Workers Press, Washington, DC, 1995.
9. Hancock, BL: Social Work with Older People. Prentice-Hall, Englewood Cliffs, NJ, 1990.
10. Hawkins, B: Therapeutic Activity Intervention with the Elderly: Foundations and Practices. Venture Publishing, State College, PA, 1996.
11. Ernts, N, and Glazer-Walsman, H: The Aged Patient: A Source Book for the Allied Health Professional. Year Book Medical Publisher, Chicago, 1983.
12. Teaque, M, and MacNeil, R: Aging and Leisure: Vitality in Later Life, ed 2. Brown and Benchmark, Madison, WI, 1992.
13. Omnibus Budget Reconciliation Act (OBRA), PL 100-203, Section 4201, Sec. 1819 (b).4. A.v., 1987.
14. Cornman, J, and Kingson, ER: Trends, issues, perspectives, and values for the aging of the baby boom cohorts. The Gerontologist 36(1):18, 1996.

15. Elliott, J, and Sorg-Elliott, JA: Recreation Programming and Activities. Venture Publishing, State College, PA, 1991.

16. Health Professions Education for the Future: Schools in Service to the Nation. The Pew Health Professions Commission, San Francisco, CA, 1993.

17. An aging society: Implications for health care needs impacts on allied health practice and education. A report of the National Task Force on Gerontology and Geriatric Care Education in Allied Health. J Allied Health 16(4): November, 1987.

18. A National Agenda for Geriatric Education: White Papers. U.S. Department of Health and Human Services Public Health Service, Washington, DC, September, 1995.

Anyone who gives you firm
prognostications about what is going to
happen is either a liar or a fool, because
the uncertainties over trends
in life expectancy, health and disability,
and retirement age are quite high.[1]
Richard Suzman
Director of the National Institute on
Aging's Office of Demography on Aging

Future Concerns in an Aging Society

Paul D. Ewald

BEHAVIORAL OBJECTIVES

Upon completion of this chapter, the reader will be able to:

1. Identify three critical age-related issues facing the United States in the future.
2. Describe ways in which the future generations of elderly are different from the elderly of today.
3. Understand and describe the respective roles of the family, the public sector, and the private sector in caring for the frail elderly.
4. Understand that populations around the world are aging at different rates and be able to explain some of the reasons for this and consequences of it.
5. Explain how societal responses to aging vary around the world because of differing rates of change as well as different social, political, and economic policies.

KEY TERMS

Age composition
Demographics
Fertility
Generational equity
Lifelong education
Migration
Mortality

Old-age dependency ratio
Public sector/private sector
Volunteerism
Work life
Young-age dependency ratio

ON THE NATURE OF MAKING PREDICTIONS

The aging of the U.S. population is not unlike a good news–bad news story. The good news is that more of us are living longer, often in better health, more independently, and with greater security. The bad news is that these advances carry considerable economic and social costs. The good news is that many of us have been, and will continue to be, the beneficiaries of technological and biomedical advances. The bad news is that we will be faced with increasingly difficult resource choices, ethical dilemmas, and political decisions. The good news is that there will be more opportunities for growth and personal enhancement in later life. The bad news is that there may likely be more years of dependency in later life.

Whether we attend to the good news or the bad news side of the story depends in large part on the social perceptions and attitudes we hold of old age, both individually and as a society. Do we think of it as a time of leisure, relaxation, reflection, and happiness? Or is it a time of greater dependency, illness, and loss? One can see elements of truth in both of these characterizations. Most of us hold dual stereotypes about the nature of old age because we can usually find validation for both the good and the bad in our day-to-day experiences: recalling our vibrant and wise grandparents one day; paying a visit to a nursing home the next.

As we come to terms with the realities of a society in which the number of elderly members is increasing steadily, our perceptions and attitudes will undergo rapid change as well. Attitudes and perceptions, however, will not likely converge into a single way of understanding our elders. From the inception of gerontology as a field of study, researchers and observers have emphasized the diversity within the elderly population and the difficulty in drawing generalizations and conclusions. As the elderly population increases, it also is becoming more diverse, with multiple sources of variation.

Gerontologists have always been future-oriented. The engine that drives the enormous expansion of interest in the phenomenon of aging is a demographic engine. Demographers have relentlessly drawn the attention of researchers, health care providers, and policy makers to the facts of a graying population. The basic facts are undisputed. The exact rates of growth and the consequences of this growth, however, are more speculative, and in some circles, hotly debated.

Demographers lay out their predictions of population growth and change on the basis of different assumptions. These assumptions most often concern fertility rates (adding new people into the population), mortality rates (subtracting people from the population), and migration (the addition and subtraction of people from the population). By examining trends over time, predictions about future growth and change can be made with a certain degree of confidence. But because future rates can never be known with absolute certainty, demographers develop multiple series of projections based on assumptions of different rates. Which series to accept, of course, becomes critically important when faced with questions of health care planning or economic policy development. Beyond predicting basic rates of **fertility, mortality,** and **migration,** other factors quickly enter into discussions of the future of an aging population.

- Will health care costs continue to escalate at the present rates?
- How will family structures change as a result of divorce, separation, and an increasing number of never married?
- How secure is the Social Security system?
- Will older adults continue to retire at relatively early ages?

- Will Americans' savings rates improve?
- Will the U.S. economy continue to expand?
- Will young adult and middle-aged women continue to enter the full-time work force at current rates?
- How will the demand for other federal expenditures change over the next 50 years?

The answers to these questions are often a great deal more speculative than fertility and mortality statistics, and yet, each will have a profound effect on the quality of the lives of elder Americans in the next century—and consequently, the quality of American life. Thus, the task of prediction becomes precarious, and the careers of predictors often short. The seriousness of the concerns identified in this chapter rests on assumptions and, to a degree, on speculation. They will change as answers to some of the questions just posed change or become known. They are based on (usually conservative) demographic predictions, and should be thought of in an if/then sense. *If* things develop as we suspect they will, *then* it is likely that . . . etc. Readers are encouraged to consider the issues identified in this chapter critically and with skepticism. Consider how the concerns may or may not materialize depending on how we come to view our elders; on how future generations of Americans come to understand issues of obligation, dependency, and entitlement; on how we behave toward different age groups; and on how we vote and behave politically. Shifts in our collective behavior will assuredly influence these concerns for better or for worse.

From among the many concerns in a rapidly aging population, this chapter focuses on three main categories of issues. First, some differences between today's elderly and the elderly of the future are identified. It is this future population with which we are mostly concerned, and they are unlike their predecessors in several important respects. Second, concerns over generational equity and distribution of resources have been raised since the 1980s and are likely to become more pressing as the expected population trends unfold. Third are concerns around how the burden of economic support, and social and medical care, will be distributed. This last concern is discussed from the perspectives of several different nations.

Populations around the world are aging at different rates, allowing us to look at different levels of societal response to the problems and challenges of aging. It will become clear that these are all very complex issues and the answers to many questions are not known. In many cases the scope and dimensions of the problems and challenges are only partially understood. The goal in this chapter is to identify several of the major issues that have received the attention of planners, researchers, and the public and try to provide some context for understanding and thinking about these issues. First, demographic shifts most important to an understanding of these concerns are reviewed.

🔳 SIGNIFICANT DEMOGRAPHIC SHIFTS

Today there are about 31 million Americans older than the age of 65, and they constitute approximately 12.7 percent of the population. By the year 2030, this group will make up between 21 and 24 percent of the population, or approximately 60 million people. Within this age group, the portion that is older than age 85 numbers approximately 3 million, or 1.3 percent of the total population. This age group (those older than 85) is growing at a rate two to three times faster than the rest of the U.S. population and is conservatively expected to number approximately 6.3 million people by the year 2030.[2] Much of our interest in, and concern over, our aging society is with the group that is older than 85, whose growth is outpacing all others. This is a heterogeneous and complex age group to study. They are often characterized as the frail elderly. Indeed, the likelihood of hospitalization or nursing home placement rises considerably with advanced age. Dementias and the cognitive impairments that many of us have come to associate with advanced age do in fact increase dramatically in rate among surviving elderly. Mobility is reduced; chronic conditions multiply; impoverishment and social isolation are greater risks. There is reason for concern as we see the unprecedented expansion of this age group. And yet, there is evidence to suggest that for a substantial proportion of those who survive into their 80s, there is a sort of mortality grace period that is marked by vitality and relatively good health.[3] And as suggested in the following section, today's population of individuals older than 85 may not be the best guide to understanding the future elderly.

Readers should also be cautioned from generalizing circumstances in the United States to other parts of the world. Societies throughout the world are aging at different rates as a result of different degrees of modernization, industrialization, and economic development. In general terms, developed nations have older populations. The countries of the developing world currently have relatively young populations, but over the next half century they will be experiencing population aging at a rate unprecedented in the developed nations. Countries like the United States have had the luxury, so to speak, of slower and steadier rates of aging throughout the 20th century and with considerable foreknowledge. The dual challenges of poorer countries will be to deal with the pace of aging and, concomitantly, the problems associated with economic development.

Another statistic of interest to demographers and gerontologists is referred to as the dependency ratio. This ratio refers to those people in the population who are usually thought of as economically dependent to those who are economically productive, and can be calculated and considered several different ways. **The old-age dependency ratio** looks at the number of people in the population older than 65 as compared with the number between the ages of

18 and 64. Although all of those older than 65 are not necessarily retired or nonworking, and all of those between 18 and 64 are not necessarily working and economically productive, this ratio serves as a general indicator of the economic burden confronting the working segment of the population at any given time. The old-age dependency ratio has increased throughout this century and will continue to increase gradually until about 2020. After this date, not long after the time that the baby boom generation begins to retire, the ratio begins to increase dramatically. Today, in crude terms, 100 workers support approximately 21 or 22 elderly. In 2020, 100 workers will be supporting about 27 or 28 elderly and thus will carry a greater burden economically.[4]

Another type of dependency ratio is the **young-age dependency ratio,** or the ratio of those younger than age 18 to those between 18 and 64. Between 1970 and 1990, this ratio declined dramatically from about 61 young people to every 100 workers to 42. Between now and the year 2010, it will continue to drop, but more slowly, to about 39 young people for every 100 workers.[4]

The young-age and old-age dependency ratios can be combined for a total dependency ratio (Table 11–1). This statistic would show that in 1990, there were about 62 young and old people to every 100 workers. This number is expected to increase to 67 by the year 2020.[4] It is important to note, however, that the share of the total dependency ratio accounted for by children is declining, while the share of the total dependency ratio accounted for by the elderly is increasing. Consider also that the care of the young in the United States is considered to be primarily a private family responsibility,

TABLE 11–1. *Old-Age and Young-Age Dependency Ratios, 1970–2050*

Year	Old-Age Ratio	Young-Age Ratio	Total Dependents
1970	17.6	61.4	79.0
1980	18.6	46.5	65.1
1990	20.2	41.6	61.8
Projections			
2000	20.9	42.4	63.3
2010	21.5	39.4	60.9
2020	27.4	39.9	67.3
2030	35.7	42.2	77.9
2040	37.1	41.8	78.9
2050	36.4	41.7	78.1

Source: Statistical Abstracts of the United States: 1995. U.S. Bureau of the Census, Washington, DC, 1995. Note: Based on middle series projections.[5]

whereas the care of the elderly carries with it more of a public responsibility (primarily through the Social Security tax and other taxes imposed on the working population). This issue and the ratios of economic dependency to productivity become significant in the discussion to follow concerning generational transfers and questions of equitable distribution of economic resources. But first, it is important to consider what is known about the elderly population of the future.

FUTURE ELDERS

The elderly population of the future (today's baby boom generation) will be characteristically different than their elderly predecessors of today. Notably, they will have many more years of formal education. Higher levels of educational attainment are associated with lower mortality, better health, reduced poverty, and a higher probability of being married and hence less likely of being alone.[2] Family size will also be in flux in the coming decades. Until about 2005, family size of the elderly will be increasing, with 35 percent of the elderly with four or more children, and 46 percent with two or three children. This reverses sharply after 2005, however, with only 11 percent having four or more children, and 55 percent with two or three. Family size has important implications for social and economic support of the elderly. Some estimates are that as much as 80 percent of care for the elderly is provided by family members, often by adult children. As family size shifts downward, the availability of family care declines commensurately. The proportion of the elderly requiring institutional care may then increase.

The gap in life expectancy is narrowing. During the 1980s, women gained about 0.2 year in life expectancy and men 0.6 year.[2] If this trend were to continue, the result would be higher rates of marriage among older people in all age groups. This is because women would not be losing their husbands as soon as a result of death and thus would be spending fewer years alone. Beneficial consequences of this would probably include reduced isolation and subsequently lowered rates of depression and suicide, interdependency of intact couples, and less dependency of single elderly on societal and familial aid. It should also be mentioned that if the trends toward higher rates of divorce and separation among younger groups continue, combined with delayed childbirth and childrearing, available familial support for the elderly is likely to decline even further than would be predicted by the elderly's shrinking family size.

In the future there will be a greater number of women retiring from longer years of work force participation. This means that more older women will be qualifying for their own pensions and Social Security benefits.[2] This will have the effect of reducing poverty among elderly women and, combined with longer marriages, will increase the real income of older couples. Fewer are likely to need economic assistance. The paramount concern in this regard is how the Social Security system of revenue collection and benefit disbursement will accommodate this larger cohort of beneficiaries with a reduced number of workers.

As the elderly population grows, so too grows the share of voters who are old. Inasmuch as older people vote more than younger people, and are more politically active generally, the elderly are likely to become a more vocal and potent political force. Currently, approximately 30 percent of federal expenditures are directed to the elderly population. If these levels of expenditures are maintained into the next century, expenditures on elderly could conceivably reach 60 percent of the federal budget by 2030.[2] Age-related voting behaviors and budget expenditures 35 years from now are nearly impossible to predict. If the elderly vote in accordance with fairly narrowly defined self-interests and maximize gains for older age groups, there will be fewer economic resources available for other purposes. But if, for example, the need for defense spending, or other large federal budget items, was to decline markedly in that time, this shift in national priorities need not be a tragedy. However, there is little evidence to suggest that the elderly vote with one mind on age-related issues or any other issues for that matter. Still, age politics are likely to become more pronounced in the coming decades. This will be unavoidable if income transfers across generations become greater. Questions about the equity of shifting more resources to the elderly are exacerbated by the downward trends in the welfare and quality of life for children in the United States. This issue is examined in greater detail in the section on generational equity.

The difficulties of forecasting the future should be evident by now. Perhaps one of the greatest flaws in forecasting is in the assumption that today's notions about transitions from work to retirement will prevail into the next century. The typical pattern of working from the completion of one's education in early adulthood to one's mid-60s, often for the same employer and in the same place, and then abruptly leaving the work force to pursue leisure and pleasure pursuits in retirement is not typical now—and for most Americans, never was. This is a pattern that fit middle and upper income white men for a relatively brief interval in our history. These are powerful stereotypes against which we measure "the good life." The issues of generational equity and caring for frail elders addressed in later sections are questions of resource availability and allocation. How we think about dependency, obligation, and the distribution of resources is influenced by whether we see others as needy, deserving, or a burden. In the United States, such determinations are made largely on the basis of what we believe one has earned through their own merit. Merit is awarded in our culture on the basis of education and training attained, work done, and contributions made. To what degree can we ascertain whether the future elderly will merit the benefits they reap? Are the elderly cutting productive work lives unnecessarily short through early retirement? Could the elderly stay on the productive side of the dependency ratio longer, thereby relieving some of the burden on younger generations?

WORK LIFE

Answers to these questions come from two very different directions that might be thought of as the supply and demand of work for older workers. On the one hand, retirement trends over the last several decades are clear. Most elderly retire as soon as they are able. They determine ability to retire primarily on the basis of finances and health, factors that may work as incentives or disincentives depending on individual circumstances. By and large, the favorable balance of these two factors have provided great numbers of older workers with sufficient incentive to take retirement at the earliest possible time. The percentage of older workers in the work force has declined steadily. It currently stands at about 3 million, the same number as in 1950, despite enormous growth in the elderly population.[6] There is evidence to suggest, however, that decision making about retirement is changing. Until recently it was believed that many of the elderly retired prematurely or against their will. In fact, those who wished to extend their work life beyond traditional retirement age were few. This group, made up largely of professionals and those who owned their own businesses, could extend their working lives as long as health allowed. But most retired as soon as they could afford to and while still in good enough health to enjoy it. In other words, the demand for work among older workers has not been great.

As the American economy and the labor market shifted in the 1980s and 1990s, downsizing and reduction in force (RIF) became familiar terms to American workers. Older workers were often targeted because of savings that would result from eliminating their higher salaries and the belief (often incorrect) that their health insurance and benefits were more costly to employers. The Age Discrimination in Employment Act (ADEA) was introduced into law to protect older workers from arbitrary and discriminatory hiring and firing practices. The effect of downsizing is amply illustrated by the fact that between 1980 and 1987 one fifth of all Fortune 500 company's employees were eliminated.[7] In the early 1990s, it was estimated that 2 million people between the ages of 50 and 64 were able and wanting to return to work.[8] Workers in this age group often opt for "early retirement" after they have exhausted their work options. Those older than 65 years of age, generally in better health than previous generations, also show interest in continued employment, but more often in part-time or flexible employment opportunities.[8] These facts would suggest that currently the demand for work among older workers exceeds the available supply. Contrary to stereotypes, older workers have been found to be punctual, reliable, conscientious, and sensitive to coworkers, have fewer sick days for acute problems, are loyal to employers, and are experienced.[6]

In response to the displacement of older workers and the interest of retirees in extending work life, a number of corporate and governmental initiatives have attempted to increase the supply side of work for older workers. The Environmental Protection Agency has made deliberate efforts to recruit workers older than 55 for short-term projects. The Days Inn Corporation targeted workers older than 55 for recruitment and consequently reduced its absentee rate by 80 percent. Companies such as AT&T, NCR, Dow Jones, and the U.S. Postal Service have begun utilizing older workers for mentor programs. Gamse[6] reports on a number of large scale job fairs and job clubs designed to assist mid-life and older workers who are changing careers or unemployed. These efforts constitute a mix of paid and unpaid work and affect workers in the 55 to 65-year-old age group as well as those past the traditional retirement age. We have still not seen significant change in the number of older workers in the work force. There are signs, however, that demand among the elderly for work opportunities is increasing, and efforts are being made to provide more work opportunities.[6]

As in most other respects, the future elderly will be considerably different than their predecessors with respect to interest in work, their work availability, and skills and talents. Gamse describes older workers in the next century as a group that will have little loyalty to a single employer or career path; their interests will be in finding work that, above all, gives them satisfaction; they will be better educated, more computer literate, and more comfortable with diversity; they will be in second and third careers relative to their earlier work histories; they will be more interested in flexible work opportunities that can be integrated with educational, leisure, and retirement activities; and they will also be more likely to protest or litigate if treated unfairly.[6]

It is important to note that powerful determinants of work and retirement patterns are the lifelong expectations we hold of each. As family structures change, as women participate in the paid work force longer, as maternity and paternity leaves become more commonplace, as education and retraining become more necessary, it is likely that older adults will become more accustomed to a mixed pattern of work force entry, exit, and reentry. The expectation of a single sharp transition from work life to retirement will become less compelling. Combined with delayed benefit eligibility for Social Security, as well as general uncertainty about the stability of the Social Security system, adults will plan differently for retirement and alter their expectations of what is typical. Work, education, and volunteer service are likely to become more integrated in the lives of older adults.

LIFELONG EDUCATION

The growth of secondary and postsecondary education in the United States since World War II has been dramatic and impressive. Although the G.I. Bill created opportunities for returning veterans to obtain college credentials and marked the beginning of an educational expansion that continues today, not all segments of the population (those slightly older or women, for example) benefited equally or at the same time in their lives. In 1985, the median years of schooling for those older than 65 was 11.3. As we prepare to enter the next century, that figure has risen to 12.4. In 1965, slightly less than one fourth of the elderly were high school graduates. In 2000, that figure will stand at two thirds.[9] Still, there continue to be barriers preventing today's elders from fully participating in educational pursuits, including low skill levels due to limited educational opportunities in earlier life and beliefs and attitudes that educational attainment is not necessary for survival.[10]

Later adult education takes many forms and, compared with the lock-step model of traditional early life education, is much more fluid and open-ended. Elderhostel has become a well known national and international program offering thousands of short-term courses of study each year. Geared to the college level and cultural enrichment, Elderhostel tends to appeal to those that are already well educated.

At least a quarter of community colleges currently target elders for particular kinds of course offerings. Those most commonly offered tend to be in the areas of financial planning and management, health and cultural enrichment, and contemporary civic issues.[9]

Increased enrollments of elders in college and university courses have been a boon to institutions that had been bracing themselves for declining enrollments during the 1980s. At that time, there was a decline in the pool of graduating high school seniors on the order of 25%. Yet, college enrollments went from 12 million to 13.4 million during this same period as a result of older adults returning to school.[11] Among the adult college population, there are more women than men, whites dominate on the order of 90%, and 85% of older students work, mostly full-time. In order of frequency, the most common reasons given for returning to school are life transitions, learning as a satisfying activity, an opportunity to meet people, and a way to fill up free time. The kinds of transitions precipitating a return to the classroom differ for older and younger adults. Those in the 25- to 65-year-old age group cite career transitions. Those older than 65 more often cite leisure transitions and family transitions.[11]

It has been observed that adult education increases during periods of rapid social change. Changes in the economy, the age composition in society, technology, the family, and the roles of minorities and women all would appear to call for an increase in both traditional and less traditional forms of educational participation among the elderly for some time to come.

VOLUNTEERISM

In 1965, 11 percent of persons older than age 65 served in some capacity as volunteers. By 1987, that figure was estimated to be 38 percent.[12] This increase in volunteer activity has been attributed to several factors. Formerly, middle-aged women were the most active participants in volunteerism. With more women either returning to work in midlife or working more after their children are grown, volunteer organizations have begun recruiting from older age groups more aggressively. Today, women older and younger than 65 are more similar in educational level than was the case three and a half decades ago. Chambre[12] has noted that popular magazines for seniors, such as *Modern Maturity,* often advocate volunteerism as an important source of meaning in later life, and this has no doubt contributed to the value placed on these activities. Despite this considerable growth in volunteerism, older adults are still seen as a largely underutilized resource relative to the potential contribution they could make. In a 1986 National Research Council report, for example, it was estimated that for every five older adults that volunteer, there are two others that are equally able and interested who do not. Many of those that do currently volunteer would be interested in increasing the amount that they volunteer.[13] Today there are many examples of effective volunteer organizations, networks, and programs. Those referred to in this chapter include some of the better known, but they are merely illustrative and by no means exhaust the possibilities currently available.

Volunteer programs exist for most skill levels and interest areas. Those described here span income and educational levels as well. The Older Volunteer Program of the ACTION Agency is an umbrella organization that includes the Retired Senior Volunteer Program (RSVP), Foster Grandparents, and Senior Companion Program. RSVP volunteers tend to be geared toward human services such as refugee services, literacy programs, long-term care, and youth counseling. Foster Grandparents and Senior Companion are targeted for low-income volunteers and provide small hourly wages. RSVP allows for expense reimbursement. These programs are funded mostly with federal dollars, with some state and local contributions.[14]

The American Association of Retired Persons (AARP) operates a Volunteer Talent Bank (VTB). The Bank is set up for the purpose of matching volunteer interests and skills with agency and community needs. Set up originally to provide staffing for AARP volunteer needs, VTB now makes referrals to many outside agencies including the American Red Cross, the U.S. Fish and Wildlife Service, and the Peace Corps.[14]

The Service Corps of Retired Executives (SCORE) provides consulting and presents workshops for small business management assistance. By the early 1990s, SCORE had 13,000 volunteers providing voluntary assistance at 750 locations. Consulting services are free of charge to client businesses and managers, and a small fee is charged for workshops to cover expenses.[14]

The National Retiree Volunteer Center (NRVC) is underwritten by corporate sponsors and recruits from among corporate retirees. This program originated in the Minneapolis area and led to community initiatives ranging from food distribution centers, to board assignments with nonprofit institutions such as libraries and museums, to nutritional and childcare educational programs for young mothers. These initiatives are determined, staffed, and directed by senior volunteers with supporting corporate funding.[14]

There is every reason to believe that volunteerism will continue to grow and become an important part of late adulthood for many of us. When asked their reasons for volunteering, the most common response given by older adults is self-esteem.[14] To the extent that retirement from paid work results in loss of social roles, influence, and sense of identity, older adults are left to their own devices to restructure their lives. Volunteer work does not provide meaning if it is perceived as busy work. When good matches are made between talents, energy, and real needs, elders have the opportunity to do what elders in traditional societies have always done—mentor, educate, assist, and guide the next generation. This has the potential for providing a renewed sense of purpose in late adulthood, and especially so when volunteer activity is widely valued by the community and society. It should be recognized, however, that the effective mobilization of volunteer activity requires recruitment, organization, supervision, and recognition.[14] These efforts often require money and support from the public and private sectors and the community. An expanded volunteer ethic in the United States could have many unforeseen benefits, including the modeling of generous and altruistic behavior to younger generations and a cooperative spirit, which in decades past has seemed to have been absent in a culture that so relentlessly emphasizes individualism and self-reliance throughout adulthood.

THE QUESTION OF GENERATIONAL EQUITY

Substantial gains have been made among the elderly segments of the population in terms of income and living conditions. The percentage of elderly living below the officially defined poverty line in the United States declined from 24.6 percent in 1970 to 12.4 percent in 1993.[15] In contrast, the percentage of children younger than age 18 living in households below the official poverty line has increased from 14.4 percent in 1973 to 22.7 percent in 1993, making children the largest poverty-stricken group in America.[16] Given children's dependency on the adults around them for survival and well-being, this fact is alarming and, some would argue, should be a source of national shame in as wealthy a country as the United States. These opposing trends have become the basis for the charge that the elderly have become an overbenefited group at the expense of the young. There is concern that as the elderly population grows it will draw even more of our national resources away from an increasingly needy younger population. The way to remedy this circumstance and reverse the trend is to recognize the importance of investing in young people. This would involve setting limits on ex-

Gerontology for the Health Care Professional

penditures and investments in the older population and redirecting those resources toward America's youth.

At first glance this argument is a powerful one. It is indeed alarming to observe these opposing trends. It has been my experience that when even the
most sympathetic students of gerontology become aware of these facts they
quickly condemn the system that takes from children to benefit the old. The
observation that the country's oldest adults are enjoying an increasingly
comfortable standard of living while the most dependent and vulnerable segment of the population is at greater and greater risk carries with it images of
selfishness, disregard for the future, and moral culpability. There are reasons
to be cautious of these charges, however, and a need to examine the situation much more carefully. Researchers and gerontologists have argued that
these impressions are misleading when taken out of context. Minkler[17] has
summarized many of these contextual considerations and counterargu-
ments.

The way in which "poverty" is measured is sometimes different for the
young and the old owing to estimated adjustments in living costs. Minkler
argued that if the same levels are used for the two groups, the poverty rate
for the elderly climbs from 12.4 percent to about 15.4 percent. By any standard, income levels used to distinguish those in poverty from those not in
poverty are artificial and set very low. When, for example, we consider 150
percent of the poverty level as true poverty, sometimes described as poor and
near-poor, the poverty rate for the elderly nearly doubles. In other words,
while it is true that many of the old are no longer living below the poverty
line as defined by the various government agencies, at least one third of them
are still living in extremely modest circumstances and would be considered
by many to be poor. All of this is to suggest that poverty is more subjective
and more complex than a magic cut-off number, and taken out of context
these statistics can be misleading.[17]

More important is the idea that the generational inequity argument
strongly implies that monies are being taken away from the young and given
to the old. In fact, the causes of childhood poverty and the causes of improved living standards for the old are independent and unrelated to one another. At the risk of oversimplification, the rise in poverty among children is
attributable in large part to market forces. There has been a decline in real
wages among workers in the 1980s, an increase in substandard wage work
and loss of high-paying jobs in such areas as manufacturing, unfavorable employment trends for many, and an increase in single parent, female-headed
households. In other words, children are poor because young adults have
been having more difficulty than ever before obtaining well-paying jobs and
maintaining families. The declining poverty level among the old is primarily
the result of changes in government policy in the 1970s. In 1972, Social Security payments were increased 20 percent and tied to annual rises in the

Consumer Price Index to protect against inflation. If Social Security were reduced to its pre-1972 levels, this would both increase real poverty among the old and do nothing to alter the changes in markets and family structure that have affected the young with such devastating consequences.[17]

Much of the cost burden of supporting an aging population is directly related to the costs of increased demand for medical care and health care resources. Those who argue for greater generational equity imply that this cost is inflated because of the demands for high-technology medical care among the elderly. In fact, much of the crisis in health care is a result not of high technology but of the failure to control the costs of health care generally, costs that affect all ages. The cost of hospital care, for example, grew from $14 billion in 1965 to $167 billion in 1985. Health care costs increase at a rate roughly twice that of the Consumer Price Index.[17]

Another flaw in the generational inequity argument is the suggestion that the distribution and redistribution of resources is a zero-sum game. This is not true of the political process generally, and there is no reason to believe that it should be true as the needs and demands of society change in a dynamic and fluid manner. The population is getting older. That calls for more resources of a particular kind. The Cold War is over. That requires fewer resources of another kind. As needs change and as the composition of society changes, so too, the rules of resource acquisition and allocation change. This is evident in changes in tax laws, in retirement rules and benefits, in proposals for flex time for workers, and in uses of volunteer resources and energy. Corporate tax rates, for example, declined from 4.2 percent of the gross national product (GNP) in the early 1960s to 1.6 percent of GNP in the early 1980s. Although politically unpopular, perhaps we can no longer afford to forego those sources of government revenues. Just as the causes of childhood poverty and reduction of old age poverty are independent, so too are solutions likely to be unrelated.[17]

Related to the generational equity debate, and a large area of study and concern in its own right, is whether age is being scapegoated when, in fact, there are sources of inequity within age groups that are greater than the inequities between age groups. It is important to not lose sight of the fact that the elderly are certainly the most diverse age group in the population and that the aging experience varies enormously by race, sex, and class. To a lesser degree, this can be said of children as well. The likelihood of growing up in poverty, for example, is many times greater for an African-American child in the United States than for a white child. The best predictor of poverty in old age is poverty throughout life. The study of aging from a lifecourse perspective underscores the fact that economic resources and assets in old age result directly from continuous progressive employment throughout adulthood that has been the predominant traditional life pattern only for white men.[18]

PROVIDING FOR THE ELDERLY

An analysis of the future of an aging society results in the recognition that the elderly population is growing at a rapid rate, and the segment of that population that is most frail and in need of greatest support (i.e., those 85 and older) is growing at an even faster rate than the rest. In response to that growing need, we can look to essentially three sources of resources and support. These include the family, the public government sector, and the private business sector. A brief review of the current system of resource provision and support in the United States follows. The U.S. system is then contrasted with the system currently in place in Sweden. Sweden is chosen for two reasons. It has one of the oldest populations in the world and, in that sense, offers a glimpse of the future. It also has among the most elaborate public sector support systems for the elderly in place anywhere. For that reason, it does not offer a probable glimpse of the future in the United States, inasmuch as few would suggest that the United States would or should adopt so extensive a social welfare arrangement. Finally, general conditions in the developing world are described. These conditions differ enormously from those in the developed countries of Western Europe and North America. These countries will experience a period of explosive old age population growth in a relatively brief time.

Based on these three sketches, we see three different scenarios for the future of the elderly population. The United States is in a state of flux right now, and the aging of its population is a political football. It is unlikely that younger generations can sustain substantially more of the burden of care for its elders both in terms of familial care and in tax support. Growth in the **private sector** is probable, but there is reason to be skeptical of the quality and sustainability of private sector options for the general elderly population. **Public sector** support involves a long-standing social contract that must minimally be sustained near current levels and, some would argue, should be strengthened in certain areas.

In contrast, Sweden's system is impressive, but at a cost that would not be palatable to most Americans. In the future, need will continue to expand in Sweden, although at a slower rate than in recent decades. As need expands, it is unlikely that the Swedish public sector will expand any further. The difference is more likely to be made up by families and growth in the private sector.

The developing world, by far, faces the greatest challenges. Most countries are ill equipped to cope with the growth in the elderly population. Governments in developing nations assume, out of necessity, that the traditional family structures will absorb the care of their elderly family members. Traditional family structures in the third world, however, are undergoing significant changes as a result of urbanization and shifting labor markets, leaving families unable to provide the kind of support they might have in stable social systems or on the scale anticipated. In some countries the public sector recognizes this and is responding accordingly with the initiation of a variety of public economic programs. A more detailed picture is sketched below.

As described in Chapter 8, some of the care for the very old involves what is described as long-term care. This is a level of care usually needed for chronic and ongoing conditions that are more prevalent in the oldest old. These chronic and ongoing conditions often limit mobility, functioning, and self-care. In many respects it is medically low-technology care, including social care and supervision. As disease conditions progress, the level of care intensifies and for some may require around-the-clock care and supervision as well as more intensive medical care. Long-term care may be provided in homes or in institutions, primarily nursing homes.

THE UNITED STATES

In the United States, funding for long-term care comes from a combination of individual resources (or out-of-pocket payment), public health insurance, and a welfare approach. All Social Security recipients are eligible for basic Medicare coverage. Medicare is a public health insurance program for the elderly. Medicare beneficiaries have some allowances for long-term care but only on a short-term basis. Only 4 percent of Medicare expenditures in 1988 went to long-term care, clearly suggesting that it is not a major source of funding for this form of care.[19] The major source of funding for long-term care, beyond private self-pay, is Medicaid. Medicaid eligibility is income-based and provides payment for health care for all those, regardless of age, who do not have the private resources to pay for medical care. Medicaid was never intended to be the primary source of funding for long-term care for the elderly, yet nearly half of nursing home revenues come from public funds, most of this from Medicaid.[4] Established in 1966 along with Medicare, Medicaid is jointly funded through state and federal funds, and by the 1980s it had become the biggest item in many state budgets, precipitating more stringent cost-containment measures.[19] Since about 80 percent of nursing homes are privately owned and operated on a for-profit basis, the United States has the unusual, or at least unique, circumstance of having private sector nursing homes heavily subsidized with public funds. Critics have argued that this has created a two-tiered class system of care.[19] Since government funding sources are income-based and favor institutional care, institutions end up providing for an inordinate number of poor or impoverished elderly. Many of these elderly require more social than medical care but have neither the family nor other social support or financial resources to elect any other option than nursing home care.

Olson has argued that through the arrangement of publicly subsidized "private" homes that quality, access, and affordability have been compromised. Studies of nursing homes within the United States[19] as well as cross-national studies[20] paint a grim picture of conditions. Quoting Olson:

The vast majority of homes fail to provide for the basic health and safety needs of the occupants. Most are substandard facilities that do not comply with even minimum federal and state standards of care; many violations are serious and life-threatening, including lack of food, proper administration of drugs, and decent personal hygiene. Due to a scarcity of physicians, a significant percentage of patients do not receive needed lab tests or adequate medical attention. Many suffer from poor nutrition, insufficient nursing care, and generally squalid conditions.[19]

Although this description may fit many nursing homes, if not a majority, there are also many high-quality, well-run nursing homes in the United States. Many of these better facilities, however, are expensive, may not accept Medicaid payments, and may have long waiting lists for admission. They may also not be equipped to meet the needs of the very sick or the very poor, thus reinforcing the two-class system.

Noninstitutional alternatives to nursing home care fall into either formal or informal service categories. Informal care refers to that which is provided by immediate family members or other relatives. Estimates are that approximately 80 percent of all care is provided by family members.[21] Most of the caregiving burden is carried by one family member, most often a woman. Estimates are that 70 percent of all family caregiving is provided by women. Approximately 30 percent is provided by adult daughters; 23 percent by wives; 20 percent by other female relatives, including daughters-in-law and sisters; 13 percent by husbands; 9 percent by sons; and 7 percent by other male relatives.[22]

Formal support services pick up where family care leaves off or is unavailable. The availability and array of noninstitutional services vary considerably by community but may include in-home assistance with meals, homemaker services, home health aides, transportation, telephone monitoring, respite for family members, day care, and legal services. These services have been designed largely to complement or aid family caregivers and less to replace them or sustain completely independent living conditions for elders. Older people may first recognize the need for some form of long-term care during or after a hospitalization. Older people require hospitalization at about four times the rate of younger people. Approximately 20 percent of all older people use inpatient facilities in a given year.[4] What distinguishes the institutionalized from the noninstitutionalized elderly is the availability of family help. Where family help is limited or unavailable, formal in-home and community services are intended to fill the gap and forestall institutional placement. Restricted availability, lack of awareness and use of community services, fragmentation, and cost containment measures, however, reduce the effectiveness of institutional alternatives. Findings from studies of demonstration projects comparing the costs of community care and institutional care have been mixed. They have not provided clear evidence that home-based care is more cost effective. There is considerable consensus, however, that it is preferred, more humane, and less dehumanizing.[23-26]

A long-standing criticism of formal in-home and community services has been the fragmented nature of the service delivery system. This fragmentation is largely a function of the financing mechanisms in place. Eligibility is usually income based, with the major funding sources being Medicare, Medicaid, Social Services (Title XX of the Social Security Act), Supplemental Security Income (Title XVI of the Social Security Act), the Administration on Aging, Veterans Administration, and Housing and Urban Development.[4] In addition to low-income requirements, many of the services are limited in volume per year or over the lifetime of the client. Other criticisms include limited access to services and a work force that is unskilled, untrained, underpayed, and overworked.[27]

In her review of care provision in the United States, Olson[19] argues that the public sector falls short in providing for the eldest and neediest members of society. Access to in-home and community-based services is limited and fragmented. Roughly 90 percent of all public funds go to nursing homes, which provide care of variable quality to 5 percent of the elderly population. With its emphasis on individualism and self-reliance, the United States places the primary financial obligation for care squarely on the elderly themselves. When care providers are needed, family members take on the large majority of the responsibility. The public sector takes over only when there are no resources and no family.

The early years of the next century will be years of political positioning and renegotiation of the social contract between society, the elderly, and the family. Action has already been taken to prolong the work life, and thus reduce the dependency, of the next generations of elderly. Cutbacks in Social Security benefits are being discussed seriously. Shifts in the dependency ratio make it unlikely that any expansion in public sector financing and services will take place. More and more one hears arguments for increasing family responsibility for care of elderly family members, but this ignores demographic trends that predict a reduction in the availability of care to the family, to say nothing of the economic, emotional, and psychological costs associated with prolonged caregiving. We are likely to see significant growth in the private sector. How well a free market approach to elder care will meet the needs of the elderly and the medical and human goals of an aging society remains to be seen.

SWEDEN

In many respects it is not possible to fairly compare Sweden with the United States. With 8.5 million people and a land mass equivalent to a midsized state in the United States, Sweden offers a very different model of elder care based on very different social and political philosophies. Sweden, therefore, is being offered in contrast to the United States to present an alternative approach. Whether it is one that the United States can or should emulate is a question that goes beyond my purpose in this chapter. The other feature that makes Sweden a fascinating example is that it is ahead of the United States, as well as most of the rest of the world, in the aging of its population. Almost 18 percent of Sweden's population is older than 65, compared with about 13 percent in the United States. Four percent are older than age 80. Sweden has one of the highest life expectancies in the world, and like other developed countries, its old-old population is the fastest growing segment. Much of Sweden's policy covering the elderly is not age specific. In 1982, Sweden passed its Social Services Act, which provided municipal social services to all persons who needed them regardless of age. In the passage of this act, access to social services were established as a right of all Swedish citizens. The explicit goals of the act were to sustain self-determination and normalization by allowing for maximum choice and supporting the individual in remaining in their normal environment. The Health and Medical Services Act was passed in 1983, and provides health care and services to all members of society regardless of age. Like social services, medical care and services are nearly all in the public sector. These publicly supported services available to all members of the society are supported through a tax system that takes about one half of a working person's income. Approximately one third of public expenditures goes to social insurance and social welfare programs. Of this expenditure, approximately 40 percent is used for various forms of old age support and care, mostly pensions and housing. There is widespread public opinion support for these policies in Sweden.[28]

Despite this generous public sector support directed toward independent living, Sweden does not differ from the United States in the proportion of its elderly that are institutionalized. It stands at about 5 to 6 percent of those older than 65 at any given time, with lifelong chances of being institutionalized being about 25 or 30 percent. The pattern of institutionalization for the elderly, however, does differ somewhat. Generally, the older person is more likely to have a short-term stay in an institution and return home, possibly going back and forth several times. Trends are also for these stays to occur among the very old, near the end of life, and for shorter periods of time. The official policy goal is to keep people in their own homes to as great an extent as possible. The result has been that more are spending their final days in institutions but for a shorter time and at older ages. Also as in the United States, Swedes' chances of spending time in an old-age home or nursing home are greater if they have no family.[28]

Sweden has one of the highest proportions of elderly who live independently. Estimates are that about 46 percent of Swedes older than 70 live alone. In Stockholm, 7 of 10 women older than 80 live alone. These rates are among the highest in the world. About 15 percent of the elderly receives regular Home Help services. The trend in recent years has been toward more services being provided to fewer clients among the old-old. These services include cleaning, cooking, washing, and personal hygiene. The client pays a co-payment of 5 to 10 percent, with the balance publicly subsidized.[28] The services are need-based and the overall effect has been to reduce differences in use across classes. Studies have demonstrated that when health is controlled for, class differences in use disappear.[28]

Subsidized community-based services that are not subject to needs assessments include municipal transport services, food services, meals on wheels, hairdressing, snow cleaning services, and district daycare centers. Most of these services are used by less than 10 percent of the elderly population.[28]

Studies of the Nordic countries generally find a ratio of formal caregivers to family caregivers of between 1:4 to 1:3. In Sweden it is estimated that family and friends provide about two thirds of all care.[28] Sweden's population is continuing to age and need will grow. It is unlikely that the public sector will expand any further. Sundstrom and Thorslund[28] anticipate that the increased need will be met by a combination of increased family support and growth in private sector alternatives that, up until now, have not been common in Sweden.

THE DEVELOPING WORLD

The expansion of the elderly population is a worldwide phenomenon, and the greatest increases by far will be in the developing world. The challenges this represents to societies in the developing world are compounded by the short time frame in which these changes will take place. For example, Guatemala, Singapore, Mexico, the Philippines, and Indonesia will all experience a tripling in the proportion of their elderly populations between the years 1985 and 2025. By comparison, growth in the United States in those years is estimated at 105 percent; in Canada, 135 percent; and in Sweden, only 21 percent.[29] In the next century, China will age faster than any other country. Official policy in China has led to sharp reductions in birth rates, which, if continued into the next century could result in a population which is 40 percent elderly.[29] So while the entire world is experiencing a shift in the age composition of its population, this is happening at very uneven rates. Currently, Western Europe, North America, and developed countries in other parts of the world are the oldest countries with respect to age composition and will be aging at a relatively slow rate in the years to come. The developing world is very young in this sense, with Guatemala, for example, currently having fewer than one fifth the proportion of old people in its population as Sweden. In addition to this rapid rate of increase, developing countries will face the challenges of aging while still dealing with all of the attendant problems of economic, social, and political development. The rapid aging apparent in these countries is, in fact, due to past successes in the area of nutrition, vaccinations, and sanitation. Life expectancies in developing countries have increased from an average of about 40 in the 1950s to almost 62 in 1990.[30] The world population of people older than 65 increases by 800,000 every month. Seventy percent of these elders are in developing countries.[30]

It is not clear how the old will be provided for in many countries. Old-age pensions are not common in the developing world. In China, for example, only 10 percent of the work force have pensions; in India, only 8 percent.[30] As economic development accelerates, traditional family patterns of care are disrupted. With urbanization, younger people move to the cities, often leaving elders alone in villages and rural areas and without support.

In the developing world, health care provisions and expenditures are a fraction of those in the developed countries. According to World Bank figures, the United States per capita spending on health in 1990 was $2763. By comparison, in Latin America, it averaged $105. In the world's poorest countries the average was $16.[30] As the populations of developing countries age, they will experience what demographers have referred to as the "epidemiologic transition" to the kinds of diseases and chronic conditions common to older age groups. This will occur while these countries are still grappling with infectious disease patterns common in younger age groups and developing countries. Hospitals, already available to only a fraction of the populations in these countries, may be overwhelmed with admissions, or demand for admissions, for cancers and cardiopulmonary diseases. Competition for resources could result in sharp class differences and age-based inequities.

Some of the wealthier countries in the developing world are initiating economic programs to reduce some of these problems. Taiwan, for example, has initiated a national health insurance system. Some Asian and Latin American countries have begun to look at mandatory pensions and savings plans.[30] But these sorts of reforms are still the exceptions rather than the rule. The more likely immediate solutions will be family and community based and emphasize low-tech, low-cost efforts to as great an extent as possible.

SUMMARY

Much has been said in this chapter about the way we might find the future as we grow older. Few of these claims are certainties. What is certain is that there will be many more elderly members of our society in the coming years and that the future cohorts of elderly will differ in significant ways from today's elderly. There are still gains to be made, although slight, in life expectancy, particularly among men. We can expect better overall health and greater independence. In the United States, the elderly of the future will be better educated as a group and, perhaps to an unprecedented extent, actively engaged in ongoing educational pursuits and community activities through both paid and unpaid work for longer periods of time. Despite this generally optimistic portrayal, the United States cannot afford to lose sight of the fact of heterogeneity in old age. This includes both a healthy diversity and a concern that aging is a very different experience for historically marginalized subgroups within the population. The aging population often magnifies the cumulative effects of inequality and inequity that have spanned lifetimes.

The major challenges facing our aging population in the future are the perennial concerns of today: care for those that cannot care for themselves, and the resources necessary for all persons to live their lives with dignity. These concerns will grow commensurate with the growth in the elderly population. To address these problems effectively, it is essential that they be reframed as shared national concerns, not as the problems of the elderly. Younger generations, who must share the burden of growing costs and care, must be convinced that the elderly merit their concern and their support and be assured that the same support systems and mechanisms will be there for them when they are old. This attitude toward the elders of our society and confidence in the future is undermined by the divisive pitting of generations against one another in a falsely constructed zero-sum game. Such constructions must be rejected by an educated voting populace.

In terms of both age composition and ability to address the problems of aging, the United States finds itself on a middle ground relative to other nations of the world. Sweden was discussed as an example of an advanced and comprehensive system of care provision for one of the oldest populations in the world. Sweden's solutions, however, are not necessarily a good fit for the United States. In the years to come the United States will be confronted with political and economic challenges in this arena that are unprecedented. Effective policy formation and decision making will test our economic and political systems in unexpected ways. Solutions will call for creativity and probably the willingness to break with past patterns and expectations. Patterns of work, leisure, caregiving, and collective actions may all take forms not commonly practiced today. The uneven rates of change throughout the world will be one more strand in the complex web that draws us further into a global economy and worldwide network of associations. Just as the United Nations Children's Fund (UNICEF) was a global response to the needs of the world's children, there may also be the need for global responses to the concerns and problems of rapidly aging populations at a high risk for dependency.

Despite the uncertainties, the opportunity to live long, productive, and fully engaged lives in the United States is probably greater now than ever before. As aging becomes a more visible national phenomenon and more central to the national fabric, elders will more often come to be seen as involved in all important aspects of public and private life. Attitudes among younger generations may well become more age-blind. And we will probably become more adept at determining when and where age itself is or should be the significant criteria for sorting people into categories. What are age-related problems versus simply problems with living? When are age-based solutions called for versus need-based solutions? In what ways are the old and young alike rather than different? What do we share in common? These questions have not been prominent in the discussion thus far. They could mark a productive starting point for confronting some of the challenges that face us.

REVIEW QUESTIONS

1. For future elderly Americans, family caregivers will:
    A. Be more available to assist with care than they are today.
    B. Be less available than they are today because of decreasing family size.
    C. Be less available than they are today because of a declining willingness to help.
    D. Be more inclined to provide financial support but not actual care.

2. The number one reason older adults give for obtaining additional education is:
    A. Boredom
    B. To socialize with younger people
    C. Life transitions
    D. Low cost

3. The most common reason elders give for volunteering is:
    A. To fill time
    B. To stay involved
    C. To meet new and interesting people
    D. Self-esteem

4. Recent trends suggest that older workers and retired persons are:
    A. More interested in continued work than in the past.
    B. Less interested in continued work than in the past.
    C. More likely to be absent from work as a result of illness.
    D. Less collegial and cooperative than younger workers.

5. Childhood poverty in the United States:
    A. Has been eliminated in the 1990s.
    B. Has increased because of the growing elderly population.
    C. Is restricted to rural areas.
    D. Is caused primarily to market forces and the problems of young adults.

6. In economic terms, the elderly today are:
    A. Better off than they were 30 years ago.
    B. Much worse off than they were 30 years ago.

C. The same as 30 years ago.
D. All quite wealthy.

7. The proportion of care for frail elders that is provided by families is estimated to be about:
   A. 10% of all care provided.
   B. 25% of all care provided.
   C. Half of all care provided.
   D. 80% of all care provided.

8. According to Olson, the majority of nursing homes in the United States:
   A. Are clean, safe, and well-managed.
   B. Are going to grow in number as the elderly population grows.
   C. Do not meet the basic needs of the elderly.
   D. Are inexpensive and accessible.

9. Worldwide, future growth in elderly populations is most dramatic in:
   A. The United States and Canada.
   B. Sweden and the Scandinavian countries.
   C. The most industrialized countries.
   D. The developing countries.

10. Compared with the United States, care for elders in Sweden has _____ support from the public sector (government).
    A. Greater
    A. Less
    C. About the same
    D. Almost no

⬛ LEARNING ACTIVITIES

1. Discuss ways in which corporations could design work schedules to better serve their elderly employees. Discuss possible contributions elder workers can offer their employers.

2. Describe potential models for work-to-retirement transition in the next century.

3. Develop a curriculum for an elder college. In addition to possible course offerings and student services, design a physical environment suitable for these elder students.

4. Describe challenges faced by developing countries in caring for these growing elderly populations.

5. Discuss ways to achieve intergenerational harmony. What can the young offer the old and vice versa?

6. Interview three middle-aged individuals about what future concerns they have as they become elders in an ever-aging society.

✻ REFERENCES

1. Roush, W: Live long and prosper. Science 273:42, 1996.

2. Spencer, G: What are the demographic implications of an aging US population from 1990 to 2030? American Association of Retired Persons and Resources for the Future, Washington, DC, 1993, p 8.

3. Perls, TT: The oldest old. Sci Am 00:70, 1995.

4. Kart, CS: The Realities of Aging: An Introduction to Gerontology, ed 5. Allyn and Bacon, 1997, p 53.

5. U.S. Bureau of the Census: Statistical Abstract of the United States: 1995, 115 ed. U.S. Government Printing Office, Washington, DC, 1995.

6. Gamse, DN: Work and second careers: Executive summary and commentary. In Resourceful Aging: Today and Tomorrow, Conference Proceedings, Vol IV. American Association of Retired Persons, Arlington, VA, 1991, p 9.

7. Rupert, P: Contingent work options: Promise or peril for older workers. In Resourceful Aging: Today and Tomorrow, Conference Proceedings, Vol IV. American Association of Retired Persons, 1991, p 51.

8. Patten, CW: Second careers: New challenges, new opportunities. In Resourceful Aging: Today and Tomorrow, Conference Proceedings, Vol IV. American Association of Retired Persons, 1991, p 47.

9. Feldman, NS: Lifelong education: The challenge of change. In Resourceful Aging; Today and Tomorrow, Conference Proceedings, Vol IV. American Association of Retired Persons, 1991, p 17.

10. Halnon, T: Older Americans and federal vocational and adult opportunities. In Resourceful Aging: Today and Tomorrow, Conference Proceedings, Vol IV. American Association of Retired Persons, 1991, p 35.

11. Aslanian, CB: Adult learning and life transitions. In Resourceful Aging: Today and Tomorrow, Conference Proceedings, Vol V. American Association of Retired Persons, 1991, p 45.

12. Chambre, SM: Volunteerism by elders: Demographic and policy trends, past and present. In Resourceful Aging: Today and Tomorrow, Conference Proceedings, Vol II. American Association of Retired Persons, 1991, p 33.

13. Institute of Medicine, National Research Council: Productive Roles in an Older Society. National Academy Press, Washington, DC, 1986.

14. Costello, CB: Resourceful aging: Mobilizing older citizens for volunteer service. In Resourceful Aging: Today and Tomorrow, Conference Proceedings, Vol II. American Association of Retired Persons, 1991, p 15.

15. U.S. Bureau of the Census: Statistical Abstracts of the United States, 113. Commerce Bureau, Washington, DC, 1993.

16. Cornman, JM, and Kingston, ER: Trends, issues, perspectives, and values for the aging of the baby boom cohorts. The Gerontologist, 36:15, 1996.

17. Minkler, M: Generational equity and the public policy debate: Quagmire or opportunity? In Homer, P, and Holstein, M (eds): A Good Old Age. Simon and Schuster, New York, 1990, p 222.

18. Stoller, EP, and Gibson, RC: Advantages of using the life course perspective. In Stoller, EP, and Gibson, RC (eds): Worlds of Difference: Inequality in the Aging Experience. Forge Press, Thousand Oaks, CA, 1994, p 3.

19. Olson, LK: Public policy and privatization: Long-term care in the United States. In Olson,

LK (ed): The Graying of the World: Who Will Care for the Frail Elderly? Haworth Press, New York, 1994, p 25.

20. Kane, RL, and Kane, R: Long-term Care in Six Countries: Implications for the United States. Department of Health, Education, and Welfare, Washington, DC: 1976.

21. Stone, R, et al: Caregivers of the Elderly: A National Profile. Department of Health and Human Services, Washington, DC, 1987.

22. Brody, EM: Women in the Middle: Their Parent Care Years. Springer Publishing, New York, 1990.

23. Caro, FG: Relieving informal caregiver burden through organized services. In Pillemer, KA, and Wolf, RS (eds): Elder Abuse: Conflicts in the Family. Auburn House Publishing, Dover, MA, 1986, p 283.

24. Edelman, P, and Hughs, S: The impact of community care on homebound elderly persons. Gerontol 2:570, 1990.

25. Pepper Commission, U.S. Bipartisan Commission on Comprehensive Health Care: A Call for Action: Final Report. U.S. Government Printing Office, Washington, DC, 1990.

26. Stephens, SA, and Christian, TB: Informal Care of the Elderly. Lexington Books, Lexington, MA, 1986.

27. Cantor, MH: Family and community: Changing roles in an aging society. The Gerontologist 31:337, 1991.

28. Sundstrom, G, and Thorslund, M: Caring for the frail elderly in Sweden. In Olson, JK (ed): The Graying of the World: Who Will Care for the Frail Elderly? Haworth Press, New York, 1994, p 59.

29. Cockerham, WC: This Aging Society. Prentice Hall, Englewood Cliffs, NJ, 1991, p 35.

30. Holden, C: New populations of old add to poor nations burden. Science 273:46, 1996.

◫ EPILOGUE

This is not the end; this is the beginning. In the preceding pages we hope we have presented you with useful information to guide you as a health care professional working with and for older people; however, there is much more to be learned. Each chapter has a list of references at the end. With a little time and ambition, you can start on your journey of lifelong learning and delve a little further into areas that are pertinent to you and your clients, patients, friends, or family.

We hope that this book has done its share to dispel some of the myths of aging and to eradicate ageism. While acknowledging that our bodies show signs of wear and tear as we age, nonetheless, most people do remain vital, productive, and lovable until the end of their lives. Resilience does not decrease with age; it often tends to increase. The next time you encounter

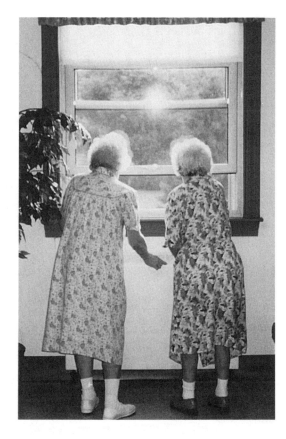

Photograph courtesy of Darby I. Northway.

someone elderly with multiple medical conditions, who you might think is at death's door, hold out hope for him or her. In rehabilitation, we are often surprised at what sheer determination and inner strength can do to restore the quality of life. Amazingly sometimes this happens even without physical progress.

So slow down, have patience, open your ears and your heart, and learn what the wise will teach you. Most of all, enjoy the ride along the way!

Regi and Walter

P.S. We welcome comments and questions. You can reach us at rrobnett@mailbox.une.edu or wchop@smtc.net

▨ APPENDIX

CHAPTER 1 — ANSWERS TO REVIEW QUESTIONS

1. B	5. D	9. C
2. E	6. D	10. A
3. B	7. D	
4. C	8. A	

CHAPTER 2 — ANSWERS TO REVIEW QUESTIONS

1. A	6. C	11. D
2. B	7. B	12. E
3. B	8. D	13. D
4. D	9. A	14. C
5. B	10. B	

CHAPTER 3 — ANSWERS TO REVIEW QUESTIONS

1. C	5. D	11. E
2. C, B, F, A, H, E, D, G	6. E	12. D
(in order, from top to	7. B	13. B
bottom)	8. B	14. A
3. A	9. B	15. B
4. C	10. B	

CHAPTER 4 — ANSWERS TO REVIEW QUESTIONS

1. C	6. A	11. B
2. A	7. A	12. C
3. B	8. B	13. A
4. B	9. D	14. A
5. D	10. C	15. D

CHAPTER 5 — ANSWERS TO REVIEW QUESTIONS

1. C	5. A	9. D
2. C	6. D	10. B
3. B	7. B	
4. C	8. B	

CHAPTER 6 — ANSWERS TO REVIEW QUESTIONS

1. A	5. B	9. A
2. D	6. D	10. C
3. C	7. B	
4. C	8. C	

CHAPTER 7 — ANSWERS TO REVIEW QUESTIONS

1. D	5. A	9. C
2. B	6. D	10. D
3. A	7. B	
4. C	8. A	

CHAPTER 8 — ANSWERS TO REVIEW QUESTIONS

1. C	5. A	9. D
2. B	6. D	10. A
3. A	7. B	
4. B	8. C	

CHAPTER 9 — ANSWERS TO REVIEW QUESTIONS

1. D	5. B	9. C
2. D	6. C	10. D
3. B	7. A	
4. A	8. B	

CHAPTER 10 — ANSWERS TO REVIEW QUESTIONS

1. B	4. D	7. A
2. A	5. B	8. C
3. A	6. C	

CHAPTER 11 — ANSWERS TO REVIEW QUESTIONS

1. B	5. D	9. D
2. C	6. A	10. A
3. D	7. D	
4. A	8. C	

INDEX

*Page numbers in italics indicate figures; page numbers with *t* indicate tables.